DATA PARADOXES

Infrastructures Series

Edited by Paul N. Edwards and Janet Vertesi

A list of books in the series appears at the back of the book.

DATA PARADOXES

THE POLITICS OF INTENSIFIED DATA SOURCING IN CONTEMPORARY HEALTHCARE

KLAUS HOEYER

The MIT Press
Cambridge, Massachusetts
London, England

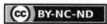
The MIT Press would like to thank the anonymous peer reviewers who provided comments on drafts of this book. The generous work of academic experts is essential for establishing the authority and quality of our publications. We acknowledge with gratitude the contributions of these otherwise uncredited readers.

This book was set in Stone Serif and Stone Sans by Westchester Publishing Services. Printed and bound in the United States of America.

Library of Congress Cataloging-in-Publication Data

Names: Hoeyer, Klaus, author.
Title: Data paradoxes : the politics of intensified data sourcing in contemporary
  healthcare / Klaus Hoeyer.
Description: Cambridge, Massachusetts : The MIT Press, [2023] |
  Series: Infrastructures series | Includes bibliographical references and index.
Identifiers: LCCN 2022019995 (print) | LCCN 2022019996 (ebook) |
  ISBN 9780262545419 (paperback) | ISBN 9780262374163 (epub) |
  ISBN 9780262374156 (pdf)
Subjects: LCSH: Medical informatics—Denmark—Case studies. | Medicine—
  Denmark—Data processing—Case studies. | Medical policy—Denmark—
  Case studies.
Classification: LCC R858.A3 H64 2023 (print) | LCC R858.A3 (ebook) |
  DDC 610.28509489—dc23/eng/20220830
LC record available at https://lccn.loc.gov/2022019995
LC ebook record available at https://lccn.loc.gov/2022019996

10 9 8 7 6 5 4 3 2 1

CONTENTS

PREFACE

Data permeate contemporary healthcare: everybody seems to be relentlessly asking for more data, of better quality, on more people. With this book, I explore the drivers for and implications of such intensified data sourcing. It has ended up as a treatise about *data paradoxes*. I think of paradoxes in the sense of opposing stories that are—each in their own way—true, although they superficially seem to preclude each other. People often use the same data to produce very different, sometimes opposing, stories about the state of affairs in healthcare. Besides paradoxical ways of telling stories *with* data, it is also possible to tell seemingly opposing stories *about* data—stories about why data are collected and how datafication affects healthcare. Although such stories appear paradoxical, they make sense when we accept that intensified data sourcing are transforming the way that we should think about data. Data are not simple pieces of information. They are ontologically multiple: parts of several coexisting networks, dynamics, and practices that simultaneously inspire and affect people in diverse ways. I invite readers to contemplate data paradoxes because I think that it can help both scholars and practitioners to use data wisely, with greater awareness of what data do and for whom.

It is impossible to study any social phenomenon without understanding it in a specific context. The stories I tell about data unfold primarily in Denmark. Why Denmark? The Danish healthcare system has one of the most advanced and integrated data infrastructures in the world. It is therefore the place to go when wanting to explore intensified data sourcing in practice. The integrated data infrastructures in that system create fantastic research opportunities, ensure many seamless clinical interactions, and confer administrative benefits, and the data resources are increasingly seen by the medical industry as business opportunities. The Danish data infrastructures therefore inspire policymakers in healthcare systems around the world.

What is rarely spoken about, however, is that the Danish experience with integrated data infrastructures also gives rise to a number of concerns. Data integration is far from straightforward, and unintended consequences proliferate. My aim with this book, in all its simplicity, is to use the admittedly extreme Danish experience with data integration to inspire a longing for *better* use of data instead of the current global urge for just *more* use of data. The first step toward better use is to acknowledge the need to look *at* data practices, not just look *with* data at the world. The second step is to ask, "Better for whom?" and "Better according to which criteria?" and to seek answers by analyzing the diverse implications of intensified data sourcing for different people, or the same people over time. This book does just that.

The book is based on a project that has received funding from the European Research Council (ERC) under the European Union's Horizon 2020 research and innovation program (grant agreement number 682110), as well as the Velux Foundation (grant agreement number 36336). The ERC grant allowed me to gather a group of excellent scholars to study data intensification as it unfolds in various health settings. This has provided a much more comprehensive understanding of the data politics involved than I could ever have achieved alone. I composed the ERC project so that I personally focused on the politics of integrating data infrastructures, while others engaged closely with a range of clinical practices affected by this data integration. In this way, we could combine breadth with depth and compare data intensification initiatives prompted by a range of actors, including researchers, clinicians, politicians, administrators, and people working with data for the pharmaceutical and medical device industry. We also covered initiatives among patients belonging to different age groups, literally from the newborn to the dead, and in different healthcare areas with different degrees of specialization, from municipal homecare to frontier genomic medicine.

The subprojects were carried out by an amazing group of scholars. Mette Hartlev took the lead on mapping legal controversies about data, partly in dialogue with Jens Schovsbo. With Sarah Wadmann, I studied data analysis initiatives covering general practice, hospitals, and psychiatry; and with Christoffer Bjerre Haase, I learned about the introduction of data tools in general practice.

Malene Nørskov Bødker helped me gain more knowledge about data practices in municipal home care. Through Francisca Nordfalk, I learned about data sourcing in the course of a newborn screening program. Together with Maria Olejaz, Francisca and I also explored an initiative to carry out genetic research on dissection donors. Francisca and I also looked at opt-out registries for research participation and how they work in practice. Without Francisca, I would not have experienced firsthand the thrill and dread of dealing with registry data. Anja MB Jensen shared her deep understanding of the organ transplant field and gave insight into the use of data in donation practices. With Lea Skovgaard Larsen, I have had the pleasure of studying public perceptions of data sourcing. Aaro Tupasela studied European integration initiatives and artificial intelligence (AI) projects. With Aaro, I also studied the enrollment of citizens in research through a genetic register tracking people with specific genetic variations. This research initiative involved samples from Pakistan, and Zainab Sheikh went into detail with this particular collection practice as an example of how a Danish urge for data provides opportunities and risks for people in a less affluent country like Pakistan. In its last stages, Sofie á Rogvi joined the project funded by an emergency grant from the Velux Foundation to help understand the COVID-19 pandemic as a data-political event. All this research informs this book, but the book is not a compilation of the articles we have produced. It is written as an independent argument, although I do sometimes reuse particularly telling quotes or passages from published articles.

The ERC group opened up our biweekly meetings to other colleagues who were also studying data practices ethnographically. We called ourselves the Data Group. It has made it possible to compare and contrast our ERC findings with other people's work. I have learned immensely from the discussions about data practices that unfolded in this group. Henriette Langstrup, Sara Green, Olsi Kusta, Anna Sundby, Nina Rud Rasmussen, Margit Anne Petersen, Aja Smith, John Brodersen, Rikke Torenholdt, Ivana Bogovic, Claudia Bagge-Petersen, Rosie Collington, Nikoline Nygaard, Line Egede Clausen, and Jette Holt have in various phases joined and fertilized discussions and debates. This book could not have been written had I not had the chance to learn from the Data Group. My first, deep-felt thanks therefore go to this marvelous group of scholars: the ERC project members and the wider Data Group.

Second, I wish to thank the many interlocutors in healthcare, in Denmark and beyond, who gave me their time to be interviewed and who have enlightened me about their perceptions, practices, and priorities. I am truly grateful. Many of them have felt that it was a risk talking to an outsider about how data *really* are used, not just how they are *said* to be used. I appreciate your trust. Others have enrolled me as an interlocutor in their deliberations about new data initiatives, and I have learned a lot from these dialogues. I hope that those who have shared their hopes and concerns see them reflected in this book.

Outstanding international scholars have also joined our meetings for shorter periods, or sometimes just once, and helped us along with comments, questions, and suggestions. It has been incredibly stimulating and a true testimony to academic generosity! Among them are (listed in alphabetical order) John Burnett, Annamaria Carusi, Sarah Cunningham-Burley, Susan Erikson, Susi Geiger, Lisa Guntram, Ilpo Helén, CF Helgesson, Linda Hogle, Sonja Jerak-Zuiderent, Jane Kaye, Thomas Lemke, Jake Metcalf, Timo Minssen, Lynn Morgan, Anna Pichelstorfer, Katie Pine, Violeta Argudo Portal, Jenny Reardon, Minna Ruckenstein, Tamar Sharon, Karoliina Snell, Heta Tarkkala, Linnet Taylor, Sally Wyatt, and Teun Zuiderent-Jerak. Each visitor has been a great source of inspiration.

Sarah Cunningham-Burley and Mette Hartlev deserve special mention for their insightful advice in the early phases, when I was applying for the ERC project, and Mette for her continued help with understanding legal intricacies; Linda Hogle for encouraging me to pursue the idea of paradoxes and for being a continued source of inspiration; and Ina Willaing Tapager and Hans Okkels Birk for suggesting important case material.

I am also deeply indebted to all the people who have commented on earlier drafts—sometimes several times—and helped me articulate my arguments. The text has benefited so much from your careful readings. My colleagues at Section for Health Services Research, University of Copenhagen, commented on the introduction, and John Brodersen, Amy Clotworthy, Sara Green, Christoffer Bjerre Haase, Linda Hogle, Jette Holt, Dorthe Brogård Kristensen, Olsi Kusta, Henriette Langstrup, Steffen Loft, Francisca Nordfalk, Ezio di Nucci, Naja Hulvej Rod, Sofie á Rogvi, Zainab Sheikh, Lea Larsen Skovgaard, Sarah Wadmann, Ayo Wahlberg, Brit Ross Winthereik, and three anonymous reviewers have generously read and commented on various chapters, or even the whole book. I remain indebted to your immense generosity! I would also like thank the editor, Justin Kehoe, and series editor, Paul N. Edwards, for daring to take on board a book about data practices in a small European country.

Elements of chapters 1, 2, and 3 have previously been published in *SSS* (Hoeyer 2019), in *Economy and Society* (Hoeyer and Wadmann 2020) and a chapter in a book edited by Susi Geiger (Hoeyer and Langstrup 2021). Special thanks go to Henriette Langstrup and Sarah Wadmann for allowing me to reuse elements of our shared work, but even more for being such extraordinary companions throughout all of these years in the quest to understand intensified data sourcing. Thank you!

Every project involves administration—a type of data work that rarely inspires happy feelings. With Janne Sørensen as project administrator, however, even these tasks have been a worthwhile enterprise. A group of excellent student assistants have been transcribing interviews and taken care of all sorts of relatively dull data work: Ida Ege Biering, Rosie Collington, Line Dyhr, Emilie Funch Nielsen, Nikoline Nygaard, Sofie Amalie Olsen, Nina Rasmussen, and Sif Vange. Sofie and Nikoline have also conducted some of the interviews for chapter 6, just as I have been allowed to quote an interview conducted by Sofie á Rogvi. Thank you for your dedication to even the less inspiring tasks involved in academic work. I am also grateful for Julie Dyson's efforts to correct my English.

Thinking is a social act. This book has been nurtured by all the brilliant minds of the people mentioned here, just as it has benefited from the ideas of many other scholars who have inspired and helped me over the years. I cannot mention every one of you. While each one of you deserves part of any praise this book might receive, I am very much aware that I retain the responsibility for all errors. I am grateful for your generosity and intellectual nurture, even though you might think I should have come to other conclusions.

There is another kind of nurture that it is also paramount for me to mention—that of the love and care of my family and friends. They have had to bear with me many times as I have posed insisting questions about mundane data practices, often in the course of us doing something completely different. They have allowed me to pursue my weird curiosities–and yet also brought me back into the circles of social life from which all important values arise. One man, more than anybody else, serves as such a point of gravity in my life: my husband, Jesper. While you never cease to support me in my work, you always also know how to make me put it aside. Thank you for sharing your life with me. Thank you for being the very center of mine!

Copenhagen, January 2022

INTRODUCTION: DATA POLITICS

Copenhagen, October 2018: "I would prefer a statistician to a doctor anytime." These words are spoken quietly by a person sitting near me, a healthy-looking man in his early twenties. I notice the wearable devices on his wrist: he seems to be collecting data on his own health. I'm attending a meeting framed as "an opportunity to discuss the prospect of data-driven healthcare." It is not the first time I hear someone at meetings, seminars, and conferences on this topic say that they would prefer a statistician to a doctor—about which I cannot help but feel puzzled, not least because of my profound respect for both doctors *and* statisticians. In my experience, practitioners of both professions tend to appreciate each other's skills, and yet they rarely wish to replace each other. What kind of future healthcare is in the minds of people who prefer a statistician over a medical doctor? What do they think they can achieve with data?

It was around 2014 that I began regularly attending such events about data and the future of medicine. By now, I have become accustomed to people telling me that we are at the cusp, or even in the middle, of a revolution. Informally during breaks, or formally as part of silver-tongued presentations, they foretell an imminent state where ubiquitous computing means that practically any activity will give rise to data, it will be possible to gather enough data on individuals to predict the advent of most diseases, and such predictions will facilitate the prevention of disease. Instead of waiting for symptoms to manifest themselves, people will be warned of future disease by data-profiling devices. Personalized regimes will replace standard treatments. Big data will replace evidence-based medicine (EBM). AI—artificial intelligence—will replace human interpretation. Apps will sideline doctors on many issues. As a consequence, the story goes, healthcare will be cheaper, more efficient, and people will live longer and healthier lives.[1] On top of this, old-fashioned administration and governance will be cast aside, to be replaced by smart algorithms designed to optimize performance. In these prophecies, data just need a bit of statistical help to do the job.

Many of the people who attend seminars on the prospects of data-driven healthcare have experienced firsthand how data-intensive technology can bring about significant changes in their own lives or their professional practice. For them, this feels like more than a prophecy. Now they want to see data used to optimize healthcare at large. They have observed how data-intensive companies have disrupted several business areas. Innovative technologies have changed how they search for information, and data-driven social platforms have made people connect socially in new ways (van Dijck, Poell, and De Wall 2018). Why should not healthcare be next? Companies like Google, Apple, and IBM are moving into health research. They are using big data methods to build decision support tools, and they are aiming for new ways of generating medical evidence (Prainsack 2017; Sharon 2016). Other big tech companies such as Amazon are experimenting with data-intensive ways of providing healthcare and dispensing drugs (Lewis 2016; Wakefield 2017; Shah 2020; Son 2021).

However, in the business area of health technology, big news quickly turns into old news. Promises fail to materialize, and business plans change. Apparently, there is something about healthcare in high-income countries that is remarkably resistant to change. Still, high-ranking civil servants, influential politicians, and chief executive officers (CEOs) continue to discuss data-driven healthcare as not only desirable, but inevitable. Data have moved to center stage of healthcare politics. What do these data promises entail? What is happening within healthcare? How does the pursuit of data-driven healthcare affect people on the ground: patients, clinicians, medical researchers, administrators, policymakers, and people in the pharmaceutical and medical device industries?

With this book, I explore what is driving the data surge and how it affects healthcare. The high-flying promises inspire concrete policymaking. Policymaking interacts with healthcare practices, giving rise to new experiences among patients and staff. How do these policies, practices, and experiences relate? Promises do not trickle through layers of practice and permeate everyday experience in the way that water soaks through cloth. Promises interact with practices and experiences—and practices and experiences bounce back. In my venture to understand the drivers for, and implications of, intensified data sourcing in healthcare, I take Denmark as my primary case. It is because Denmark is in many ways extreme. It is a country with thoroughly digitized health services, pervasive data sourcing, highly integrated data infrastructures, and personal identity numbers that make it possible to track citizens across sectors and throughout and beyond their individual lifespans. It is a country eager to be at the forefront of the prophesied data revolution. Denmark is the perfect place to explore the politics of intensified data sourcing.

DATA PROPHECIES: GLOBAL PROMISES AND LOCAL PRACTICES

The buoyant promises of digital disruption that I have outlined thus far are part of a more general societal change. In the whirlwinds of the twenty-first century, data promises have come to pervade policy environments in all corners of the world—not just in healthcare, but also in education, social service, and transportation. Across these sectors, data are referred to as gold mines or the new oil. First concentrated in relatively small circles in Silicon Valley on the American West Coast and around places like the Massachusetts Institute of Technology (MIT) on the East Coast, ideas about how the world *could* be governed based on computational calculation are rapidly turning into ideals for how the world *should* be governed. These ideas, however, are not simply travelling to other parts of the world: they are reinvented, entrenched, and made powerful by interacting with local histories, opportunities, and desires.

Though apparently attuned to positivist ideas of "evidence," the ideals of a data-driven society also exert a form of spiritual appeal. Informatics scholar Morgan Ames describes Silicon Valley ideals as exerting a *charismatic* authority of the type that Max Weber spoke about in relation to religious leaders (Ames 2019; Weber 2003a). Historian Yuval Harari literally designates the type of "dataism" that these ideals promote as a *religion* (Harari 2018). Social scientists such as Susi Geiger and Richard Tutton describe the expectations of data in big tech circles as a *mythology* operating at the intersection of capitalist extraction and promissory gospel (Geiger 2020; Tutton 2017). Some computer scientists genuinely discuss a messianic future state of "singularity," wherein human life is transposed into an eternal state of information and where machines and humans are one being (Shanahan 2015). For people believing in singularity, this concept implies a transcendence of death. If everything is data, the reasoning goes, then everything can live forever as just that: data. Influential voices in the movement promoting data have even founded a company called the Singularity University, where policymakers from all over the world take courses and engage with their thinking (Bernsen 2019).

Expectations as to data and digital technology are intertwined;[2] the one shapes the other. Elements of the buoyant belief in the power of data can be traced to a hopeful counterculture that emerged with the Internet in the 1980s. It was a culture where people experienced the informatization of social interaction as a liberation. The early users of the Internet spoke about access to data as empowering. In 1995, the computer scientist Nicholas Negroponte announced the coming of an era where bits would take over from atoms (Negroponte 1995). Humanity was to be freed from its material prison. What would be important would be information. In 1996, John Perry Barlow from the Electronic Frontier Foundation even presented a "Declaration of the Independence of Cyberspace," in which he said about state power: "You have no moral right to rule us nor do you possess any methods of enforcement we have true reason to fear" (Barlow 1996: 2). For people like Barlow, the Internet represented a sphere beyond state power, despite the fact that the American military held a key role in building it.

In the 1990s, Negroponte had begun serving as a government advisor, along with other tech-savvy geeks. Those in government circles were attracted to their hopeful forecasts and saw in their vision something other than a reason to abandon state power: it was to be reinvented as a seamless, supportive force. Ideas about a digital makeover of public service began to sizzle in policy environments all around the globe. Today, people with very different levels of authority—from low-ranking information technology (IT) specialists to high-ranking civil servants, from well-paid consultants in companies like Gartner, McKinsey, or Deloitte to incredibly wealthy business owners such as Tesla founder Elon Musk—have become voices in a choir singing about a data-driven future. In this future, everything is information and information is everything. Each through their own path of discovery, people in very different positions have come to see data as a solution even when dealing with very different problems. How, then, do data prophecies perform on the ground? How do these prophecies affect contemporary politics?

Data are high on the health policy agenda everywhere, not just in Denmark but also in the European Union, the United Kingdom, the United States, and beyond. China is developing an integrated data infrastructure in the form of a social credit system (Lengen 2017; Liang, Das, Kostyuk, and Hussain 2018), and India has launched digital smart cards connecting citizens to colossal biometric databases (Nair 2021; Dahdah and Mishra 2020). To facilitate data (re-) uses, most policymakers focus on investments in *data integration*. The money goes to infrastructure building. In its *Data Strategy* document from February 2020, the European Commission identifies an ongoing digital transformation of the European economy and society "affecting all sectors of activity and the daily lives of all Europeans. Data is at the centre of this transformation and more is to come" (European Commission 2020b: 1). In the same document, the Commission suggests investing in data infrastructures. Then, just after its publication, the COVID-19 pandemic struck, and the sense of crisis gave rise to a record-high stimulus plan emphasizing investments in what is green and digital. The ideas from the *Data Strategy* could now be backed with significant funding (European Commission 2020c): as much as 20 percent of the greater than 700 billion euros for this stimulus plan will be used to support digital integration. By November 2020, the Commission had proposed a Data Governance Act (Vestager 2020) setting up a legal framework for data sharing in eight sectors, including health. Specifically, the plans in the European Union of building a European Health Data Space, where all types of data (including medical records, genetic data, and patient-generated data) can be stored, exchanged, and reused for governmental planning, research, and cross-border care (European Commission 2020a). These ambitions reflect a form of geostrategic rivalry in which the European Union seeks to use its existing health data resources to gain territory in the global market for data analysis, which is currently dominated by American and Chinese companies.

The political attention to data meant massive investments even before the pandemic. Again, most investments have gone into digital infrastructures. The EU Data Strategy involves ensuring the "interoperability of health data through the application of the Electronic Health Record Exchange Format" (European Commission 2020b: 30)—an ambition that was repeated in the pandemic recovery plan and is to inform the European Health Data Space.

This is not the first time that a crisis has led to a call for integration of health data infrastructures. In the United States, President Barack Obama sought to combat the financial crisis of 2007–2008 by investing in the interoperability of electronic health records, among other things (Wachter 2017). The investments went into the development of what was described in the Act—known as the stimulus package—as a "Health information technology architecture that will support the nationwide electronic exchange and use of health information in a secure, private, and accurate manner" (US Congress 2009: 132). A budget of around 30 billion US dollars was allocated to health data integration. With its support of personalized medicine, the Obama administration also worked to ensure "secure access to the electronic healthcare information of more than 125 million patients" (US Food and Drug Administration 2013: 40).

In 2015, the Council of the European Union similarly adopted a strategy paper on personalized medicine according to which member-states should work to "support the standardisation and networking of biobanks to combine and share resources" and "promote the interoperability of electronic health records to facilitate their use for public health and research" (General Secretariat of the Council: Working Party on Public Health 2015: 7). In January 2019, the European Union invested an additional 21 million euros in the construction of an interoperable electronic health record through the Horizon 2020 program (https://www.smart4health.eu, see also Felt, Öchsner, and Rae 2020), and in its 2020 data strategy paper, "the development of national electronic health records (EHRs) and interoperability of health data through the application of the Electronic Health Record Exchange Format" was again a priority area receiving an additional two billion euros (European Commission 2020b: 30). As these examples illustrate, the integration of health data has been subject to investment for some time now. Yet apparently it is not as easy and smooth to ensure data flows as the data gospel suggests. In fact, it seems to be extremely difficult to make data do what the optimistic prophecies otherwise suggest is "inevitable."

Nevertheless, low-income countries are following suit to ensure good data flows. A highly influential United Nations (UN) report, *A World That Counts*, states that "[i]mproving data is a development agenda in its own right" (The United Nations Secretary-General's Independent Expert Advisory Group on a Data Revolution for Sustainable Development 2014: 3). The report even articulates a new vision for global public health: "Never again should it be possible to say, 'We didn't know.' No one should be invisible. This is the world we want—a world that counts" (3). Along with their multilateral investments, nongovernmental organizations (NGOs) such as the Bill and Melinda Gates Foundation donate significant amounts to create data infrastructures. Data almost seem to comprise a new form of, or an alternative to, development aid. Dreams of data ubiquity have captured the imagination of policymakers even in countries still fighting to fulfill basic health needs (Adams 2016b; Erikson 2016; Hoeyer, Bauer, and Pickersgill 2019). This is, in the most literal sense, a world that *counts*—a world that does its counting before it acts (Jensen and Winthereik 2013).

Policymakers clearly *aim* for data ubiquity all around the world. Therefore, there is a need to know more about what integrated data infrastructures can imply in practice. Where can you go if you wish to observe such an integrated data infrastructure? A typical choice for policymakers is a study trip to Denmark. This tiny EU country of just 5.8 million inhabitants receives numerous delegations from North America, Europe, Asia, and Australia. They visit the offices of a platform called *sundhed.dk*, which gives all citizens online access to their electronic health records; they visit an organization called MedCom, known for setting standards for data exchanges between individual health suppliers; or they go to the National Biobank, containing blood samples on most citizens—samples that can be linked to healthcare, social, and educational data. The biobank alone has in recent years received delegations from all corners of the world, including 156 delegations from Japan and 59 from the United States (Tupasela 2021b).

Why do they visit Denmark? At the turn of the millennium, Iceland, another Nordic country, was seen internationally as the epicenter for genomic research. A national biobank and a genealogical database were established, and a company was commissioned not only to run the two databases, but also to build a national electronic health record system and combine all three for research purposes. The company attracted investments on a scale affecting the overall gross domestic product of Iceland (GDP). However, it also created much controversy (Almarsdóttir, Traulsen, and Björnsdóttir 2004; Árnason and Simpson 2003; Fortun 2008; Pálsson and Rabinow 2001; Potts 2002; Sigurdsson 2001; Thorgeirsdóttir 2004). As a result, the company did not complete the electronic medical record system.

Today, Denmark is one of the most fiercely digitized countries with one of the most integrated health data infrastructures in the world (Aanestad and Jensen 2011). For decades, Denmark has been competing with the other Nordic countries to be the most attractive place for medical research (Tupasela 2017b; Tupasela, Snell, and Tarkkala 2020; Tupasela 2021b). In Denmark, there are tissue samples, medical records, registries, and quality databases available on practically all citizens, and they all can be used for research (Bauer 2014). Most of them even with informed consent exemptions. When the Obama administration began investing in the digitization of healthcare records, Denmark had already long been using digital health records and established centralized national databases. In Denmark, all pharmacies receive prescriptions electronically, and drug data are stored on individual profiles that can be accessed by patients and health professionals regardless of institution or place. Similarly, referrals to specialized care are placed on central servers where hospital wards or specialists fetch them. Most Danes take this level of integration for granted and can hardly remember how it was to fiddle around with a paper prescription or referral. This is why delegations go to Denmark to see what integrated data infrastructures look like in practice. Denmark has become a key site for studying health data integration.

Data are used for ever more purposes, and not just in Denmark. Besides treatment and research, they are used for monitoring clinical quality, for achieving administrative objectives, and for facilitating remuneration. Each of these purposes draw upon increasingly complex algorithms depending on multiple data sources. In the past, an ostensibly simple activity, such as remuneration, operated in relatively uncomplicated data loops (combinations of diagnostic and treatment codes), but they are now increasingly qualified with data sources meant to represent treatment *outcomes*, such as data on employment, sick leave, educational status, patient satisfaction, patient-rated outcomes, and so on (Hogle 2019). The data landscape has become a site where multiple goals, all dependent on more data, converge. To reach these many goals, the need for speed has come to the fore: researchers, clinicians, administrators, and industry all want what they term "real-time" data. When prophecies hit the ground, they hit multiple grounds, as it were. Each data promise may sound feasible, but in practice, each one interacts with many other uses of data. The many purposes generate friction (Edwards 2010; Pellegrino and Mongili 2014; Edwards, Mayernik, Batcheller et al. 2011).

In the chapters that follow, I show what happens when the data promises from American big tech and the circles around the Singularity University interact with a local healthcare system, which is in some ways far more advanced in terms of digitalization and data integration than the fragmented American healthcare system. I believe that experiences from the Danish experiment in health data infrastructuring can illuminate some of the challenges faced by other healthcare systems. Still, all healthcare is local. Unique local circumstances find ways of bouncing back. My study of Danish data infrastructures is meant to help raise awareness of the importance of locality. My hope is that this awareness can help both policymakers and researchers to reconnect policy, practice, and experience. They need to explore the specificity of their own cases and exert judgment instead of importing standard answers.

THE POLITICS OF INTENSIFIED DATA SOURCING: A BOOK ABOUT PARADOXES

In this book, I will put aside assumptions about the disruptive effect of big data and instead explore who wants which data and what they use them for. I take as my point of departure the basic empirical observation that more actors want more data, of better quality and about more people—while the actors often disagree about who should be allowed to use those data, and for what purposes. I call this phenomenon *intensified data sourcing*. My interest revolves around the *data politics* characterizing this development. Again, my guiding curiosity is: What drives intensified data sourcing in healthcare, and what are the implications for the governance of healthcare, for health professionals and for patients?

I have used this term, "intensified data sourcing," several times now, and I should explain why. It is, I admit, less seductive than its more popular cousin, "big data." Big data has become, effectively, a buzzword (Vincent 2014). It is typically associated with high-tech solutions, AI, and organizational "disruption." Sometimes it is defined as a methodological shift to work with velocity, variety, and volume (the three Vs), but in policy discourse, it remains vaguely defined (Boyd and Crawford 2012). The high-tech association turns the gaze toward future applications and potential impacts that have not necessarily materialized yet. I wish to capture the interplay between policy, practice, and experience and therefore do not wish to be constrained by the preconceptions bound up in the term "big data." I thus focus on intensified data sourcing to explore both blinkering high-tech solutions and the type of low-tech manual data collection that the push toward becoming data-driven also, in some areas even predominantly, has set in motion. Intensified data sourcing is a way of naming that which can be observed empirically in health services: a range of people (from clinicians and researchers to politicians and industry representatives) wanting more data, of better quality and on more people—while disagreeing on how these data should be used. I prefer "data sourcing" as an alternative to more established terms such as "data mining" because the mining metaphor is entirely inadequate to capture the *type* of data work involved. Data are not dug out of the ground—they are made. Intensified data sourcing includes the dynamic processes of creating, collecting, curating, and storing data, while simultaneously making them available for multiple purposes.

When I explore the interplay between policy, practice, and experience in intensified data sourcing, it is because it has important consequences for the options people have for pursuing health. Health is a basic condition for human beings in their pursuit of whatever matters to them. Illness causes suffering, pain, and sorrow. How societies respond to such agony is important. Even measures of prevention can become sources of grievance. It is important to understand how intensified data sourcing affect these very intimate aspects of people's lives. I focus on the data sourced through healthcare services because the relations people establish when seeking help from a health professional typically relate to something of outmost importance to them—something that they would not necessarily share with just anybody. Healthcare data matter to people.

As I have become interested in the stories we tell—and those that we ought to tell—about the consequences of intensified data sourcing in healthcare, I have found that the drivers are manifold and the implications *paradoxical*. I have noticed that patients, clinicians, and administrators sometimes use similar data to tell almost contrasting stories. Even more important to my interests in the drivers for and implications of intensified data sourcing is the fact that my interlocutors—the wide range of people I have met and interviewed—often tell almost opposing stories about why data are needed and the effects they have. As a consequence of this experience, this book has come to revolve around paradoxes. For some reason, I had not anticipated this. The opposing stories were causing me many a headache: I could not make the stories align. Gradually, I realized that this was a key point.

Paradoxes are classic figures of Western thought. Philosophy has grappled with paradoxes for thousands of years, such as pondering the truth value of statements such as "I am a liar" (Schad 2016). More recently, technological developments, and digitalization in particular, have been seen by some scholars as generating paradoxes. The philosopher Ezio Di Nucci talks about "the control paradox," where AI and other technologies simultaneously provide enhanced control and give rise to loss of control (Di Nucci 2021). The STS scholar Judy Wajcman makes similar points about digital time management and observes further how these technologies save time—or are supposed to save time—yet also generate new sources of time pressure (Wajcman 2015, 2019).

The Greek etymology of the term is *para*, meaning "contrary to," and *doxa*, meaning "opinion." According to Merriam-Webster, the term "paradox" can mean any of several things, including "one (such as a person, situation, or action) having seemingly contradictory qualities or phases." Contradicting stories can often run counter to *doxa*, common opinion. Drawing on this understanding, I refer to paradoxes in this book as situations where ostensibly contradictory stories are both (partly) true. Or, at least, they appear equally true to different stakeholders. In short, I am interested in the societal effects of people subscribing to different, but coexisting, truths.

Like philosophy, organizational psychology has also held a keen interest in paradoxes, albeit not for quite as long. Rothenberg (1996) analyzed the creative processes of outstanding thinkers like Niels Bohr and Albert Einstein and suggested that an ability to think in opposites in tandem lay at the root of their creativity. Bohr, for example, tried to resolve how energy acted both like waves *and* particles. Organizational psychologists today talk about "paradoxical frames" as a form of mindset that enhances thriving and creativity in complex organizational environments full of tensions between competing demands (Miron-Spektor, Ingram, Keller et al. 2018; Liu, Xu, and Zhang 2020). Paradoxical frames are understood as "mental templates that individuals use to embrace seemingly contradictory statements or dimensions of a task or situation" (Miron-Spektor, Gino, and Argote 2011: 229). Personally, I am not suggesting any particular psychological benefits of a paradoxical mindset (nor that such a mindset exists as a measurable disposition), but I do believe that paradoxes are part and parcel of contemporary healthcare organizations.

Paradoxical thinking has also found its way into management theory as a response to "competing demands that cannot be resolved by making trade-offs" (Henriksen, Nielsen, Vikkelsø et al. 2021: 1; see also Luscher and Lewis 2008). Poole and van de Ven noted that when "organizational theories attempt to capture a multifaceted reality with a finite, internally consistent statement, they are essentially incomplete" (Poole and van de Ven 1989: 562). They therefore encouraged organizational analysts to build better theories by embracing paradoxical claims. According to organizational paradox theory, managers often need to do both A and B and adhere to multiple versions of truth to find solutions that work for all organizational actors (Lewis and Smith 2014).

Paradoxical thinking implies embracing ambiguities. Ambiguity contrasts with contemporary policy ambitions around data-driven healthcare systems that promulgate ideas about simple and unambiguous answers. The policy ambition is typically to resolve uncertainty with data and give an answer about effect (yes/no) and efficiency (low/high). Instead of promoting answers of that type ("either/or"), I encourage a willingness to think in terms of "both/and." It is stimulating to consider paradoxes. Schad and colleagues even quote the philosopher Søren Kierkegaard as an incentive for those inclined to retreat from paradoxes: "The thinker without paradox is like a lover without feeling: a paltry mediocrity" (Schad et al. 2016: 4).

Throughout this book, I thereby point to drivers for and implications of intensified data sourcing that sound like contradictions, but which nevertheless coexist. I will discuss, for example, how data intensification has created both less work and more work; how data both empower and disempower staff and patients; how data both uncover patient concerns and cover up patient concerns; and how data intensity both tightens organizational control and generates new forms of organizational disintegration. In formulating each of these paradoxes, I use the term "data" as shorthand for "intensified data sourcing" because the stories my interlocutors tell about data often set them up as agents in their own right. Indeed, data can exert agential powers, but what they do depend on the types of sourcing and use that they inform. Sometimes a paradox is solved simply by realizing that the same data initiative produces almost opposite effects in different places, or for different people, or during different periods of time. On some occasions, it is a case of the old adage: one person's meat is another's poison. In other instances, the paradox becomes a reason for rethinking the phenomenon at stake—for example, what counts as "patient concerns" if these concerns are both uncovered and covered up? More generally, however, I use the figure of the paradox to ponder on the productivity of apparently exclusive stories. If we accept several propositions as all conferring something partly true, what do their coexistence allow or produce in the given setting? Toward the end of each chapter, I will reflect on this question. The curious reader can peep at the full list of paradoxes that I discuss throughout the book by skipping ahead to table 7.1 in the conclusion, but otherwise I develop them chapter by chapter.

For people inhabiting data-intensive environments, there is also the more experiential dimension of the paradoxes relating to opportunity and risk. The ambiguity that I have described as a matter of contradictory stories about data also reflects something more general in our contemporary engagements with data and digitalization. If the Internet was a liberating space for the competent few in the 1990s, it has now permeated most aspects of everyday life, including that of people who are not the least tech-savvy. And the Internet is clearly no longer a space of freedom, but rather a zone of state power and big business.[3] In his memoirs, the whistleblower Edward Snowden, who became known for revealing the data-collection practices of the US National Security Agency, described coming to the uncanny realization that Barlow's Declaration of Independency had given sway to pervasive surveillance (Snowden 2019a). Today, he claims, anyone with an uncovered camera might have an intelligence officer looking at her or his face when typing. Shoshana Zuboff and others have described how big tech's accumulation of data assets have become instrumental in the global economic system in ways that also encroach on freedom and privacy (e.g., Zuboff 2019). Any Internet search now provides an opportunity to collect data not just on the object of the search, but on the citizen looking for information. Should I look up a disease online, my search history constitutes a data point about me (or, rather, my Internet Protocol address). Such data can be offered for sale. The infrastructures in place have generated an explosion of opportunity and a wide range of new risks. Living in data-intensive environments is living with the paradox of being simultaneously enriched and exploited, empowered and disempowered.

For the remainder of this introduction, I reflect on the vocabulary that I will use in this book to understand the paradoxes involved in the politics of intensified data sourcing—"data," "infrastructures," and "data politics"—and how this book situates itself in the literature on these topics. I then present some additional reflections on what it implies to see paradoxes as the analytical product; and then I end by introducing the individual chapters.

DATA: EVERYBODY SEEMS TO WANT THEM . . . BUT WHAT DOES THE WORD MEAN?

"Data" is a peculiar word. It is derived from the Latin *dare*, meaning "to give." The American pragmatist John Dewey once noted that it would have been more appropriate to talk about what is *taken* (Dewey 1929). Data are not given but *"selected* from this total original subject-matter which gives the impetus to knowing; they are discriminated for a purpose:—that, namely, of affording signs or evidence to define and locate a problem, and thus give a clue to its resolution" (Dewey 1929: 178, emphasis original). Dewey's point was epistemic, but it has gained new political relevance as big tech companies now thrive on data accumulation and ways of transforming these traces of our everyday lives into capital accumulation (van Dijck et al. 2018; van Dijck 2013; Sadowski 2019; Zuboff 2019). As financial assets, most data are taken rather than given (Fourcade and Kluttz 2020).

To dwell a little longer on Dewey's epistemic point, "data" can refer to anything used to inform an understanding. The geographer Rob Kitchin, in his acclaimed book *The Data Revolution*, refers to data as "numbers, characters, symbols, images, sounds, electromagnetic waves, bits—that constitute the building blocks from which information and knowledge are created" (Kitchin 2014: 1). With a similar emphasis on knowledge making, the information scholar Christine Borgman (2015) writes: "Data are representations of observations, objects, or other entities used as evidence of phenomena for the purpose of research or scholarship" (28). Data, it seems, are "building blocks" and "representations" that can take practically any form—so long as they can be made subject to computation. I use the plural form of "data" in recognition of this "building block" view, which in turn characterizes the quest for "more data" to be accumulated as assets (Pinel 2020, 2021; Birch 2017; Birch, Cochrane, and Ward 2021). In healthcare, however, data are no longer just used for "research or scholarship," as Borgman's and Kitchin's definitions suggest. As I will argue throughout the book, this changes how analysts must think about data.

Data always have histories (Loukissas 2019). They are made, not found (Leonelli 2016); they are cooked, never raw (Biruk 2018; Gitelman and Jackson 2013). Data are "inscribed," as Latour would say (Latour 2014), through processes of computation that make them at the same time exchangeable as stable objects and flexible in the sense of being open for multiple interpretations. They come into being through datafication. One of the most widely circulated books about big data defines "datafication" in this way: "To datafy a phenomenon is to put it into a quantified format so it can be tabulated and analyzed" (Mayer-Schönberger and Cukier 2013: 78). Anthropologists similarly discuss "datafication" as a "conversion of qualitative aspects of life into quantified data" (Ruckenstein and Schüll 2017: 261). I, conversely, think we need to distinguish between datafication and quantification. To explain why, I will have to say a bit more about how the term "data" is used in practice.

I had worked with intensified data sourcing for some time and thought a lot about these academic definitions before realizing that I had forgotten to ask what the word "data" meant to the people I was interviewing. When I began asking this question, "What does the word 'data' mean when you use it here in your organization?" my interviewees often looked puzzled. As Rosenberg notes, the word "data" is used to discuss other concepts, but not in itself seen as a concept worth exploring (Rosenberg 2013). I now wish to use some of the responses I received to my question to illustrate the evolving meanings of the concept of data. In *Philosophical Investigations*, Ludwig Wittgenstein (2001) argued that words acquire their meaning through familiarity with situations already known to the user. No word carries any inert meaning; the meaning of a word emerges in its *use*. To understand what words mean, Wittgenstein therefore suggested studying actual language-games—the ways in which language is used—as a meaning-producing practice.

In policy papers, at conferences, in interviews, and when directly asked, people mostly refer to data as something digitally recorded, often providing registry data as examples. Anne, from a regional quality assurance organization, first said, "I actually think we have a fairly broad conception of what data are." She then added that "we talk about both data and metadata." As I remained quiet, waiting for her to continue, she resumed: "We call it 'data' as soon as it can make up a data set with some rows and columns." For her, data were something to be registered in a structured manner, ready for computation. The definition was not so broad after all—it fitted well with the common focus on quantification in the literature.

Clinicians, conversely, often talk about how "data cannot capture every-thing." One general practitioner, Frederik, felt slightly overwhelmed by my invitation to define "data": "That's a really big question! When does some-thing in the world turn into data? Well, it involves some kind of registra-tion, I guess. To make it documentable. It is an attempt to turn real-world experiences into something transferable." Again, data relate to the *transfer* of information, but first and foremost they are about documentation. They need not constitute numbers presented in rows and columns. Clinicians are very aware of the legal aspects of documenting clinical practice, and those data need not be subjected to calculation in order to matter.

At the governmental level, the civil servant Ninna first said that "data" meant "a technical piece of information," but then spoke about a historical development leading to an expanded understanding of data, where data is more akin to an amorphous mass of information (which is why in this quote, I translate "data" in the singular):

> It need not be just a numerical value anymore. It used to be, when people spoke about data, but not anymore. It can be free text and everything. All of this we do see as data today, whereas earlier it needed to fit into a spreadsheet. Today, it is all types of information (. . .) on a continuum to what is really close to something like knowledge.

Here, we see not only an expanded notion of data, but also a slippage from data into knowledge. I asked: "When did this happen?" And Ninna responded:

> I'm not sure. (. . .) Traditionally, we made a distinction between pieces of infor-mation out in the health services, in the physical health record, health informa-tion, also legally. And then, when it was turned into something electronic, for example through entry into our registries, then it became data. But the world isn't like that anymore. There are no paper records from which selected pieces of infor-mation are turned into data. Today, everything is information that circulates.

Today, every piece of clinical documentation is digital right from the start, and thereby it already is an object of potential transfer. It need no longer be "in rows and columns." When I asked: "Is there anything which isn't or can't become data then?" Ninna laughed, then paused, and after a while, said: "Of course, there must be something which isn't turned into data. I just can't think of it. (. . .) What matters is traceability. Everything traceable is data."

Two elements of Ninna's reflections are particularly worth noticing: the emphasis on traceability/exchangeability and the conflation of data and knowledge. To have data about someone (or something) is seen as *knowing* something about them. Interestingly, when I interviewed people from patient organizations, they were very aware of this move toward ubiquitous transferability. Hanne, who chaired one of several cancer patient organizations in Denmark, said that "data are something you gather somewhere so that others can go and look at them." Lone, who suffered from diabetes and who had worked for years in promoting patient rights and giving a voice to patients with chronic conditions, similarly emphasized the exchangeability of data, but she added that it could feel like surrendering parts of her life: "It's actually my entire life history they ask for. It's there somewhere [in the digital archives], and they can access all of it." She thereby conveyed how she, as a patient in a fully digital and integrated system, felt little control over who gets to know what about her.

The pharmaceutical industry and the medical device businesses are also among the actors currently wanting more data. I interviewed an experienced lobbyist, Bent, one afternoon in his organization's beautiful offices in the capital region of Denmark. He had worked for years to promote industry access to public health data. When I asked which "data" he and his colleagues were lobbying to access, he said:

> everything that's in the registries, the admittance registry, cancer registry, cause-of-death registry and so on (. . .). And then it is everything that the Regions [responsible for running the hospitals] have got. The quality databases (. . .) on a continuum to health records, which are not that structured, but contain information all the same (. . .). And then there are the biobanks. Wet data. (. . .). What I hear industry say, is that they want the knowledge in all of those data.

Bent talks about data as "tools" for capturing "everything," or else as a "totality" akin to what Zuboff (2019) sees as typical for the big US data companies. This involves conflating many different types of information, in many different media, created for many different purposes, and repurposing them in line with business strategies. Like Ninna, he conflates data and knowledge. He does not talk about numbers: *everything*, in his view, can be turned into information, decontextualized, and transferred to new users who will find a way to make value out of it.

Taken together, these musings on the meaning of "data" show—in line with Wittgenstein's notion of meaning emerging through language-games—how people associate the word "data" with what they do in the course of their daily work. Running through most of these quotes, these "language-games" in Wittgenstein's sense, is a dominant sense of something traceable that can be subjected to computation, decontextualized, and transferred to other users. In this sense, datafication and digitalization are twin developments: digitalization turns all types of records into data. In short, *data are all the many types of information that are traceable, decontextualizable, transferable, and reusable*. Still, in everyday conversation, the sense of data as being what is coded and countable often takes precedence.

Note how people, in these musings on data, often speak about the same data (same in the sense of being a particular entry of, for example, a diagnostic code into an electronic health record), but they want to use them for different purposes (clinical memory, quality assurance and other more administrative goals, research, or to generate economic growth). Infrastructural integration turns the same data entries into elements of very different projects directed toward different objectives (Winthereik 2010). Data are thereby not just different representations in the epistemic sense suggested by Borgman and Kitchin; rather, they are ontologically *multiple* in the sense suggested by Mol (2002): aspects of several things at once. In short, with data intensification, data are not only multiplying; they are becoming multiple.[4] The people I have interviewed do not recognize this multiplicity. I think they should. In the chapters that follow, I explain why.

Another thing that people rarely acknowledge when talking about data is the materiality of data. The notion of data as "pure information," which can be found in the thinking of, for example, Negroponte, permeates both policy circles and practitioners. Still, I insist on thinking about how we encounter data in material forms. The media scholar Kate O'Riordan (2017) points out that data always necessitate a medium, however fluid it might be: "Information, like humanity, cannot exist apart from the embodiment that brings it into being as a material entity in the world; and embodiment is always instantiated, local, and specific" (127). Similarly, the science and technology studies (STS) scholar Paul Edwards (2010) notes that "data always have a material aspect. Data are *things* (. . .) with dimensionality, weight, and texture" (84, italics in original). This observation points in the direction of the next analytical concept: infrastructure.

INFRASTRUCTURES: MATERIAL, POLITICAL, AND MORAL

I could have outlined how my interlocutors discuss and make sense of the concept of infrastructure—their language-games—in the same way as I just did with data. I will not do that. Among the people building health data infrastructures in Denmark, there are anthropologists, information scholars, and people with training in STS. In conversations with me, many of them talk about infrastructures as sociotechnical accomplishments: an interplay of people and technology. Still, these insights tend to be forgotten when investments are made. Policy papers mostly describe infrastructures as "things" that someone will "build." I will therefore elaborate on how I approach infrastructures analytically to explicate both the thinking that informs my own analysis and a mode of thinking that circulates among some people working in the field I study, but is sidestepped in many investment plans and strategy papers.

Inspired by Star and Ruhleder's seminal paper (1996) on research infrastructures, I think of infrastructures as *activities* rather than things. They are activities in the sense that they are not stable. What they are depends on what they do, or what people do with them. Everyone and everything connected through an infrastructure can engage in different relations; hence there is not one infrastructure, but many interrelated infrastructures that come into being through different social practices. Unlike large-scale material infrastructures encountered in the public space, such as roads, electricity, and water supplies (Larkin 2013), information infrastructures are difficult to observe empirically. Perhaps this is why Bowker and Star (1999) note how infrastructures are typically invisible until they cease to work. Breakdowns make them stand out and demand attention. Just like roads, data infrastructures need repair. They are never finished (Gupta 2018; Howe, Lockrem, Appel et al. 2016). Infrastructures are more than wires and software: they are what people do with them and because of them.

In her influential work on biological research infrastructures, the philosopher Sabina Leonelli (2014) suggests exploring infrastructures by way of observing the work practices and standards that make up a "data journey" in steps of de-contextualization, re-contextualization and re-use for new purposes. Leonelli focuses on research uses of data, whereas I follow data journeys in multiple directions that reflect the many different uses of data, including research but also administration, clinical use, and industrial profit making. It is a classic insight that any form of coordination demands some kind of work (Strauss, Fagerhaugh, Suczek, and Wiener 1997), and it remains a special task for STS to create awareness of all the tacit work (French 2014; Jensen 2022a), as well as the values and priorities (Carusi and De Grandis

2012), that shape data flows. Infrastructures in healthcare are important. They interact in a most literal sense with bodies, they affect life-and-death decisions, and they can inspire hope, shame, and sorrow (Johansen and Andrews 2016; Langstrup 2013; Petersson 2019). They are means of politics.

DATA POLITICS: THE INTERPLAY OF POWER, KNOWLEDGE, AND TECHNOLOGY

Although I could make people discuss the meaning of the words "data" and "infrastructure," "data politics" is not a term used by policymakers and practitioners. Some of my informants even juxtapose data and politics, as if they belong to opposite domains. When I say that intensified data sourcing has *political* implications, it stems from my analytical interests—it is not how the people I study frame it. So what do I mean by "data politics"?

Intensified data sourcing is political because data sourcing intervenes in people's possibilities for achieving their aims. The political scientist David Easton (1953, 1965) famously defined politics as "the authoritative allocation of values for the society." I aim for something less confined to the processes of state power, something more distributed. Still, I can use Easton's classic definition to explain what I am thinking of with the term "politics" because intensified data sourcing potentially intervenes in each element of his definition—"authority," "allocation," "values," and "society"—along with affecting what these terms even mean. *Authority* in data-intensive organizations asserts itself through the creation of particular claims to knowledge and by seeking to control access to this knowledge (Lyon 2019). Data are increasingly used to *allocate* resources through performance measurement regimes and algorithmic automation of decision making (Lury and Day 2019). Data also establish and certify *values* as well as communicate them (Prainsack 2019; Sharon and Zandbergen 2016). Finally, it is through data that populations are constructed in ways that make *societies* emerge as governable entities (Grommé and Ruppert 2020; Ruppert 2012; Desrosiéres 1998; Didier 2009; Tupasela, Snell, and Cañada 2015).

I am not the first to use the concept of data politics. Annelise Riles (2013) refers to data politics as a mode of power where there is ever more data, but with no increase in certainty. Evelyn Ruppert and colleagues discuss data politics as materially mediated interventions in the lives and rights of citizens (Ruppert, Isin, and Bigo 2017). They emphasize the performative power of data—the ability of data to conjure the objects and relations that they are said to portray. I am fully in line with this approach. The media scholar Tim Jordan (2005) defines a related concept, "information politics," as "a complex antagonism that is driven by a social and cultural relationship, understood as a dynamic of forces of care and capture, in which some benefit is gained by extracting some kind of value that is lost, and hence impoverishes others" (11). Like Jordan, I want to explore forces of "care and capture" and their uneven effects. Unlike Jordan, however, I do not see data politics as focused on resources alone. Politics, for me, is not a zero-sum game.

Intensified data sourcing affects intimate aspects of people's identity, emotional struggles, and relations to others. Data politics operates at the knowledge/power nexus. The interconnection between power and knowledge was at the heart of Foucault's interest in biopower (Foucault 1973, 1991, 2002), and along with the emergence of forms of governing at a distance, this interconnection has been explored in great detail and with incisive elegance in governmentality studies (Dean 2010; Miller and Rose 2008; Rose 1999, 2007). Data serve this ambition of governing at a distance.

Data politics sweeps across many social arenas, not just healthcare. It is changing societies. Datafication almost serves as a label for our current moment in time (Maguire, Langstrup, Danholt, and Gad 2020). In recent years, I have attended many conferences called things like the "Data Moment," "Data Times," "The Age of Data," and so on. The academic literature is inundated with social diagnostic labels trying to capture our time and age: "metric society" (Mau 2019), "audit society" (Power 1997), "dossier society" (Laudon 1986), "evaluation society" (Dahler-Larsen 2012), "risk society" (Beck 1999), "network society" (Castells 2010), "platform society" (van Dijck et al. 2018), "algorithmic society" (Peeters and Schuilenburg 2021), and of course, the popular terms used in politics and media such as "information society" and "knowledge society" (Webster 2002).

Each of these diagnostic labels has been used to describe social developments that are intimately connected with data practices, as well as with wider power struggles revolving around forms of knowing. These labels have been proposed by scholars of astute vision who have contributed with incisive insights into the forces at play in data politics. Nevertheless, it is not my aim with this book to suggest one more diagnostic label. I am not planning to diagnose society. Diagnostic labels are too one-sided in their description to fit the developments I observe. For example, I could say that we live in a society governed by data with equal conviction as I could claim that we live in a society where emotions hold greater political strength than ever before (Durnová 2019). I therefore aim for a different type of generalization than an overarching "diagnostic". I believe that data politics cannot be known in an abstract and generic way, but just as important, I believe that thinking with paradoxes can be much more analytically stimulating. What do I offer the reader with this book, then?

THINKING WITH PARADOXES: QUESTIONS AS ANALYTICAL PRODUCTS

This takes me back to why I believe that thinking with paradoxes can be helpful. In place of *one* diagnostic label, they attune analysts to think about several coexisting developments. Paradoxes go beyond simple answers. With my insistence on paradoxes, I aim to stimulate better questions, while at the same time avoiding definite answers that preempt local curiosity. My ambition is in line with Fortun's (2008: 288) reflections after studying genomic promises in Iceland: "What is needed is an analytical adroitness, a tolerance for contradictions and paradoxes [. . .] and sustained critical involvement."

Many STS scholars will understand my view of knowledge as an ability to pose relevant questions. It is, however, important to be explicit about this when studying organizations that aim to become *data-driven*. These organizations are permeated by ideas about knowledge as *answers*—answers of positivist certainty. Data projects thrive on a lure of "evidence" without explicating the type of transferability between contexts that should constitute that evidence. The contemporary rhetoric about data makes it necessary to be much more explicit about what you can learn from a specific study of a data practice. There is a lot to learn from case studies. They can make us understand mechanisms of more general significance. We just never know for sure what is relevant in a new case. All situations have unique features. It does not mean that scholars, policymakers, or administrators should abandon the use of data or stop learning from experience. On the contrary, it should make them more curious about which data they should request locally.

If I propose better questions as my main contribution, how did I myself arrive at those questions? Data science typically relies on either hypothesis testing or pattern recognition. As I wrote this book, I did something very different. I conducted a form of ethnographic fieldwork at home. For more than five years, I have participated, observed, interviewed, and collected cases from news and networks, traced cases, and looked into their background. These types of research data are very different from those data that make it into public registries and health records. They are hermeneutic and phenomenological, discursive and reflective. I kept recalibrating my curiosity with my informants (Marcus 2021). The methodology is elaborated in chapter 4.[5] I compared notes from various sites to look for commonalities and differences, tensions and contradictions. In this way, I gradually produced lists of drivers and implications. In the course of this, I noted opposing stories about such drivers and implications and then thought about how and why they might all be at least partly true. Seeming opposites coexisted side by side; similar drivers could be related to seemingly opposite effects. In short, I identified perplexing paradoxes. A paradox does not close a case. It is a *both-and* that invites the analyst to linger, contemplate, and explore what remains unruly (Ballestero and Winthereik 2021). I hope the paradoxes I have compiled can inspire people to look for similar complexities in other settings without being simply lost in nuances.

With awareness of paradoxes, I aim to create a more cautious as well as more playful attitude to data. Why playful? As C. Wright Mills (2000 [1959]) once argued, it is important to avoid using methodological rigor as a reason to stop thinking. I think that awareness of paradoxes can help creating the needed playfulness. My hunch is that paradoxes do a better job of sparking curiosity than p-values and confidence intervals. The point is not to replace or downplay the relevance of p-values and confidence intervals; but to let these methodological tools serve the sense of judgment. Clinicians, administrators, and policymakers should be no more data-driven than researchers. They should use data to exercise their judgment.

Furthermore, those working with data initiatives need to study data practices. As I noted earlier, policymakers rarely define what counts *as* data: they encourage people to *see with* data, but do not *look at* data. With this book, I turn the gaze around to look *at* data rather than just *with* data. We have to care about how data are created, collected, curated, stored, and exchanged, and look at what those processes do. To use data well, those in charge of data analysis in each organization need to take into account the social and political dynamics of data. One of the most striking things about the many reports and strategy papers that propel data promises is probably the absence of discussion of such sociopolitical dynamics. I have read countless consultancy reports and strategy papers claiming to outline opportunities and risks associated with new data initiatives, and not one of them have mentioned well-known insights such as Berg and Goorman's "law of medical information" or Markus's "theory of knowledge reuse" (Berg and Goorman 1999; Markus 2001). In 1999, well before any of the strategy papers referred to previously in this text, Berg and Goorman presented their iconic observation on data work in healthcare."The further information has to be able to circulate (i.e. the more different contexts it has to be usable in) the more work is required to disentangle the information from the context of its production." They used this observation to pose a very relevant question concerning the sociopolitical dynamics of health data: "who has to do this work and who reaps the benefits?" (Berg and Goorman 1999: 52).

The information systems researcher Markus drew together available insights on the reuse of data sources back in 2001, identifying four types of reuse that all depend on tacit knowledge about what data mean if users are to arrive at accurate conclusions. She also suggested that to successfully reuse data, the organization needs to analyze its costs and incentives, as well as how it interacts with professional roles among those affected. Insight into the sociopolitical dynamics of data reuse is really not new; it just seems to have escaped the preachers of the messianic gospel about becoming a data-driven society. There is an important role for the social sciences and humanities in recovering this type of lost knowledge (Hoeyer and Winthereik 2022).

THE CHAPTERS

The first five chapters in this book present different aspects of intensified data sourcing. Taken together, they tell a story about what is driving intensified data sourcing and what the implications are for policymakers, staff, and patients. Each chapter develops a conceptual approach to the given aspect: promises, living, work, experiences, and wisdom.

Chapter 1, on *data promises,* gives an introduction to the political promises associated with data intensity and data integration sweeping across all healthcare systems. It outlines how global drivers for intensified data sourcing interact with local opportunities and struggles, describes what makes data appealing to so many people in and around the health services, and presents a categorization of dominant goals with data that the rest of the book draws upon. Data are used for *research, clinical, administrative-political,* and *industrial* purposes. These purposes relate to four goods: *knowledge, health, good governance,* and *wealth.* I also argue that it is important to accept the gravity of the problems people face—their proclaimed data needs—without necessarily accepting the claimed power of the proposed solutions. Rather than buying into the narrative of the technological power characterizing contemporary data promises, I suggest that in many instances, the political power of data revolves less around what data can actually do and more around what it *promises* to produce in the present. Data tools do not always deliver. Instead, they buy time. They make it legitimate to postpone initiatives aimed at helping citizens. Often, data are left unused.

Chapter 2, on *data living,* moves from the high-flying promises to the more mundane implications on the ground. It gives insight into the everyday experience of living in Denmark as a place characterized by a high degree of data integration. To understand what data intensification produces at the level of everyday living involves appreciation of context. I present five types of contexts: new conceptions of health and illness, global rankings, descriptions of key data infrastructures, and narratives of living in the web of a civil registration system assigning a number to each individual. I also argue that global trends in data-intensive medicine acquire local form and meaning as they interact with national infrastructures and the hopes and concerns of local communities.

Chapter 3, on *data work,* describes four types of work that all proliferate in health services as a consequence of data intensification: *production, analysis, instruction,* and *use.* Despite promises of less work and more automation, many data initiatives involve more work or shift around who does the various types of work. Whereas chapter 2 focused on patients and other citizens, this chapter focuses on health professionals and how increased amounts of data work affect the clinical gaze. Health professionals often consider data work as meaningless and frustrating. Nevertheless, it is not uncommon for clinicians to respond to these frustrations by setting up their own data-gathering initiatives—and produce even more data. I suggest that data have become the lens through which they see their own work, and this makes the grinding data mill accelerate.

Chapter 4, on *data experiences,* continues the discussion of drivers for and implications of intensified data sourcing by focusing on the embodied and emotional reactions to data work. It thereby goes beyond assessing data for their epistemic values (the information they convey or fail to convey) and power effect (what they do as governance tools), and suggests exploring the experiential dimensions of working with data in a phenomenological sense. In relation to each of the four types of data work discussed in chapter 3 (production, analysis, instruction, and use), people have embodied and emotional experiences. They are affected by their data work. They react emotionally to representations of data, such as to graphs, tables, and color-coded maps. When data are seen merely as epistemological tools, the human engagement with them is reduced to matters of data literacy. The best route to awareness of a more phenomenological understanding of data, I believe, is by working reflectively with our own engagement with data. I therefore build the point on an introspective approach to my own methodology and my own data. Readers who are curious as to my methodology can go directly to this chapter. I conclude the chapter with a presentation of five lessons about data experiences of relevance to researchers as well as practitioners.

Chapter 5, on *data wisdom,* returns once again to the list of purposes with datafication from chapter 1 and addresses the epistemological and normative challenges with reaching these goals. It describes various forms of knowledge and how clinical work depends not only on data, but also on knowledge forms that cannot be datafied. I provide examples of potential errors in a data analysis and use. Wise data use requires forms of expertise beyond what is offered by data scientists. STS, anthropology, and related disciplines can contribute in important ways to build such expertise, and thereby help form "Data Wisdom."

Chapter 6, *data pandemic,* takes the COVID-19 pandemic as a case that exemplifies the themes and paradoxes from the preceding chapters. The pandemic constitutes a tumultuous and globally significant period where data predictions came to put their mark on societies all over the world. Many citizens became data consumers in new ways, discussing curves and interpretations of test results, death tolls, and even data lingo such as the "R-number." With colleagues in epidemiology, I initiated a collaborative research project with questionnaires in Denmark, the United Kingdom, Netherlands, and France (for a total of 200,000 respondents) to map the impact of the pandemic. We also did telephone interviews with Danish citizens from the beginning of the lockdown in March 2020 and onward (Clotworthy, Dissing, Nguyen, Jensen et al. 2020; Varga, Bu, Dissing, Elsenburg et al. 2021). I draw on this material to revisit each of the themes from the previous chapters (promise, living, work, experience, and wisdom) and reflect on how the pandemic both confirmed and challenged some of my previous findings. I gradually came to realize that I had hitherto primarily viewed data as depoliticizing instruments, but the pandemic now clearly showed that attempts of governing through data opens up a Pandora's box of moral and political contestation. We are likely to have to live with the political repercussions of this moment of data politics long after the virus has ceased to dominate everyday life.

The conclusion of this book sums up the themes as a set of data paradoxes. Data intensification revolves around integration of information infrastructures, and this integration implies interactions among various domains, many of which have not previously been connected. If the drivers for and implications of intensified data sourcing give rise to paradoxical stories, how then are policymakers and administrators to anticipate what a data initiative might produce in their organization? To inspire curiosity (and a healthy dose of caution), I suggest a new metaphor to replace the current preference in policy papers for seeing data as "oil" or "gold mines." The linguists Lakoff and Johnson (1980) taught us how metaphors shape our actions, desires, and analytical frameworks. Data are abstract and intangible; metaphors make them more like things—more comprehensible for the human mind. Metaphors such as "oil" or "gold," however, direct the attention to the creation of wealth. It is limiting. I therefore suggest a rather different metaphor: "drugs." If we analyze (and regulate) data with the same care and attention as we analyze and regulate drugs, I believe we can learn to pose more relevant questions than when we think of them as hidden sources of wealth to be mined or drilled out of the ground. I end the conclusion with a critique of the ethics of intensified data sourcing and a call for new ways to think about regulation. The dominant ethics discourses have tended to focus on individual choice (and thereby individual responsibility). I believe that we need to rethink how patients and citizens can gain from the benefits of intensified data without succumbing to the risks.

By exploring the policy, practice, and experience of data-intensive medicine, the entire book represents an ethnographic engagement with data, and like all ethnography, it needs to embrace the ambiguities. As an ethnographic engagement with data, the book draws on and inscribes itself in an emerging corpus of work in anthropology documenting the effects of datafication on healthcare (Adams 2016a; Biruk 2018; Cool 2016; Erikson 2012; Hogle 2016, 2019; Mason 2018; Merry 2016; Storeng and Behage 2017; Taylor-Alexander 2016), while being equally informed by, and intended as a contribution to, work in STS on the role of data in the health services (Hedgecoe 2004; Prainsack 2017; Pickersgill 2019a, 2019b; Sharon and Zandbergen 2016; Sharon

2016; Greene 2007; Tupasela et al. 2020), and data-intensive knowledge practices (Moriera and Palladino 2011; Leonelli 2016, 2012b; Strasser, 2019; Sætnan, Schneider, and Green 2018). The book can thereby be read as a contribution to what various scholars have called critical data studies (Iliadis and Russo 2016), critical (big) data studies (Wyatt 2022), the anthropology of data (Douglas-Jones, Walford, and Seaver 2021), and anthropology of (big) data (Levin 2019). Still, the ambition is not disciplinary: the book is written for anyone interested in how intensified data sourcing affects contemporary healthcare. My ultimate aim with this book is to pave the way for a carefully balanced approach to intensified data sourcing that dares to reach out for new opportunities—while remaining aware of unintended risks.

1   DATA PROMISES

October 2017: "We need to disrupt all value chains!" It is said with conviction, and it comes from a high-ranking civil servant in the Danish healthcare system. The feeling of being given an order makes me straighten up in my chair in the audience. Without explaining what "all" these "value chains" are, nor what this "disruption" will involve in practice, she continues: "We have the most amazing data resources in Denmark, but if we do not act now, we will fall behind!" She is speaking at an annual meeting called the Health Observatory, a gathering of approximately 500 people working with digital health in Denmark. She recounts with agitation and delight what she has learned from a study trip to the United States (and, it seems, particularly from speaking to "a guy doing those algorithms for Amazon and Uber"). It is the third talk during that conference where the speaker mentions a study trip to the United States, and I am feeling increasingly puzzled. I cannot follow how her take-home messages logically connect. I am aware that though the setup looks like an academic conference, talks at this type of meeting adhere to different criteria of success than research presentations, but still: How do "amazing data resources" become an obligation to "disrupt"? I am also beginning to wonder: Who are they visiting on these study trips, and why?

It is not my first time attending these Health Observatory meetings—typically referred to by the participants as "family gatherings" because it is more or less the same group of people coming every year (see also Lindholm and Lerche 2019). I love the welcoming atmosphere, as well as the frank and forthright introduction to what is going on in digital health in Denmark. During lunch later that day, I learn that several of the civil servants who are attending the meeting have taken courses at Singularity University in Silicon Valley. One man says with profound gravitas as he is leaning over the table toward me: "The world will never look the same to you again!" Apparently, these trips help the prophecies of digital disruption travel from circles in Silicon Valley to Danish hospital wards and administrative corridors. Singularity University also had opened a branch in Denmark just months earlier that year (called SingularityU because "university" is a legally defined name in Denmark that can be used only by those acknowledged by the authorities as such). Study trips to the United States are not the only recurring topic in the talks this year. The very same five PowerPoint slides appear in several talks. These slides were even sent to me by a kind informant a few weeks earlier. They are used to explain the investment of half a billion Danish kroner (DKK) into something called "the health data program." They represent some of the recent investments that were done, so that Denmark does not fall behind.

When I first received these slides, I was thrilled! I thought they contained just what I needed to know about ongoing initiatives aimed at intensified data sourcing in Danish healthcare. The slides mention a 2013 Organisation for Economic Co-operation and Development (OECD) report in which it is pointed out that "the goldmine [of Danish data] is only partly exploited" (OECD 2013: 18). Danish hospitals, the report observes, collect many data that are left unused. The next slide explains that, based on this report, the government asked the consultancy group Deloitte to advise on how to optimize health data use. Deloitte (2014) suggested centralizing data flows to facilitate easier data reuse. The consultancy described the overall purpose as a matter of "supporting a culture in the health services, where the point of departure for medical and health economic actions is *based on data and knowledge about what works*" (6, emphasis added).

In the years that follow, I realize that the Health Data Program was just one investment among many. The slides did not *explain* the ongoing intensification of data sourcing in Denmark. They represented just one particular assemblage of consultancy reports, investments, and perceptions of data needs that all feed into the same overall impetus toward intensified data sourcing. Even the talk about the "need to disrupt all value chains," which first confused me, begins to make sense when seen as part of this wider discourse. The various talks convey the same eschatological sense of being on the verge of something both frightening and attractive. These consultancy reports and talks embody potent *data promises*.

In this chapter, I explore data promises and how they interact with data infrastructures on the ground. Data promises are paradoxical drivers of intensified data sourcing. They are justified by a need for—and promise a future of—decisions based on some sort of "evidence," *but they are not themselves supported by evidence*. First, I reflect on existing studies of promissory politics and how these studies can help us understand data promises as they come across in reports and strategy papers. I then turn to how local infrastructures and political histories interact with global developments by turning to the actors requesting more data for four overlapping purposes: research, clinical use, governance, and economic growth.

PROMISES: THE WORK OF CONSULTANCY REPORTS AND STRATEGY PAPERS

Promises lie at the heart of contemporary data politics. Sociologist Alan Petersen (2019) suggests that digital health is consistently promoted through promissory discourses where statements about what *will* occur become arguments for not only letting it occur, but for *investing* in making it happen. Callahan (2009) finds in such techno-optimistic promises a motor for escalating healthcare costs. Science and technology studies (STS) scholars have had a long-standing interest in the social lives of technological promises and expectations (Koch 2006; Rapp 2011). They have pointed out that though expectations announce the future, their political power operates in the present (Hedgecoe 2004; Brown, Kraft, and Martin 2006; Brown and Michael 2003; Vezyridis and Timmons 2021). While some dismiss optimistic promises as hype and call for more realistic expectations (Löfgren and Webster 2019), STS has warned against searching for the truth behind the buzz (Vincent 2014). The most urgent task is to explore what promises to do—here and now—in the environments where they circulate. This is also my goal when exploring how promissory policies interact with practice and experience.

As stated in the introduction, data promises generate investments in infrastructure. Investments in infrastructure "signal the desires, hopes, and aspirations of a society, or of its leaders" (Appel, Anand, and Gupta 2018: 19). These signals can easily overrule any documented need for such infrastructures. They depend on narratives and metaphors, and when effective, Annas (2014) argues that they "can make even out of control and extraordinarily expensive quests seem much more reasonable and supportable in theory than they are likely to be in practice" (226). Promises can be too big to fail, as it were, in the sense that they raise expectations that cannot be cogently evaluated in the same way as everyday requests for financial support for more limited projects. Therefore, big infrastructural investments are sometimes more likely to receive funding than small projects; or, rather, they acquire their funding based on rather fluffy claims and arguments (Davies, Frow, and Leonelli 2013). Morrison argues that because all innovation by definition springs from an infrastructure, it has turned out to be rhetorically effective—though not logically necessary—to claim that investments in infrastructure will lead to innovation (Morrison 2017). Lee (2015) suggests that infrastructural investments are also politically appealing because different actors can align them with very different hopes. Infrastructural investments carry great appeal.

With metaphors for data such as the new oil and gold mines (Nord-Forsk 2014; Palmgren 2017), it should not seem strange that data promises tend to revolve around profit and national growth (Vezyridis and Timmons 2021). Consultancies are often commissioned to quantify a potential profit: they tend to offer a number. Their estimates typically evade academic standards of transparency, but such numbers can make thoughts about a future return on infrastructural investments acquire an aura of factuality (Merry 2016; Espeland and Stevens 2008).

To give an example, I have several times heard policymakers at conferences and during informal meetings reference a particular report from McKinsey when arguing the need to invest in digital data infrastructures in healthcare (McKinsey & Company 2016). The report claims that Sweden would be able to cut its healthcare expenditure by 25 percent through digitization. In its argumentation, it makes a comparison to Denmark—as Sweden's "more digitally advanced" neighbor—although healthcare in Denmark is not 25 percent cheaper. The report has a brief "Methods" section that simply says that the claims are based on a reading of the literature (yet it provides no references), on statistics (but it does not specify which ones), and on 100 interviews (without clarifying with which types of actors or providing any quotes). It is all the more curious that *Danish* policymakers mention the report as proof that Denmark could save 25 percent through digitalization, thereby disregarding the fact that according to the report, Denmark should already have achieved the savings (in a period of digitization when healthcare costs went up). In short, it is a report with numbers that provide rhetorical strength, but with no clear evidence to support the claims it is used to propagate. Still, most policymakers know how such consultancies work. When I complained to a civil servant about the lack of documentation of the 25 percent (in the course of a meeting where it came up), she laughed and said, "You know, we always say, 'if you need a higher number, then call McKinsey.'"

Data promises encourage investments for fear that the country will fall behind. Speed consistently comes across as a necessary parameter (Jackson 2017). The recurring articulation of "falling behind" that I also heard at the conference with which I opened this chapter has made me wonder: Behind *whom*? In most talks and reports, the nature of the competition remains blurred (Digitaliseringspartnerskabet 2021; Regeringen 2021). Although people go on study trips to the United States and marvel at the growth of its big tech companies, few people consider the US healthcare system worth copying. It is certainly not leading with respect to data integration. The same people who return with a sense of thrill from their US study trips typically remark that American healthcare is scattered and expensive and has left data integration to data brokers. In a 2016 report called "Digitizing Denmark. How Denmark Can Drive and Benefit from an Accelerated Digitized Economy in Europe," commissioned by Google and written by Boston Consulting Group, I finally find some competitors mentioned by name:

> Looking outside of Europe, several Asian countries (Hong Kong, China, Taiwan, Singapore, and South Korea) are highly digitized and/or are undergoing rapid digitization. There is a risk of Denmark being rapidly surpassed by these more digitally proactive economies, leaving the nation in a digital backwater on the global scene, with capital, talent, and growth being focused elsewhere. The value at stake for Denmark . . . translates into a potential 150,000 net full-time equivalent (FTE) positions and more than 200 billion DKK added to the GDP by 2020, an 83% increase in the GDP growth rate. (Alm, Colliander, Gotteberg, et al. 2016a, 4)

"Digital backwater" does not sound very nice, and although the calculation of FTE positions remains opaque, it sounds scary. However, it also sounds like a very generic description of economic threats. The narrative of falling behind Asia has been around since the 1980s (Deming 1986). There are no references to support the claim. Singapore is highly digitized, and yes, South Korea is too, and China is investing in an integrated tracking system, but the rest of Asia is far below the Danish level of digitization. Furthermore, how will competition in this form of digitization between countries affect an 83 percent increase in the gross domestic product (GDP) growth rate?

Numbers again seem to serve as rhetorical devices that give effect to the narrative, rather than as evidence in an academic sense. The report sums up its recommendations as follows:

> Denmark must make faster and broader digitization a national top priority. It is essential for the country in order to secure future GDP growth and create new jobs, as well as to stay competitive in a global and increasingly digital world. (3)

This conclusion lays the groundwork for a nice market for information and communications technology (ICT) companies like the one financing the report. I cannot imagine how digitalization could be given higher priority than it already has, but the report insists that "being in a good position today does not mean Denmark can relax its efforts" (3). Still, the Boston Consulting Group is firm enough in its convictions to have made a whole series of *very similar* reports. One of them carries the title "Digitizing the Netherlands" (and the same subtitle as the one on Denmark). It notes—with a strikingly similar narrative—the following:

> The Netherlands, as one of the leading digital frontrunner nations in Europe, must make further digitization a top priority . . . to secure growth and jobs in a rapidly changing digital world. (Alm et al. 2016: 3)

Yet another report called *Digitizing Europe*—surprise!—recommends similar investments for all of Europe. Much as Ferguson (1994) once noted with respect to policies for development aid, the framing of the problem and solution often remains the same, regardless of context. It might incite us to view the Boston Consulting Group as selling *data promises* with this report; not "data and knowledge about what works" (to use the phrase from Deloitte). Consultancy reports seem to be relatively free to make such authoritative "recommendations" without documentation, at least when they serve already powerful agendas. Pollock and Williams (2010) use the term "promissory organisations" for consultancies that are themselves relieved from keeping their promises. When policy priorities change, they can write a new report.[1]

Data promises are fed not only by consultancies, but also by computer scientists. Domingos (2015), for example, talks about a Master Algorithm that designs itself and cuts itself loose from human interference, an algorithm that

> can derive all knowledge in the world—past, present, and future—from data. Inventing it would be one of the greatest advances in the history of science. . . . The Master Algorithm is our gateway to solving some of the hardest problems we face, from building domestic robots to curing cancer (xviii).

Computer scientists discuss this idea because they already now work with algorithms that develop other algorithms, so that humans do not know how the latter algorithms work (Tegmark 2017). Because digital data analysis is associated with great power, data promises also provoke warnings. Hope and fear go hand in hand (Mulkay 1993). Some computer scientists now fear that such a Master Algorithm will take control of all life (Tegmark 2017). They fear a digital power that will erase the human world as we know it. The sociologist Richard Tutton observes how the old utopian vision of progress more broadly has acquired a dystopian outlook in the inner circles of Silicon Valley, where private investments are now made to facilitate escape from the Earth to settle on Mars following potential disasters (Tutton 2017; Tutton 2020). In interesting ways, the dystopian scare just adds to the gravitas of the digital challenge and, for many of the people I have met, underlines the pivotal importance of being part of the "data-driven" future. If a Master Algorithm is about to take over, it is better to be prepared. Fear can also be a mobilizing promise.

The politics of data promises may fly on the wings of eschatological gospel, but the changes they install strike real people in the present. The implications are often a lot more mundane and low-tech—less sophisticated and less accurate than the consultancy promises suggest. This is why I keep insisting on relating the policy visions to the practices and experiences that patients and health professionals have with contemporary healthcare. For patients, the quest for evidence is much more than a rhetorical game or a business opportunity (Rabeharisoa, Moreira, and Akrich 2014; Rabeharisoa, Callon, Filipe et al. 2014). They are confronted with suffering and despair (Novas 2006; Petersen and Tanner 2015). It is because of them that we need to keep questioning which types of investments data promises stimulate. Patients depend on responsive healthcare systems (Lomborg, Langstrup, and Andersen 2020). Who, then, are the people wanting more data, and what do they wish to do with them? Why do they believe that healthcare needs more data?

DATA MULTIPLE: MANY ACTORS, MANY PURPOSES

To understand the drivers for intensified data sourcing, we must understand why local decision makers think they need more data. Regardless of the problem, global gospel does not rule the world simply by sounding exciting. Promises must speak to local concerns and perceptions of problems (Kieser 1997; Røvik 1996). At the same time, nobody just "needs" data. An urge for data is not like thirst or hunger. It is an acquired taste—one nurtured through university training and organizational interactions. So what have people learned to desire?

I have compiled the most common purposes that are said to justify intensified data sourcing in table 1.1. This table does not exhaust the calls for more data, but it does serve to illustrate types of purpose. I have organized it into four groups of data users: *researchers, clinicians, administrators/politicians,* and *industry.* Users do matter (Oudshoorn and Pinch 2003; Hyysalo, Jensen, and Oudshoorn 2016). Some individuals occupy several or all of these roles but may approach the data with different affordances over time, depending on their institutional setting and how it is governed (Pine and Bossen 2020). I propose the four groups as a way to reflect on how data are supposed to serve purposes associated with four types of good: *knowledge, health, good governance,* and *wealth.* These purposes weave into each other, just as individuals occupy multiple roles. Winthereik and colleagues have described how purposes often multiply when medical information is digitized: the digital form facilitates new ways of thinking about legitimate data usage (Winthereik, van der Ploeg, and Berg 2007). In that sense, we might say that purposes are not defined by human collectives alone. I return to the multiple purposes throughout this book because the simultaneous pursuit of several *different* goods—using the *same* data sources—is a key feature of intensified data sourcing. The most striking aspect of such a list is that so many people want to use data, practically all of which are produced, or will be produced, in the clinic or by patients.

What does this talk about "multiple uses" mean in practice? It means, for example, that when a hospital doctor sees a man with arthritis, a diagnostic code is used to describe the disease. In Denmark, the current computer systems use the international diagnostic manual, ICD-10, which is translated into a coding language. Codes are integrated into so many systems that updates to the international manual such as the ICD-11 (adopted by the World Health Assembly) are not immediately implemented (Green, Carusi, and Hoeyer 2022; Lie and Greene 2020). The diagnostic code specifies the type of arthritis in a taxonomy of disease. This code is combined with a code for the type of visit or health service and then used when communicating with other health professionals and when reporting to central registries.[2]

Table 1.1

Purposes for which actors want more data

Actors/Goods	Stated Purposes Claimed to Justify Intensified Data Sourcing
Researchers Knowledge	Clinical research, such as the use of patient data to • Document the effect of changes in clinical procedures and evaluate the effects (and side effects) of treatments • Identify patients for randomized clinical drug trials or experiments with precision medicine Health services research focusing on • Usage of patient data to identify, e.g., patient needs or patterns of inequality • Usage of patient data to assess, monitor, and compare, e.g., different forms of organization Epidemiological research, such as the use of patient data to • Monitor and predict disease burden and distribution • Identify population health problems and potential causes of disease Laboratory research, such as the use of patient data and samples to • Validate new laboratory methods • Carry out -omics research to understand mechanisms of disease Big data research using population data sets, also beyond health-care, to • Identify patient pathways and interactions • Identify patterns of disease or raise new hypotheses based on unexpected correlations
Clinicians Health	Systematic approaches to ensure consistency when dealing with, for example: • Screening, triage and assessment of needs • Follow-up (e.g., discontinuation of drugs, side effects, chronic care, polypharmacy) Optimized treatment options • Use of experiences from similar patients to make targeted treatment plans (e.g., in personalized medicine) • Enhanced monitoring of patients at risk Coordination and easy information exchange • Communication and coordination between clinicians, across units and sectors • Communication between clinicians and patients Monitoring of quality, such as by using patient data to • Identify safety problems (e.g., infection rates) and unusual patterns (e.g., in prescriptions or deaths) • Document progress or achievement of goals Public health surveillance, such as • Pandemic surveillance • Preventive measures

(continued)

Actors/Goods	Stated Purposes Claimed to Justify Intensified Data Sourcing
Politicians and administrators / Good governance	*Political Level*
	Establishment of goals and assessment of whether goals are reached, such as • Less use of physical force in psychiatry, or shortened waiting times • Equality in health provisions and outcomes • Medical error Preparation for negotiations with external actors, such as • Unions • Pharmaceutical companies and other suppliers Preparation of governmental reforms, such as • Financing and remuneration models • Creation of new units of administration Prioritization between areas, such as • Psychiatry or cancer • Documentation of effect of services Initiatives to cut expenditure and change routines, such as • Optimization of resource use disruption of routines (e.g., using big data to predict, prevent, and plan) Change of power balance • Political management allowed access to the same knowledge as clinical staff • Patient empowerment: patients are given access to their own data
	Administrative Level
	Remuneration and budget control • Service per fee (e.g., general practitioners, pharmacies, and specialists) • Value-based care Accountability • To avoid fraud • To ensure quality Efficiency and value for money, including "LEAN thinking" and measurement of effect
Industry / Wealth	Create more efficient products, such as • Personalizing treatment and prevention and achieving better effect • Developing data tools that patients can use for monitoring and intervening in their disease Expand innovation and lower research and development (R&D) cost, such as • Use data as cheap "sandboxes" • Minimize costs associated with RCTs • Develop new products, including digital devices Monitor effect of drugs postmarketing, such as to • Identify side effects and drug interactions Expand markets (and profits) with real-world evidence (RWE), such as by • Moving indication thresholds or documenting off-label uses to enhance marketing • Instigating value-based pricing through documentation of effect to differentiate prices To use data as assets in their own right such as by • Delivering data access and analysis to other companies

The registries are used for research and planning. The code is the basis for reporting to quality databases used to document organizational performance. It is also used to produce lists of patients for organizational LEAN work. It is used for remuneration purposes, as well as to identify potential trial subjects for the pharmaceutical industry wishing to do randomized clinical trials (RCTs). This is what I meant when, in the introduction, I wrote that data have become *multiple* (Mol 2002): they are data on many things and come to produce (and form part of) very different phenomena than clinical care.

I now turn to examples from each of the four purposes that involve intensified data sourcing. I will show how data promises in relation to each of the four purposes are characterized by a peculiar temporality: the burden of evidence rests with the future, while "data and knowledge about what works" means relatively little in the present. Still, I also want readers to understand why people think they need more data. It is important to understand the challenges that researchers, clinicians, administrators, and industry representatives face to appreciate the drivers for intensified data sourcing.

RESEARCH PURPOSES: DATA AS TOOLS OF KNOWLEDGE

Researchers are not one group with one set of interests, and the same data are used for very different types of research (cf. table 1.1). Still, across various fields, there is a push for data to gain statistical strength, capture complexity, and capture new aspects of phenomena or even establish new phenomena. There is also, for each research field, increased interest in accessing data for educational purposes. Data are crucial for career opportunities in an ever-more-competitive research world (Biagioli and Lippman 2020; Pinel 2021).

Medical researchers often work in the clinic, and they use patient data to identify patients for inclusion in trials or to document and publish the effects of local innovation. Health services researchers also depend on data generated in the clinic or by patients in order to explore the function and effect of the healthcare system, but often these researchers work elsewhere, in universities, semigovernmental, or independent research institutions. Similarly, epidemiologists must have access to population data to identify disease patterns and problems relating to, for example, inequality or discrimination. Epidemiologists also use data to identify agents of disease related to pollution or behavioral dispositions, among other topics, and to promote and document the effects of societal strategies of prevention. Patient data are also used for laboratory research, as when new laboratory methods are validated, and in Denmark, clinically derived samples are also used for various forms of -omics research at the population level (Nordfalk and Ekstrøm 2018). On top of all these existing research forms, computer scientists now wish to explore amorphous clinical data sets with big data methodologies. They all need more data to generate future evidence.

Here, I wish to focus on just one instance of how investments in the creation of "future evidence" do not themselves necessarily involve using existing evidence in the present. My example revolves around the call for more data to enable what in the United States is typically called "precision medicine" and in Europe is known as "personalized treatment." The call for "personalization" is not new. Clark (1937) raised the problem of individual variation in drug responses as early as the late 1930s, and the shortcomings of RCTs being conducted primarily on white males have been addressed by policymakers and patient activists for decades (Epstein 2007). Nevertheless, this ambition has served as a lever for data integration projects throughout the Western Hemisphere from the 2010s onward, as laid out in the introduction. So how do researchers document their "need for more data"?

I have attended numerous scientific, industrial, and political conferences on personalized medicine. They are organized and attended by academic researchers, industry representatives, and healthcare system representatives. These actors also publish reports and strategy papers. The organization responsible for specialized care in Denmark, Danish Regions, drew up several such strategy papers, and based on one such "action plan" for personalized medicine (Danske Regioner 2015), a national project was launched (Sundheds-og Ældreministeriet and Danske Regioner 2016). This could be seen as a long process of consultations that leads to a synthesis—a perfect example of building on the best-available evidence. However, the project strategy endorsed by the health authorities provided few details on content, no work packages, and no methods (Skøtt, Rasmussen, Kruse et al. 2015). What the project strategy lacked in specificity was made up for in terms of the gravity with which the authors argue the urgency for investments in personalized medicine. One graphic in particular, which I will discuss in some detail, communicates this urgency.

The graphic is presented not only in reports, but also at conferences and in workshops, sometimes by several speakers during the same event—to the

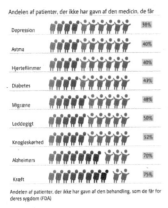
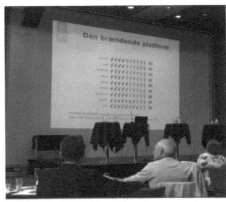

FIGURE 1.1

The burning platform. A photo from one of the conferences displaying the graphic (reproduced on the left) that lists "Share of patients who gain no benefit from drugs" (referencing the FDA report). The graphic is used in reports and in an endless number of talks to argue the need for personalized medicine, here with the heading (in Danish): "The burning platform." (Credit for figure: Ulla Hilden. Photo: author)

point that it is introduced with variations of "you probably all know this figure," and often with the heading "The burning platform" (see figure 1.1).

The graphic lists "the share of patients who gain no benefit from drugs" in relation to nine diseases. It is said, for example, that 43 percent of Danish diabetes patients and 75 percent of Danish cancer patients gain no benefit from existing treatment options. It is an astonishing set of claims, especially considering that patients live with diabetes (and other diseases on the list) for many years. Why is nobody questioning these claims?

If lack of evidence for existing treatments is said to explain the urgency of investments in personalized medicine, a more pressing point, in my view, is that the graphic itself lacks 'evidence.' The Danish report from 2015, in which it first appears, references a US Food and Drug Administration (FDA) report as the source (US Food and Drug Administration 2013). The FDA report (and a very similar graphic) was used by President Barack Obama to promote personalized medicine in the United States. The FDA sounds like an authoritative source, but in support of the claims contained in the graphic, this report merely references an article from 2001 (Spear, Heath-Chiozzi, and Huff 2001). One perhaps could have expected more recent documentation on which to build the future of medicine. When reading the 2001 article, however, the evidence base dwindles even more. The study presents no methodological explanation and actually just lists some numbers in a table in relation to an argument about what it would take to develop pharmacogenetic tests (see Senn 2015 for criticism from a statistician). Furthermore, there are some interesting leaps in each translation. The 2001 article referred to "response rates of patients to a major drug for a selected group of therapeutic areas," whereas the FDA report uses the caption "for whom drugs are ineffective." The leap from "response rates to *a* major drug" ("drug" as the singular) to the FDA phrasing "for whom drugs are ineffective" ("drugs," plural) to the Danish claim of "no benefit" is remarkable. In essence, this means that the claim that there is no evidence for the effect of existing treatments is itself being made without supporting evidence. Apparently, proponents of personalized medicine can make do with a narrative that merely *appears* to rest on data and a *promise* of better evidence in the future. The burden of evidence rests with the future; in the present, a good narrative will do.

The absence of interest in understanding the problem (the evidence base today) in order to promote a solution (personalized genomic medicine) involves a particular temporality. The solution is so grand that it becomes unnecessary to probe the problems supposedly haunting the present. And, really, why should scientists who are working in the nexus of science and policy want to debunk a graphic that might help raise billions in research funding for a large-scale data-gathering project? Despite all my reservations, I acknowledge that there are valid scientific arguments for embarking on large-scale projects aimed at a more data-intensive form of research. Researching clinicians rarely feel certain that a treatment will work: they sincerely want better predictions. I understand and appreciate their desire for data. My point is that the political process does not depend on "data and knowledge about what works" (as Deloitte suggested), and even the researchers involved in raising the funding do not seem to care. Researchers, clinicians, and policymakers coalesce in their pursuit of *future* sources of evidence while demonstrating tenuous relationships with *existing* evidence.

CLINICAL PURPOSES: DATA AS TOOLS OF HEALTH

Like these researchers, most clinicians agree: They need more data! When you ask the clinical staff, at least in Denmark, they require data to ensure consistency (e.g., in screening, triage, and treatment), optimize treatment options (precision medicine and monitoring techniques), ensure coordination (e.g., better documentation and communication), monitor quality (e.g., identify safety problems or document progress), and carry out public health surveillance (e.g., for prevention and pandemic preparedness). In short, they desire data and find them helpful when they facilitate action that optimizes patient care and prevention (cf. table 1.1). It is worth explaining some of these interests and the tensions they involve in just a little more depth.

Data in the form of code (e.g., diagnostic code) complement narrative documentation by delivering options for working systematically across patient populations, such as by identifying outliers in drug prescription patterns or medication errors. Codes are easy to search. They make it easier to schedule systematic checkups. GPs typically have around 1,600 patients, and they need tools to locate those in need of special attention. Similarly, in municipal care, hospital wards, and even screening programs, coded data help to build systematic routines. There are numerous examples of mistakes reflecting faulty routines or forgetfulness (Donaldson, Corrigan, and Kohn 2000). Anyone with responsibility for the life and death of patients is scared of making a mistake: data and digital support tools can help in establishing procedures to minimize this risk.

Another reason for clinicians desiring data in the broader sense of digital documentation is that should anything go wrong, they have documentation that can prove their innocence. Though Denmark does not have the same level of litigation as the United States, there is a driver for data intensification in what is called *defensive medicine*—data aimed at protecting the health professional rather than treating the patient (Wang 2017).[3] Clinicians are aware that data serve multiple purposes and cannot afford to think of them *only* as therapeutic tools. In clinical work, data are also legal tools.

Many clinicians also support infrastructural integration in the hope that it will ease their work with ensuring seamless patient pathways and coordination between units. As I will describe in more detail in chapter 3, they mostly loathe spending time on producing data. Very few health professionals got their education in order to make data for all the other users in table 1.1. Many clinicians, therefore, request better digital systems that can reduce the amount of time they must spend on data work. With a raised eyebrow, one doctor said to me during a break at a seminar about data tools in clinical practice: "It makes no sense that I can take this," he pulled an iPhone out of his pocket, "and find a pizza restaurant in a second. But if I want to find any piece of information on one of my patients [in the electronic health record], I need to spend at least ten minutes!" Rikke, a civil servant working on the national integration of information technology (IT) systems, was painfully aware of these complaints and once explained to me how deep dives into some patient records revealed how some patients' heights had been recorded more than thirty times. Her guess was that it is simply quicker to ask the patients than to find the information in the record. Investments in digital data tools thrive on the promise of making the search easier, despite the common experience of being lost in a data overload that partly results from already having access to too much information. The sense of future potential overrules the current experience because the alternative is seen as accepting the status quo. Similarly, the prospect of being able to predict pandemics and plan public health interventions through massive data collection, including social media (SoMe) monitoring, survives repeated failures to make meaningful predictions and helpful interventions (Aiello, Renson, and Zivich 2020; Caduff 2015). Again, it might be because doing nothing is not a particularly appealing option when facing problems that affect the life and death of patients. Hope needs a nest in which to place its eggs, and currently data tools deliver such nests.

In some instances, the data produced while working with patients mingle in worrisome ways with governance needs. With Malene Bødker, I looked into a new data tool introduced in Danish municipal eldercare to document whether older citizens received the home care they needed (Hoeyer and Bødker 2020). For citizens requesting home care, the municipality had decided to offer rehabilitation instead. Rehabilitation meant that older people would be trained to be able to care for themselves. The municipality then installed a data-scoring system to measure whether these citizens, after this training, could manage well enough to get along without help. Rehabilitation was said to empower these older persons. The key promise was that the data tool would enable the staff to focus on patient goals and allow the older people to determine when they reached these goals. The municipality also paid for a scientific validation of the scoring system as a commitment to "evidence." However, the data were never used. The IT systems caused problems and could not deliver data in a format that the municipality could use for its analysis. Instead, the municipality decided to use data on *reduction in home-care costs* as proof of *rehabilitation success.* The so-called success was backed with data, yes, but not data on older citizens getting the assistance that they need. In practice, older citizens were deprived of home care, and the data on their clinically measured ability to care for themselves—which were supposed to speak for them if they had unmet needs—remained silent in the databases. Despite the high-flying data promises, data meant to document clinical success and ensure accountability can be depressingly weak when confronted with strong political interests in reducing expenditures.

POLITICAL AND ADMINISTRATIVE PURPOSES: DATA AS TOOLS OF GOVERNANCE

Clinicians and administrators subscribe to somewhat different data promises. I regularly receive invitations from high-ranking administrators and politicians wanting to discuss the potential for "total disruption" of existing practices. Clinicians typically have much more modest dreams, of smart software making their everyday workflow easier. Politicians and administrators, conversely, often talk about disrupting these workflows. In contemporary administrative parlance, "agility" refers to the ability to swiftly shift work goals, not agile and seamless tools that can underpin existing work practices and goals.

Not all administrators and politicians think about disruption. Some are just deeply concerned about finding ways for optimizing governance. Public authorities everywhere are tasked with providing a factual background on which political leaders can base their decisions, and with ensuring that political goals are translated into practice (Bessette 2001). Therefore, administrative and political data requirements cannot be separated. Good governance is both a political and administrative task. In fact, many of the political aspirations around data have been most clearly articulated in my interviews with administrators. The current vision for good governance involves the following objectives (also listed in table 1.1): to set goals and see whether you reach them; to be in a strong position when negotiating (e.g., with unions or industrial partners); to build reforms on "data and knowledge about what works"; to prioritize among areas based on analysis rather than the perceptions and opinions of clinical stakeholders; to use data to find ways of cutting expenditure and reorganizing care in smarter ways; and to change the power balance in the health services by giving patients more leverage in relation to health professionals. Administrators are also inclined to think that financial control depends on a fine data grid. All of these political-administrative aspirations are in line with what is typically called "New Public Management (NPM)" (Hood 1991)—though by now, "Old Public Management" might be a more appropriate term. Politicians and administrators also consider it their job to build the infrastructures that fulfill the perceived needs of researchers, clinicians, and industry.

There is something undeniably appealing about most of these requests for data articulated by Danish policymakers (and also by politicians and administrators in many other countries), not least after four years where the White House was so ready to dismiss scientific evidence as fake news. In many ways, the essence of good governance is to emphasize accountability and efficiency. Some people might dislike authorities' interest in using data to prepare themselves for negotiations with trade unions, or for planning reforms aimed at cutting expenditures, but a public service that does not seek to spend taxpayer money with care is not particularly appealing either. Again and again, however, I have been struck by the disjunction between what data are supposed to do in the future and how they are being used in the present.

Data are said to be necessary to curb expenditures and provide better incentives. Is it through data that expenditures are currently being curbed—in the present? In some cases, perhaps, but certainly not as a general rule. For years, for example, a so-called reprioritization contribution was in place in Denmark, where operational expenses on hospital budgets were reduced by 2 percent based on an *expectation* of increased future efficiency (Højgaard 2017). This logic is not data-driven; it is a simple budget reduction. Arguably, it has made hospitals more efficient. Yet this was not based on data—it came from the necessity of running faster to care for patients with a smaller budget. Similarly, when building some new Danish hospitals, it was decided that the future buildings would be 8 percent more efficient than previous hospital buildings. This calculation was a key part of financing the investment, and yet the 8 percent reduction was not based on data or existing evidence (Ejbye-Ernst 2019a, 2019b). Similar "savings" were calculated into the budget when two administrative regions purchased a new electronic record system from the American supplier Epic (Allen 2019). This purchase is a story in its own right, and I will return to it in chapter 3, but the point here is just that the new system promised to deliver better data, and these data in turn were promised to deliver savings—yet the promises themselves lacked any supporting data (Hildebrandt 2017d; Søgaard 2021). It turned out that there were no savings with the new system: on the contrary, efficiency went down, but the administrative management continued to insist on a future potential that just had not yet materialized (Wolf 2017). In short, there is no tradition for using "data and knowledge about what works" (again using Deloitte's promissory sentence) when implementing cuts in expenditure. It is a promise for the future, not a demand on the present.

Another way to create efficient use of resources is said to be by establishing the right incentives. Value-based care is one such international trend aimed at increasing efficiency (Hogle 2019; Bonde, Bossen, and Danholt 2018). It was already part of NPM to remunerate based on added value rather than stable budgets (Hood 1991). In that sense, the core elements of value-based care have a substantial history. In 1983, when President Ronald Reagan in the United States and Prime Minister Margaret Thatcher in the United Kingdom introduced neoliberal reforms, each in his and her own way, a group of Danish civil servants prepared a so-called modernization program. It was adopted by a right-wing government wishing to reform the welfare state (Nissen 2009). The program introduced market mechanisms to make the state more responsive to citizen needs and to make service delivery more efficient. It involved creating exchangeable units that could be delivered according to market principles, where each service could be measured and accounted for (Mau 2019). NPM was seen as the solution to unwieldly growth in the public sector, and already in the 1980s, proponents of NPM saw ICT as the key to developing more efficient and accountable management (Hood 1991). The emphasis on measurable units prepared the ground for datafication. Much later, and under the telling rubric "Forgive us, for we did not know what we were doing," the small group of civil servants behind the modernization program stated that they thought they were trimming a growing bureaucracy when in fact they were starting a bureaucratic mill of increased documentation (Gjørup and Hjortdal 2007). When value-based care is now presented as a new solution to the problems of NPM, it is a rhetorical trick more than any real change. Furthermore, the reinvention of value-based remuneration is not based on new "evidence." Policymakers refer to reports from the consultancies selling them software to make new calculations of "value," but these reports are themselves without citations or anything that would count as empirical support by academic standards (SAS Institute 2017). The burden of evidence continues to rest with the future, not with the present when the investments are made.

While administrators continue to explain how data are needed to determine what is efficient, the cost efficiency of data collection is not itself considered. I asked a data analyst, Liselotte, about the cost of data sourcing, but she replied: "Basically, I couldn't care less about the cost [of collecting data]. . . . I just want [the data] that I need at my disposal." She wanted data to calculate the most efficient use of resources, but her own work did not need to be calculated on the same terms. I interviewed four civil servants from the national audit organization that works for the Danish parliament—the organization responsible for ensuring the efficient use of public resources. They all dismissed my question about the cost of data collection. One of them, Sarah, explained: "Data are not considered an expense. They are the basis for calculating efficiency."[4] In official reports and financial bills, cost items include digital tools, but rarely working hours. Clinicians just need to run faster when others want more data.

All the same, the current political conception is that accountable and efficient governance depends on having easy access to ever more data. This sense of data dependency is historically specific. Public healthcare has been governed from its inception—the question is how and by whom (Vallgårda 2003). In the early twentieth century, hospitals were in the hands of the medical profession (Vallgårda 1992). Doctors provided regular reports to the political system, but governance worked through delegation. Occasionally, doctors would request political guidance on how to make priorities (Wadmann and Pedersen 2020), but they would retain significant space for clinical judgment. Today, policymakers request Real-Time Data. Data help the administration overcome what has long been known as "the asymmetry problem," where only the clinical staff could claim to know what was happening on the ground (Kjærgaard, Knudsen, and Frølich 2008; Knudsen, Christensen, and Hansen 2008). Data thereby shift power balances and move decision-making power upward in the system, at least superficially (Moore 2018). Data promises exert political power, not because they build on "evidence" or always generate "evidence," but because they pledge a way out of the predicament—sometime in the future.

ECONOMIC PURPOSES: DATA AS TOOLS OF WEALTH

All over Europe, policymakers increasingly see medical data as sources of *wealth* and economic growth, rather than just tools for health (Tarkkala, Helén, and Snell 2018). Therefore, they listen to the wishes of industry partners. As Sunder Rajan observes, states can be important agents for establishing novel markets in the area of health (Rajan 2003, 2006). In such markets, health data become a form of asset ready for capitalization (Birch, Cochrane, and Ward 2021; Vezyridis and Timmons, 2021). In Denmark, the medical industry is the largest export sector, and politicians facilitate and sometimes even pay for forums in which the lobbying can take place (Venkatraman, Mani, and Ussing 2015; Danske Regioner and Dansk Industri 2019). They also pay consultancies to investigate data needs in industry (PA Consulting 2019). In these reports, industry partners often raise concerns about "unnecessary" data protection, particularly challenges with the European General Data Protection Regulation (GDPR), which is seen as a barrier to "growth," and they complain about difficulties with finding the relevant data. Otherwise, the industrial representatives typically express the needs listed in the lower part of table 1.1.

As the industrial lobbyist Bent explained in the introduction, industry basically wants access to everything: easy, fast, and in a manageable and machine-readable format. Why? In particular, pharmaceutical and digital device companies express an interest in being able to "play around" with data to try out and develop new ideas (LIF 2020). They want access to clinical documentation and often talk about it as Real World Evidence (RWE) (US Food and Drug Administration, US Department of Health and Human Services, Center for Devices and Radiological Health, and Center for Biologics and Research 2017), a somewhat blurry concept with several meanings (Wadmann and Højgaard 2020). RWE is supposed to fuel commercial innovation processes. "Data sandboxes" is a common euphemism for this (Bech-Bruun 2019). "Sandbox" has a peculiarly innocent and childish ring, considering that it revolves around giving industry access to intimate patient data collected in the course of public healthcare that are now supposed to be used for the purpose of optimizing commercial market shares (sometimes the sandbox metaphor refers to synthetic or virtual data which are computer-manipulated datasets, though they still originate from patient data). It is not any stranger, I guess, than using the term "cookie"—something sweet, pleasing, and gratifying—to refer to a digital surveillance tool (Bernsen 2019).

Besides "playing around," pharmaceutical companies also want access to patient data to identify side effects and drug interactions, and to expand their market by proving the value of drugs according to new pricing models associated with value-based care (where the impact on patient lives and health outcomes affects remuneration). The main pharmaceutical lobbying organization sees "a significant potential" in value-based pricing of drugs (Larsen, Hirsch, Broe, et al. 2020: 17). Some want to expand off-label use without conducting expensive RCTs, or they want cheaper alternatives to them (Eichler, Bloechl-Daum, Broich et al. 2018). Data access is also expected to help to magnify the market for drugs by finding indications for earlier diagnosis or expanded use (LIF 2020). Drug dispensing in chronic care is also increasingly dependent on data tools to monitor how patients metabolize and use drugs, and companies in areas such as diabetes care, therefore, invest heavily in digital health and machine learning to stay competitive (Karlsson 2021).

My interviews with industrial players have involved a series of rather special experiences. Few people in the private sector allow direct quotes, and I have rarely been allowed to record our conversations. In one case, I was first threatened with a lawsuit about a quote in a newspaper about surveys indicating public resistance to industrial access to patient data. However, in the end, we had several informative meetings, and I learned a lot. Another surprising instance was when a representative from one of the major global data analytics companies, a company sometimes referred to as a leading "health data broker," once invited me for coffee after I had asked a critical question at a public meeting. She wanted to know more about my work and discuss socially robust ways of using data. Having read about their notorious secrecy, I had long pondered how to approach this company—and here I was receiving an invitation from them! The commercial data world is full of surprises.

This mix of threat, openness, and secrecy says something about the ambivalent position of industry in relation to health data. It is both confident and defiant. It knows that it has the support of authorities and politicians, but also that it lacks similar support from the public. When I mentioned the term "data anxiety" in the course of a meeting (Cool 2019; Crawford 2014; Pink, Lanzeni, and Horst 2018), two commercial data analysts exclaimed with one voice: "Yes! That's it. We all suffer from data anxiety!" Partly, this anxiety relates directly to uncertainties about how to comply with the rules of GDPR (an anxiety shared by many academic researchers), but my sense was that there was a deeper, more emotional aspect of their exclamation. They constantly had to tackle conflicting expectations to health data as both a source of revenue and as something beyond economic calculation (Hoeyer 2016).

As policymakers have responded to the sense of global competition, population data are turned into brands (Tupasela 2017b, 2021b), and brands subjected to optimization by way of removing "legal barriers for use" (Tupasela 2017a; Tupasela, Snell, and Tarkkala 2020). In 2003, Denmark introduced informed consent exemptions for biobank research and endorsed registry research without ethics approval to increase its research competitiveness (although in 2020, ethics approval was reintroduced for genomic data). In 1995, a registry was established where people could sign up if they did not want to be contacted by researchers. It was called the Researcher Protection Registry. In 2014, the ministry decided that too many people had signed up, and then the registry was simply deleted so all citizens again were available for research (Nordfalk and Hoeyer 2020). The minister responsible for this at the time, Margrethe Vestager, who later, as EU commissioner, became known for fighting the monopolies of the Big Tech companies, said that she had a clear feeling that people "had not meant to opt out of research" when signing up in the registry, and their research participation was necessary to create a basis for evidence-based policymaking (Nordfalk 2015). Since the justification of the deletion of the registry was not based on any data, it again appears that evidence is something that should materialize in the future rather than informing politics in the present. Legal entitlements in the present must be sacrificed to ensure future opportunities.

The competition among countries also is used by data brokers. In an interview with a global data analytics company, I was told that they always needed to see where they could do which type of study, in light of data availability. On their home page, I had noted that they seemed to possess any type of data imaginable, from social media to prescriptions, beautifully integrated in a graphic representation. In the interview, however, I learned that data sets are not easy to combine. Different countries provide different options for research, and no country has all the data included in their integrated marketing graphic. Social media data was on their menu, but they did not necessarily buy the data from the platforms. They could "scrape" them ("we are pretty good at that," they said). Scraping has been described as a niche market in its own right (Angwin and Stecklow 2010).

Markets in health data take many forms, and these forms reflect both different infrastructures and the modes of calculating value that they facilitate (Franklin 2007; Callon and Muniesa 2005). Depending on the type, I was told, some datasets were available from the authorities, but not all types in all countries. The company expertise partly revolved around knowing where and how to get what. For example, they usually did studies depending on data from general practice in Sweden rather than in Denmark because GPs are publicly employed in Sweden. In Denmark, the majority of GPs are self-employed and not in the habit of pooling their patient data (at least not after a high-profile controversy about governmental reuse of data from general practice).[5] Sweden, conversely, is more restrictive than Denmark over access to registries and biobank samples.

Many government initiatives focus on attracting international investments (Ministry of Foreign Affairs, Ministry of Health, Ministry of Business and Growth et al. 2018; Schultz, Flyvbjerg, Thelborg et al. 2017). One government project costing 400 million DKK involved building an infrastructure for the identification of patients for clinical trials. It was meant to attract international pharmaceutical companies to carry out clinical trials on Danish patients. In an interview, the director of the initiative, Lise, explained the economic potential to me, but when I asked for data or calculations that indicated a positive return, she retracted and said: "It's actually not like we earn money on this," and then continued, "it's more about learning from industry and so on." In fact, she now wanted clinics to collect more data to document the learning value of trials. Again, the promise of economic growth does not need to be supported by "data or knowledge about what works" to ensure investment. Data are expected to deliver future evidence for the decisions already made, not to inform decisions in the present. The recruitment initiative was made permanent with additional funding. Similarly, the national audit organization did a survey of investments in digital infrastructure and found that in 23 out of the 96 projects they investigated, the risk calculation was produced *after* the investment was made (Statsrevisorerne and Rigsrevisionen 2020). Data are often produced to support what is already decided, not to inform decisions.

Some of the big American tech companies also seem to have an interest in the Nordic countries. They place data centers in Denmark, for example, in order to "green wash" their electricity drain (Maguire and Winthereik 2021). In an interview with the investigative journalist Markus Bernsen, Rob Nail from Singularity University further explained that the reason why the US big tech companies invest so heavily in Denmark is because this tiny country is considered an interesting "testbed" for their vision of "a fully automated society" (Bernsen 2019: 81). Denmark is far more digitized than most places, he said, and it also has a social security system that can ensure stability while existing societal structures are "disrupted." The companies aiming for total disruption expect some form of upheaval when people lose their jobs, and when their options become based on automated predictions in areas such as education, health, and policing. Here—as the logic goes—the Danish welfare state might stabilize the conditions for the experiment.

In the area of health, access to Nordic data resources is also interesting for very concrete reasons. These resources can be used to validate data prediction that otherwise is based on commercially available data, such as those from Facebook (or Meta), Apple's Research Kit, and FitBit. Teis, a centrally placed IT developer, knew firsthand about the interest in Danish health data among several US big tech companies. The companies, I was told, want to validate the predictions they make based on data generated on their own platforms. The health data of Danish citizen-patients are authenticated by health professionals using the same traceable personal identity numbers as Danish phone users provide to the phone companies. This type of information can say a lot about the validity of the predictions that otherwise are just based on inferences from consumer-derived data. Coming from the opposite direction, as it were, Danish researchers and clinicians dream of access to the data on people's phones and their online lives, also in order to integrate the two sources of health data.

Big tech companies and pervasive state tracking sound, to some, like a match made in heaven. The platform offering online access to health records, *sundhed.dk*, has a strategy to facilitate citizen upload of consumer data such as that from wearables. It is said that the purpose is to ensure citizens' safe storage. It also facilitates the linkage of data. The policy papers on a new European Health Data Space also promise the option of integrating consumer-generated data with public healthcare data, as mentioned in the introduction. Not everybody is content with the speed of the public initiatives, however, and several projects (e.g., something called the HedaX project) have received large amounts of public and private research funds to build infrastructures where the personal identifier number can link data on shopping from loyalty cards with activity-tracking data (e.g., FitBit), and commercially purchased tests (e.g., ancestry testing), as well as public health records. If commercially available data can be linked with hospital data, companies can claim higher accuracy of the predictions they sell—also in other countries and for persons who have never agreed to merge their FitBit data (for example) with medical records.

Finally, there are markets for health data that operate underneath the surface (Tanner 2017). Some people working with data security at the national level have told me about the black market for health records created through hacking. Apparently, medical records sell for as much as 1,000 US dollars, while credit card information can be purchased for just 1 dollar. The buyers are, ostensibly, mostly people using the information for blackmail, but insurance companies also are said to be among the customers. They want access to unfiltered health records to test the veracity of hospital invoices and patient claims (see also Rowley 2017). Unfortunately, their attempts to protect their legitimate businesses by detecting patient and hospital fraud help generate a black market for data, thereby putting other patients at risk.

PARADOXICAL PROMISES: THE EVIDENCE-FREE QUEST FOR FUTURE EVIDENCE

In this chapter, I have explored how the data promises promoted by policymakers, consultancy companies, and data enthusiasts at all organizational levels interact with perceptions of data needs among researchers, clinicians, politicians, administrators, and industry representatives. I have shown how the promise of *future* accountability based on data is a key driver for intensified data sourcing, but also how data do not deliver such accountability in the present.

Although Deloitte might proclaim an ambition of having political and organizational decisions based on "data and knowledge about what works," neoinstitutional organization theorists will describe such as vision as being slightly naive (Weiss 1986; Brunsson 1989; March and Olsen 1976). This phrase from the Deloitte report probably should be read more like a marketing slogan than a sincere ambition. A lot of organization studies have documented how organizations tend to mimic decisions from other organizations rather than conducting their own data analysis (Abrahamson 1996; Benders and van Veen

2001; Czarniawska 2005; Frenkel 2005; Kieser 1997; Newell, Robertson, and Swan 2001). It is not even obvious that organizations, or governments for that matter, *could* base decisions on data. Most of the decisions about data investments mentioned in this chapter touch upon volatile parameters and affect stakeholders with competing values. Data can inform decisions, but decisions cannot be data-driven (Rittel and Webber 1973). As the organization theorist Charles Lindblom once said, most organizational decisions build on nothing more than the "science of muddling through" (Lindblom 1959).

Feldman and March (1981) have argued that organizations tend to collect—and request—more data than they use because this enhances the legitimacy of those in power. It is easier to accuse top management of having collected too little than too much information. Alvesson and Spicer (2012) even claim that most organizations thrive on collecting data without using them. It creates what they term "functional stupidity":

> Functional stupidity is organizationally-supported lack of reflexivity, substantive reasoning, and justification. It entails a refusal to use intellectual resources outside a narrow and "safe" terrain. It can provide a sense of certainty that allows organizations to function smoothly. (1196)

Alvesson and Spicer (2012) are very clear that functional stupidity does not operate through "intellectual deficits but through political expediency" (1214). Against this background, and in light of the examples across all four intertwined domains, it is time to rethink the work of data promises.

Data investments thrive on a claimed need for future evidence, but investment proposals are rarely backed by similar evidence themselves. Data are not used in the present, but they are expected to do their trick in the future. It is a paradox where both stories are true: people like to think of their decisions as building on data and "evidence," at least in the future, and yet they also neglect using data or "evidence" in the present. I suggest that the coexistence of two truths can be productive for policymakers because it provides an aura of legitimacy and allows *postponement of action*. By claiming that it is better to wait until more data have been accumulated, data promises generate a form of temporal disruption of public accountability. In this context, data-as-promise is—politically—a more powerful resource than data-as-evidence. The paradox also is productive for researchers, who can get funding for research by playing along with popular narratives and still adhering to their scientific values, if not in the present, then—perhaps—in the future. It is productive for clinicians, who hope to get tools in the future that they are missing in the present, and who can adhere to values central to evidence-based medicine without being able to reach that threshold here and now. Further, it is productive to industry, which can use it as leverage to get access to resources.

It is necessary to take both tenets of the paradox seriously and not see the desire for data as somehow fake or akin to lying. People have good reasons for wanting data even when they do not use them for making decisions to invest in data sourcing. Their "data needs" do not arise out of the blue—they are nested in real-world problems. It is, for example, no coincidence that the tenets of New Public Management (NPM) can be reinvented again and again (Pedersen 2019a): the problems of accountable and efficient government are not solved. While the sense of data needs becomes a motor for data collection, the act of postponement makes it possible to *feel* accountable—in the present—although it does also push the fulfilment of accountability ideals into the future. Promissory data legitimize postponement of action—and *fill the waiting time* with a genuine and serious task: intensified data sourcing.

All in all, the eagerness of policymakers to attract capital and make themselves available as testbeds for digital disruption reflects the rhetoric of economic threat from the Boston Consulting Group report cited above. Consultancy reports, policy papers, and think tank statements all argue the need for ever-more-radical measures and lenient legal frameworks, "lest we lose competitiveness" (Regeringen 2019: 7). If the anthropologist Veena Das once noted that citizens in low-income countries are often forced to create an opportunity out of economic deprivation—for example, by making their bodies available for organ harvest (Das 2000)—then citizens in the Nordic countries are increasingly forced to *create vulnerability out of privilege,* "lest they lose competitiveness." It is not their bodies but their data that are up for sale, and they are not making the bargain themselves. Their governments are managing the business for them. Vezyridis and Timmons (2021) have made a similar argument about health data in the United Kingdom. Petersen (2019) suggests that the new trade in data might be a "Faustian bargain" of surrendering something as valuable as one's soul to reach out for the promised land of digital health. My point here is that the nature of the bargain is unknown because the question of which goods the stakeholders will use data to pursue remains unsettled.

I have focused on the data needs articulated in reports and by the people I interview, but I could also have included their negative counterparts. When I mention researchers wanting data to deliver new knowledge, some say that researchers just want data to boost their curriculum vitae (CV) in an academic world corrupted by metrics. When I mention clinicians wanting data to deliver health, some say that many clinicians just want their clinic to have "good quality" in malfunctioning systems for performance measurement. When I mention administrators and politicians wanting data to deliver good governance, some say that they are really trying to build structures for surveillance and control, akin to what you find in cruel dictatorships. When I mention industrial actors wanting to generate wealth for society, some say that it is an economy driven by a form of greed that, like a cancer, eats its way through the bone and marrow of medical evidence.

I have not described these negative counterparts in any detail because they are motives that people attribute to others, never to themselves. Some also point to police uses of medical data. Still, the police can access genetic data in Denmark only for investigations of terrorism cases, not for other types of crime, and it has never appeared as an official reason for any of the initiatives. The negative counterparts, these less benign motivations, are not the official reasons for wanting data. Still, once data are available, they propel new uses, and this sense of "potentiality" (Taussig, Hoeyer, and Helmreich 2013; Svendsen 2011) might very well be a driver for intensified data sourcing. In that sense, the negative counterparts can also be understood as what my interviewees see as likely implications of intensified data sourcing, although it is what they fear rather than what they desire.

How do the data promises discussed in this chapter interact with local infrastructures and affect the everyday lives of patients? This is the topic of chapter 2, which also explains the Danish health data infrastructures in more depth, and thereby also their appeal to the big tech companies and to policymakers elsewhere. By moving closer to the infrastructures shaping everyday living in Denmark, I provide a better sense of the context for the developments I describe in this book. Context is also essential for anybody who wants to understand why policymakers from all over the world, who dream about an integrated health data infrastructure of the Danish type, might not get exactly what they expect when investing in digital infrastructures.

2 DATA LIVING

October 2017: Cramped in my office one afternoon, Lone, Henriette, and I are sitting with some fruit and coffee and a recorder on the table between us. Henriette is a colleague of mine, and we have for years shared an interest in data and what it means to be a patient in a data-intensive healthcare system.[1] We were therefore extremely pleased and grateful when Lone agreed to be interviewed about her experiences both as a chronic diabetes patient and as an influential activist. Lone is known for her work with promoting data at what has been called the "nexus" of clinical, regulatory and industrial objectives (Gottlieb 2013). She has worked tirelessly in patient organizations, served on committees, and advised various agencies and companies. Now is our chance to hear why.

Over the course of three hours, while the dim daylight outside the office windows turns into the type of grayish October darkness that you only find far from the equator, she conveys her conviction that in a data-intensive healthcare system, patients must learn to communicate their concerns through data: "We [as patients] won't be recognized anywhere if we can't measure our experiences and priorities in ways that are acknowledged as evidence." She underlines her point by saying: "We've all felt ignored when things don't appear in a formalized questionnaire!" Lone happily admits that health services are already flooded with questionnaires and other forms of data gathering. These are typically integrated into digital platforms, accessible from phones and laptops, coming in as pop-ups, and later stored in the electronic health record (Langstrup 2013). What Lone wants, however, is to use them for giving her own concerns more leverage. As an example of what Rabeharisoa, Moreira, and Akrich (2014) call "evidence-based activism," Lone wants patient concerns to be presented convincingly and scientifically.

During the course of the interview, a sense of paradox gradually transpires. Lone explains how she works to design questionnaires that datafy patient concerns and interests, and then laments how questionnaires often end up consuming the time of health professionals to such an extent that there is no time left for thoroughly engaging and working with a patient's identified concerns and interests. When Henriette and I ask her to reflect on this, Lone looks back on how it used to be:

> When I was diagnosed in the 1980s, there was very limited data collection, but ample time for the clinical dialogue. [Whereas today] there isn't [ample time] anymore, because you prioritize talking about data today, and you collect so much data. There's just ten minutes for the consultation and you need to go through all the data. The clinician is obliged to focus on these things.

Time pressure makes it even more important to focus on the right topics. This is why Lone wants *good* data. However, data steal time from the explorative dialogue. Data simultaneously uncover *and* cover up patient concerns and interests.

Lone's concerns speak to topics that have been articulated in various ways in relation to healthcare, such as how datafication distorts the clinical assessment (Petersen 2019; Verghese 2008; Wachter 2017), erodes accountability (Wiener 2000; Wiener and Kayser-Jones 1989; Sullivan 2017; Hogle 2019), and makes the patient "disappear" (Hunt, Bell, Baker, and Howard 2017). When we take Lone's perspective, however, the implications are strikingly ambiguous. She certainly does not want data collection to be omitted. She likes questionnaires! Like many patients, she wants digital data tools to be available for everyday care (Nøhr, Vingtoft, and Bertelsen 2019; Zurita and Nøhr 2004). Furthermore, data work today permeates clinical care to a point that without data, healthcare itself can be said to be eroding. Data are *part of*, not just an unnecessary addition to, treatment. Besides the questionnaires mentioned by Lone, contemporary living with disease involves a lot of monitoring of bodily functions with data. She knows that her health depends on data tools. For her as a chronic patient, living with disease has become a practice of living with data.

Enfolded into the paradox of uncovering and covering up her concerns, Lone is living with a second paradox. It relates to empowerment and disempowerment. I gradually realize this as I notice how Lone shifts between emphasizing how data enable her to monitor her health and communicate her priorities—and how she laments what she calls "data stress." Occasionally, she says, she needs what she calls a "data holiday." A concurrent sense of both empowerment and disempowerment also comes across in the way that digital datafication makes patient information travel. Lone says that she wants to use data to influence research and clinical routines. However, it was also Lone whom I quoted in the introduction as saying, "It's actually my entire life history they ask for. It's there somewhere [in the digital archives], and they can access all of it." Like other patients whom I have encountered in the past five years of fieldwork, Lone has sometimes felt uncomfortable when data have turned up in unexpected places. One example is when doctors mention things from her files that she herself finds irrelevant for the specific condition or situation she wants to discuss. Data both empower *and* disempower her.

The second paradox reflects a key dilemma for information technology (IT) once articulated by Brown and Duguid (2000) as inherent to digitalization: information becomes simultaneously "too sticky" and "too leaky." "Sticky" refers to when data are stuck and inaccessible, and "leaky" is when data circulate in uncontrolled or unexpected ways. Danes mostly complain when information is *not* accessible to clinicians needing it—that is, when data are too sticky, or when healthcare professionals have *not* checked up on their medical history prior to a consultation (KMD Analyse and Dagens Medicin 2017). Still, every time a problem of sticky data is solved for one patient, someone else is likely to experience their data as being too leaky. There does not seem to be an exact right level for all. Even without considering hacking and other types of illegal leaks, the experience of leaky data belongs on the dark side of seamless data integration. Shortly before she leaves, Lone says something that has stayed with me:

> I have a feeling that the day I got diagnosed, many years ago, I became public property. I have some kind of obligation towards my society; there is some kind of *right* to step in and pry into my life. It's a combination of all sorts of registers where you can extract all sorts of information about me that others are not obliged to deliver about themselves, as persons (her emphasis).

When data tracking becomes an obligation, data do not only leak; they drain. Cheney-Lippold (2017) argues that data-intensive living reconfigures the relationship between self and collective. Lone's notion of being "public property" shows how her position in the data collective involves ambivalent feelings. Clinical information has somehow become disentangled from the confidential clinical encounter and been made available for what Bowker (2005. P. 30) terms as "the epoch of potential memory" (see also Wadmann, Hartlev, and Hoeyer 2022). A sort of digitalized panopticon model has been established (Haggerty and Ericson 2000).[2] I have known and followed Lone for years. I have heard her powerful presentations. I know how she uses data effectively to promote her cause. It is only during the course of this interview, however, that I understood how data sometimes also disempower her. She cannot have the one without the other. For Lone, living means living with data. That is why I call this chapter Data Living.

Data living is a state of being in the world where a person's opportunities and risks are fully interwoven with the data used to represent this person. For chronic patients like Lone, data living takes on a particular meaning. Chronic patients often monitor their bodies: their biological lives are interconnected with informational lives (Langstrup 2018). This informational life is embedded in data infrastructures. Data facilitate opportunities and involve risks. Data shape everyday living. Kaziunas, Lindtner, Ackerma, and Lee (2018) talk about "lived data" as a condition of life, where data have become an "integral way of living, collectively produced and engaged with" (53). Kitchin (2021) points to the need to understand "data lives"—where and how data move—in order to understand "living with data"—how data affect the everyday lives of citizens (see also Lupton 2016b). This double move is also my ambition with this chapter. However, when Kitchin says about his own examples (mostly drawn from Ireland) that they "are equally applicable to elsewhere" (2021, p. 11), I depart from his analysis. I believe that locality matters. Context matters. It matters in particular when citizens become patients because they then have so much at stake, but very different options for pursuing a good life depending on where they live.

Lone's two paradoxes are, I wish to suggest, characteristic of contemporary data living: data both uncover *and* cover up, they both empower *and* disempower. This chapter unfolds these paradoxes, along with a deeper introduction to the particular contexts where I have encountered them. Because context is needed to understand the particularities of the types of data politics I unfold in this book, I begin with some reflections on the notion of context.

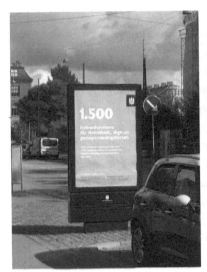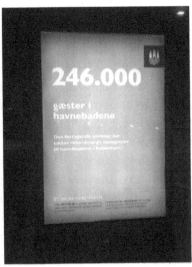

FIGURE 2.1

Data living. For some reason, Danish authorities think that ordinary citizens are interested in data on all sorts of things. It is common to see posters in the streets informing citizens that, for example, 1,500 citizens in Copenhagen Municipality are currently undergoing digital rehabilitation training (left), or that 246,000 citizens are taking a dip in the harbor (right). Data living is also to be addressed as a potential consumer of data rather than as a citizen in need of rehabilitation services or clean water for swimming. Photos: author.

LIVING: FIVE TYPES OF CONTEXT

Ayo Wahlberg (2018a) has argued that medical discoveries and epistemic regimes are always reinvented in local forms. There is not a clear point of "invention" or "discovery" followed by gradual "diffusion" (Rufo 2012). Even a phenomenon as ostensibly global as cutting-edge genetics takes on local forms reflecting particular values and ways of thinking (Taussig 2009). Similarly, data-intensive medicine takes on local forms, not just through interpretation, but thanks to how new technological options interact with infrastructures, politics, and social dynamics. As this chapter describes how an advanced healthcare system has adapted to and reinvented the data promises espoused by the global gospel associated with Silicon Valley, it similarly illustrates the importance of context. Data practices everywhere are entangled in particular historical, political, economic, technological, and social landscapes. When I speak of "Denmark," I refer to a political jurisdiction in which particular data infrastructures constitute conditions of possibility for particular forms of data living. I do not refer to a nation with any particular characteristics. Nations are imagined communities (Anderson 1983) rather than obvious contextual markers. Jasanoff has shown in her research, however, that, as legal jurisdictions, nations give rise to particular ways of dealing with both technological promise and peril (Jasanoff 1987, 2012a; Jasanoff and Metzler 2020). It can be helpful, therefore, to know about the histories and characteristics of the nations in which data infrastructures work.

Context is not a "thing" out there that you can go out and discover. It emerges through action and it is tied to practices (Dourish 2004). Context is an analytical construct (Strathern 2004). In this chapter, I play around with multiple analytical constructions, each with its own relevance and potential. Contextualization has been an important anthropological contribution to the study of technology (Carsten 2011; Lawton, Ahmad, Peel, and Hallowell 2007; Vitebsky 1993; Bruun and Wahlberg 2022) and also a key justification for the empirical turn in bioethics (Kingori 2013; Hoffmaster 2001). However, the way in which "context" sometimes has been set up as a form of explanatory meta-actor on par with "culture" or "power" (Latour 1986), has given the concept a troubled history in science and technology studies (STS; Asdal and Moser 2012). From the perspective of Actor Network Theory, the inclination has been to work the other way around and see such meta-actors as the result of associations, bottom-up—needing to be explained rather than as explanatory devices. My approach to "contexualization" in this chapter is therefore to explore forms of datafication that construe particular places and "populations." These types of contexts operate through, and have performative effects on, everyday data practices, as well as the people they engage (Grommé and Ruppert 2020; Ruppert 2012; Bauer 2013). No contextual unit can be taken for granted.

I provide five types of context here. First comes a thematic discussion of the changes in healthcare and medicine that sustain a shift toward data living. Second follows international rankings as an example of classic context descriptions that are themselves created by international datafication processes. Third are descriptions of the infrastructures that make Denmark into a site that policymakers from around the world care to visit. Fourth is the historical background for constructing these infrastructures. Finally, I describe some narratives of how it is to live one's life in the web of such infrastructures—focusing on the civil registration system providing each individual with a unique number. Each of these modes of providing context illustrates how ostensible global data promises interact with local conditions of possibility and create particular options for data living tied to place and social networks. Each of them also illustrates how Lone's paradoxes play out as contradictory stories about data living.

WIRED MEDICINE: RECONFIGURING HEALTH AND ILLNESS THROUGH DATAFICATION

Intensified data sourcing interacts with changing conceptions of health and disease. Healthcare in the Global North shares a number of overall developments that take on particular forms in different healthcare systems. Jewson (2009) famously outlined a development from the seventeenth century onward from "bedside medicine," through "hospital medicine," to "laboratory medicine." Jewson suggested that at the bedside, in people's own homes, patients were partners in defining the problem. Medical expertise, however, remained limited, and thereby so did the actual chances of receiving help. As people moved into the hospitals and researchers began using experiments and statistical methods, as well as laboratory tests that could reveal otherwise hidden pathologies, the medical ability to act on disease grew. However, the agency moved away from the patient. Today, patients are moving back out of hospitals, but they continue being connected to medical information infrastructures, as Lone exemplifies.

Jewson's account is a history of the implications of increased specialization in medicine. It is a specialization interwoven with datafication. Medical specialization has always been contested. Some clinicians fear losing sight of the whole patient. In her work on early-twentieth-century specialization of healthcare in Denmark, Signild Vallgårda (1992) notes how, for example, a doctor in 1937 feared that "each specialist focuses his [sic] attention on the single group of organs whereby patients risk not being seen as the spiritual and bodily unit each human being fundamentally is" (109). And in 1944, a general practitioner (GP) commented that it is unsatisfactory "to see people describe a blood sample, an electrocardiogram, or an X-ray without knowing anything about the actual patient" (125).

Specialization interacts with datafication by making the part stand in for the whole: a body stands in for a person; a sample stands in for a body; data stand in for a sample. Each specialty deals with only one aspect of a person. Whereas doctors in the eighteenth century could use smell—a corporal and sensory engagement with the patient—as a diagnostic tool, data have now taken the place of bodily experience as the valid basis of medical knowledge (Porter 1999).

History did not stop with what Jewson called "laboratory medicine." Today, a form of *wired medicine* has developed. It operates along with what is left of bedside, hospital, and laboratory medicine. When I use the term "wired medicine," I think of the contemporary forms of digital mediation of patient care. Digitalization implies an informatization of diagnosis, prevention, and treatment, as I suggested earlier. It opens a market for decision support tools such as IBM Watson or Google's DeepMind.

I remember my own surprise the first time I went for a meeting in a hospital ward and came to a place with no beds. Although clinically responsible for patients, the ward was situated in a plain office building, and instead of beds or clinical examination rooms, there were computers. This ward cared for its patients by monitoring their data. Such monitoring is possible only where data infrastructures are so interconnected that all care providers seeing patients in person report to the same systems—and where also patients can digitally connect to the infrastructure and upload data to, and respond to data feeds from, the ward without actually visiting it. Such wards are not an option everywhere. Data-intensive medicine does not produce the same types of data living in different locales.

Digitalization also facilitates treatment at a distance. When I write that patients are "moving back out of hospitals," I mean that they are increasingly treated as outpatients, monitored with data tools, rather than as inpatients receiving in-person care in a bed in a hospital. They are "wired." Such e-health options in many cases send patients back to their own homes while still ill (Farrington and Lynch 2018)—hooked up on what Henriette Langstrup terms "chronic care infrastructures" (Langstrup 2013). If Parsons (1951) once described disease as a temporary state that you would be cured of—or die from (chapter 10)—Wahlberg observes how most people today either live with illness or with a risk profile defining elements of their lives. Practically all of us are in a chronic state which he calls "morbid living" (Wahlberg 2018b, 2009; Wahlberg and Rose 2015). Morbid living is permeated by data, and patients have to find a way through an overload of data and maneuver between information shared with the healthcare services and what they exchange on social media with friends and fellow patients (Kingod and Cleal 2019). They can feel empowered by monitoring and sharing, but when data are used in unexpected ways or by others against them, disempowerment takes hold (Barassi 2020; Andrejevic 2005; Ruckenstein and Granroth 2020).

Another global trend in medicine is the expansion of disease categories through datafication (Green and Vogt 2016). Definition of illness becomes relegated to data thresholds rather than bodily experienced symptoms (Moynihan, Heath, and Henry 2002). People can become patients based on a risk profile, such as high cholesterol or blood pressure levels, long before developing any disease. Even common signs of aging have been included in the most recent international classification of diseases (Haase, Brodersen, and Bülow 2022; Lie and Greene 2020). Greene (2007) has coined the phrase "prescribing by numbers" as a way of describing how data take the place of actual symptoms (Greene 2007). When doctors treat patients based on data thresholds rather than symptoms, it involves a risk of overdiagnosis or, if you prefer, overtreatment (Vogt, Green, Thorn Ekstrøm, and Brodersen 2019; Brodersen, Schwartz, Heneghan, O'Sullivan et al. 2018). Pharmaceutical companies have a great interest in defining cutoff values in ways that expand their market in relation to such data-induced diseases (Wadmann 2014a; Dumit 2012). This is partly why the list of data users keeps expanding in the way I described in chapter 1.

One of the great promises of data-intensive medicine is, as also stated in the introduction, increased precision. The American biologist and tech guru Leroy Hood has popularized the term "P4 medicine"—a vision for a type of medicine that is predictive, preventive, personalized, and participatory (Price, Magis, Earls et al. 2017; Hood, Lovejoy, and Price 2015; Hood and Flores 2012). A lot of the hype around P4 medicine revolves around extremely data-intensive forms of monitoring and treatment associated with, for example, genomic medicine combined with data from wearables and sensors. The results are less groundbreaking than it may sound (Vogt, Green, and Brodersen 2018; Vogt et al. 2019), and yet it is among those people most fascinated by these promises that you find people preferring a statistician to a doctor. The P4 vision also serves as the inspiration for initiatives such as those described in the previous chapter, related to "personalized" medicine.[3] There is an irony at play here, however, and that is that *if* the proponents succeed in preventing disease through these technologies, the "patients" will never encounter the ailment for which their everyday activities are the cure. They will be patients, but they will never be ill. They will be in a state of morbid living, in the sense of living in a data-intensive treatment regime even though what can be phenomenologically experienced is no longer a disease. The patient experience revolves around prevention.

Although P4 may sound like the type of disruption prophesized by global data promises, the actual clinical practices focusing on implementing the new tools are more gradual developments than disruptive disturbances. Gjødsbøl, Winkel, and Bundgaard (2019) have analyzed the discrepancies between the discourses in policy papers and practical clinical reasoning in their understanding of genomic medicine. They remark: "Diagnoses do not 'jump out' of the genomic code as the policies of personalized medicine would have it; rather a firm diagnosis constitutes the condition of possibility for pursuing genetic knowledge" (p. 6). "Data-driven medicine" is typically more of a catchy phrase than an accurate description of clinical practice.

Another, and final, trend in contemporary medicine relating to data is patient-generated data. Many people find data tracking fun and empowering (Kristensen, Jacobsen, and Pihl-Thingvad 2017; de Boer 2020; Kragh-Furbo, Wilkinson, Mort et al. 2018; Roberts, Mackenzie, and Mort 2019). Fitness trackers can give people a sense of thrill when they successfully datafy their achievements (Kristensen and Ruckenstein 2018; Lupton 2020). From a health perspective, though, studies suggest that the effect is limited. On average, people stop using them after a year (Wise 2016). Sometimes people bring the data they generate with wearables and other devices, or that they order through online testing, to their doctors (Fiske, Buyx, and Prainsack 2020). According to one survey, 50 percent of Danish GPs have patients who come based on self-generated data (Videbæk, Geertsen, and Dam 2019). As suggested by Lone's comments, it means that the consultation can come to revolve around the data. The data they bring illuminate certain things, but they also consume consultation time. The fun that people have with data generation can sometimes come with unexpected consequences. Some have been surprised, when using direct-to-consumer genetic testing, to realize that their data have become commercial assets for the companies they thought were servicing them (Geiger and Gross 2019; Christofides and O'Doherty 2016; Lupton 2016a). At this point, people lose control over their data. The empowerment they experience is commingled with new sources of disempowerment.

I focus this book on the drivers for, and implications of, intensified data sourcing initiated within the remits of healthcare systems, and therefore I do not go into further detail with direct-to-consumer data tools. Nevertheless, there is an interesting contrast between the thrill described by sociologists studying consumers and self-trackers and the impression from studies of data practices initiated by healthcare systems: for example, when people in rehabilitation are given digital devices for training (Schwennesen 2017, see also figure 2.1). These patients are not quite as thrilled. In some instances, physical examinations in post-surgery cancer care have been replaced with patient data scores (Torenholt, Saltbæk, and Langstrup 2020). Again, such patient data work is anything but entertaining. Still, when healthcare systems offer data tools that do not conform to patients' own ambitions, some try to hack the digital devices to make them serve their own goals (Kaziunas, Lindtner, Ackerman, and Lee 2018; Pols, Willems, and Aanestad 2019). They turn disempowerment into new options of empowerment.

Each of these uses of data in wired medicine depends on data infrastructures, and because infrastructures differ, medical practices take on local forms. Several of the options for monitoring disease at a distance described here reflect a healthcare system with a high degree of digitization. If Denmark has a particularly high degree of digitization, what does such a ranking imply?

RANKINGS: THE MOST DIGITIZED—AND HAPPIEST—PEOPLE IN THE WORLD?

Rankings are common elements of descriptions of context, but why mention them in a chapter about data *living*? Rankings are enunciations of relative worth. They are applied to people, places, organizations, and even nations. They shape data living by shaping the stories we tell about ourselves and others. Furthermore, rankings are made with data. International rankings use data to make global differences stand out (Merry 2016). Rankings come in many forms—as lists, graphs, and as positions such as being first or number one. As examples of global data collection practices that explicitly compare nations, rankings are apposite tools for contextualizing Danish data practices.

Denmark has long been indexed by international organizations as an excessively digitized and data-intensive country (Kierkegaard 2013). The United Nations (UN) ranks Denmark at the top of its list of public digitization, praising the nation's level of integration across systems, as well as the level of inclusion (DR Nyheder 2018; United Nations 2020): everybody features in the systems. The online health portal *sundhed.dk* (operating since 2003, and offering online access for citizens to medical records since 2009) is ranked among the most advanced in the world (Frost & Sullivan 2017). In 2017, Denmark was the first country to try appointing an ambassador to big tech in Silicon Valley (Baugh 2017). The initiative received a lot of attention, and other countries followed suit. It happened in acknowledgment of the power of the so-called GAFAM companies (Google, Apple, Facebook, Amazon, and Microsoft): their joint value had surpassed that of Denmark's gross domestic product (GDP). The Danish government also wanted to attract investments from these companies, as described in the previous chapter (DR Nyheder 2019a). In addition, Denmark was the first country to sign a Memorandum of Understanding with the private organization World Economic Forum to try to set up data-ethics rules for big data, algorithmic governance, and cross-border data trade (World Economic Forum and Government of Denmark 2018).

Being the first, number one, or at the top of a list can become a political goal in its own right, "lest we lose competitiveness," as the reports in the previous chapter put it. The threat of being "less digitized" than, for example, Estonia (branding itself as an E-nation) or Singapore is diffuse, and yet it shapes political choices. In 2018, Denmark thus implemented an act on "digital-ready legislation," which made it into a demand that future legislation should be formulated so that its administration can be administered digitally, and in principle automated, as far as possible. As Plesner and Justesen (2021) argue, it creates a relatively obscure process where computer specialists now take key roles in formulating the laws of the country. Rankings shape the narratives we tell about ourselves and the forms of life we come to pursue.

Concerning health, the Organisation of Economic Co-operation and Development (OECD) ranks Denmark at the top among its surveyed countries in terms of coverage of core services (OECD and European Union 2018: 175). According to the Euro Health Consumer Index, however, Denmark dropped to a position as the fourth-best health service system in Europe when the organization decided to include suicide rate and means of prevention in the measures for producing the ranking (Björnberg and Phang 2019). Shifts in data practices tend to interact with such moral and political valuations, though the organizations producing the rankings rarely explicate their values (Moreira 2019; Ackerman, Weatherford Darling, Soo-Jin

Lee et al. 2016; Cruz 2017). Through indexing, "best" is presented as something measurable without specifying best-for-whom or the criteria used. It is a separate issue that Denmark no doubt has very high suicide rates—according to international comparisons some of the highest in the world—but I have often heard colleagues working with death registries exclaim with exasperation that "it's because suicides are *registered* in Denmark!" In many countries, they claim, the stigma of suicide leads to underreporting. Rankings in this way might say as much about differences in registration practices as about the phenomena they rank. Ranking organizations rarely publicize doubts about the validity of the data they use.

There are all sorts of rankings. International organizations love to rank. For instance, the World Bank publishes interactive lists, according to which Denmark ranks at the top on "government effectiveness" and "rule of law" (http://info.worldbank.org/governance/wgi/Home/Reports). The World Justice Project also ranks Denmark number one in terms of rule of law (https://worldjusticeproject.org). According to the 2019 numbers from the Social Progress Index measuring of basic human needs, wellbeing, and opportunity, Denmark ranks second in the world (http://www.socialprogressindex.com/). In a 2020 report from Transparency International, Denmark shares with New Zealand the top position in the global ranking of countries with least perceived corruption (Transparency International 2020: 2). Again, this might not say as much about corruption as about perceptions and expectations, and yet such details are often neglected when a ranking is communicated by policymakers.

There are other top rankings, which are rarely referred to with pride. Denmark shifts between having the highest or second-highest level of taxation in the OECD (OECD 2021), and it is said to be the most expensive country in the European Union in which to reside (DR Nyheder 2020). Such rankings are used politically when right-wing politicians wish to criticize the redistributive politics of the welfare state. Rankings feed into political arguments that in turn affect everyday living. Some indexing initiatives are also construed as nonprofit initiatives financed by companies such as Deloitte. As described in the previous chapter, consultancies happily use rankings when articulating data promises. Indeed, some rankings are produced to motivate action (Sauder and Espeland 2009). A low ranking can be a reason for investments to catch up, and a high ranking a reason to invest in order to stay on top. Rankings can transform multidimensional differences into a unidimensional need for change.

Rankings often have commercial impact. A ranking with a clear commercial aim—and one that is certainly more widely circulated in the media than rankings on "rule of law"—is the position as "World's Best Restaurant" on a list of the World's 50 Best Restaurants, produced by the UK media company William Reed Business Media. For some years from 2010 onward, the Copenhagen restaurant Noma has held the top position, and in 2021, Noma was first and another Copenhagen restaurant named Geranium was second on the list. It is ironic, for something as subjective as taste and as incommensurable as a restaurant experience, that a position on a unidimensional scale can become so widely circulated. I have never spent the 4,600 DKK (app. 700 US dollars) that a meal at Noma costs, but I have been struck by how many times I have been asked about Noma by people around the globe when they hear where I live. It becomes almost an element of the very identity of a city, when a certain ranking is repeatedly associated with its name. The impact of a ranking does not necessarily derive from an accurate "measurement" of sorts, but from the way it corroborates narratives about people and places. Rankings "make up" places and people (Hacking 1986). Data living is also a question of living with the stories that data can tell.

Many friends and colleagues also comment—tongue-in-cheek—on the World Happiness Report (Sustainable Development Solutions Network 2020), which for many years placed Denmark at the top of the list of the happiest people in the world (Denmark recently was supplanted by Finland). A colleague from the United States once remarked on this happiness figure during a dinner at our place. He jokingly mused about Noma, happiness, and Denmark as a "cute" country, somewhat "fairytale-like," referencing the Danish fairytale author Hans Christian Andersen, and then added that he should not have been (but he was) surprised that Denmark even had a queen. "A queen!" he exclaimed with a laugh. Denmark is a constitutional monarchy, where the royalty have no political power but the position as head of state has been held by a member of the same family for more than a thousand years. It is not difficult to relate to his sense of puzzlement; it *is* pretty strange. In an interview, Queen Margrethe was once asked what she thought about the ranking as the world's happiest people. She replied: "How big is happiness? How are we to measure it? In which units? Still, I do think it is safe to say that we are an extraordinarily fortunate people" (Trier 2016).

Just as datafication makes certain features of patient lives visible while concealing others, rankings make certain features of "Denmark" stand out, while covering up others. When we use rankings as a context for understanding the nature of intensified data sourcing in the institutions visited by policymakers from around the world, we see a thoroughly digitized and wealthy country that offers free healthcare, education, and extensive social benefits, with a stable, multiparty democracy and high respect for the rule of law. It ought to be an easy and satisfactory place to live. For many citizens, this is the case. Rankings, however, are best at conveying common (average) experiences and less good at imparting outlier (unusual) experiences. Nevertheless, what helps to create seamless interaction for some can provide obstacles for others. In the pages that follow, I will provide examples of people who do not consider themselves as fortunate as the queen suggested they were. Data ubiquity allows many patients to be seen by the healthcare system; but data also sometimes cover up or conceal what patients wish doctors could see—or, conversely, enable doctors to see what patients would like to keep hidden. It is through the type of data ubiquity indicated by several of these rankings that Lone's two paradoxes emerge. I need, therefore, to describe the highly integrated data infrastructures in Denmark in more detail. It is to this task I now turn.[4]

INFRASTRUCTURES: CURATED TRANSFERS, AUTOMATED POOLING, AND PLATFORMS

As an alternative to rankings, one can provide context via narrative descriptions of the infrastructures for healthcare data that have been built in Denmark. In a sense, it is like going behind the level of digitization measured in the rankings to describe what these rankings seek to capture: namely, which organizational and informational infrastructures are in place.

The Danish data infrastructures are highly integrated, partly because healthcare is primarily tax-financed. Public healthcare delivery is organized through three administrative layers: the state level, five regions, and ninety-eight municipalities.[5] The state coordinates legal frameworks and entitlements. The Regions are mainly responsible for specialized care. The municipalities finance primary care such as elder care and nursing homes. Taxes are paid to the municipalities and to the state, who then transfer money to the Regions through data-dependent accounting systems. The Regions organize most healthcare delivery through either public or private suppliers.[6] In Denmark, data used for running the system clinically and administratively also have been transferred to central registries and used in research for years (Bauer 2014).

In most countries, health data remain scattered. Private hospitals hold on to their own data, and individual practitioners have no routines for sharing. It makes it difficult to use data for developing healthcare services at the system level (Olsen, Aisner, and McGinnis 2007). Big tech companies have amassed enormous amounts of data, but they too keep their data in silos. The data may still flow in ways individuals have no chance of understanding (Tanner 2017; Prainsack 2020; Sharon 2016; McMahon, Buyx, and Prainsack 2019). National pooling of data provides the backbone for many of the features that make Denmark a country that policymakers wish to visit. I think it makes sense to talk of three types of pooling, which were introduced stepwise but are working alongside each other today: curated transfers, automated pooling, and platform organization.

Most registries were constructed based on an idea of curated transfer: a medical professional decided which information about a patient that needed to enter a central register. From the first half of the twentieth century, registries have been collecting information from health professionals in such structured formats. Many registries were initiated by physicians carrying out research. These registries only later became part of a national registry infrastructure. Today, the registries are managed by the Danish Health Data Authority, and some disease registries are partly automated so that registries build on other registrations.

Automated pooling made its entry with the online health portal *sundhed.dk*, which relied on full transfers of the whole medical record to a shared repository. It facilitated direct patient access, as well as access for health professionals treating someone and needing to see a medical history from another hospital. It implied abandoning the idea of curation. There was no longer somebody selecting an individual piece of data. Everything was transferred. Quality databases comprise another example of automated data pooling (though some of them still operate more on the basis of curated transfers), but one to which patients have no direct access. They are used for clinical, administrative, and research purposes.

Recently, platform organization has emerged as a new ideal of data integration. Now the ambition is to let health professionals work directly on central digital platforms. Thereby, health professionals must fetch the specific data that they need, and they can do so only when treating patients. It erases—or perhaps reverses—the curation of data. All data are centralized from the start, and doctors treating patients apply for access. National platform models are not meant to cover all data, but only those that can help facilitate coordination.

In my interviews with centrally placed civil servants, the curated transfer is referred to as the "old" way and classified as a baton race (with the information being a baton passed from one to another), while shared platforms are classified as patient-centered (everything about a patient is gathered in one place, and health professionals access only what they need when they need it). Examples of platforms are central online options of registrations of organ donor choices, opt-out of biobank research, living wills, and Do Not Resuscitate choices.

Another platform, also accessible to citizens through sundhed.dk and mobile apps and to health professionals through their local IT systems, is a shared pharmaceutical system with the Danish name *Det Fælles Medicinkort* (Pedersen 2019b). All pharmaceuticals prescribed to a patient are recorded in the same system. The GP, for example, makes out prescriptions in the system. Pharmacies retrieve the prescription directly on the platform server. Staff in the municipalities use the platform to look up what they need to supply to those in eldercare. Patients can look at their own prescriptions and ask for renewals by downloading the platform app or logging into *sundhed.dk* (the two systems are integrated). It has been widely recognized as a success, and yet a platform organization is not a stable and unitary form. The pharmaceutical platform, for example, incrementally adds modules for procedures such as automated dispensation, where robots package medicine in doses according to when they are to be consumed (Jensen 2020b). This is to help patients who take several medicines daily and find handling multiple packages difficult and confusing. It is also used to monitor unfortunate developments in dispensing in contentious areas, such as the use of opioids or penicillin. When data are centrally available, they can also be used for multiple purposes and continuously integrated in new ways. How did this level of data integration come about?

HISTORY: SMALL STEPS TOWARD BIG DATA

A fourth way to consider context is by reflecting on the historical rise of the healthcare system and its data infrastructures. In contrast to the top-down political implementation of interoperable data infrastructures seen in the United States during the Barack Obama administration, Danish data infrastructures gradually developed in a more bottom-up way (Aanestad and Jensen 2011; Phanareth, Rossing, and Vingtoft 2019). They were subject to limited opposition. The old baton model came about mostly as people in the municipalities or clinics approached a member of an organization called MedCom when encountering coordination problems. MedCom runs the health-data-net [Da; *Sundhedsdatanettet*], a service that validates and authenticates individual users' access to health data. This gradually grew out of many other coordination initiatives (Jensen and Hulbæk 2019). In a conversation with two women who had worked for decades with this form of coordination, I was told:

> Digital communication began when a GP came with a piece of paper and said, "Look, I have this discharge letter and I can see it's been printed out, and do you know what I do with it? I hand it to my secretary and then she writes it into my system. It's madness. Couldn't we join the two wires so that it enters my system directly?" And this is what we did. We've been making sure information can be shared between systems.

MedCom responded to local problems and facilitated data exchange. The two women said that it used to be relatively easy to solve such problems, but one added: "It's not that easy anymore. Everything is subject to central approval now. (. . .) It is getting very bureaucratic and slow." Both women were concerned about this development because it made the solutions they were able to provide less responsive to user needs:

> We always knew where the problems were . . . now it takes a "governance model" and "a steering committee." (. . .) Still, on the other hand, it means you have somebody who takes responsibility for everything (. . .). You don't need to cover your own ass when something doesn't work out as planned.

The sense of bureaucratization also reflects the shift from a baton model to a platform model. Platforms are centralized by design.

For other countries currently aiming for enhanced digital integration, it is important to acknowledge that the Danish infrastructures, in which contemporary forms of data living are now embedded, emerged out of millions of choices aimed at solving small, practical problems. Systems such as the Danish ones did not grow out of a master plan. There was no mastermind, no Big Brother, planning or overseeing the individual quests for data integration. In the 1960s, Denmark was far behind the digitization of American healthcare (Collen 1986, 1991; Greene and Lea 2019), partly because there was no need for billing systems, which was one of the first uses of computers in hospitals (Evans 2016; Koopman, Jones, Simon et al. 2021). It was not technological competence that made integration possible in Denmark; it was the social ambition of running a welfare state.

The welfare state, with its social benefits and public healthcare, did not appear out of the blue or without a fight. Contemporary citizen rights and entitlements reflect historical layers of conflict. As in the other Nordic countries, the Danish welfare state emerged gradually out of the people's movements of the nineteenth century. Across the Nordic countries, the workers' movement gained strength in tandem with new, collaborative economic models that encouraged shared ownership of, for example, abattoirs and dairies, as well as cooperative shops. As pointed out by Swedish ethnologists, the call for the poor to have greater influence was accompanied with a strong emphasis on self-control (Frykman & Löfgren, 1987; Qvarsell, 1986). The leading classes in government and business did not welcome these new movements. In Denmark, however, a consensus gradually emerged around a more social-democratic system, in particular during the recession in the 1930s. The totalitarian regimes situated south (Nazi Germany) and east (Soviet Union) of Denmark provided more collaborative forms of governance with a certain appeal, even for conservative observers. The consensus settled on welfare provision—as well as a collaborative system for negotiations between labor unions and employers. The negotiation system with unions became known as the Danish model (Marcussen and Ronit (eds.), 2010).

It takes many small steps to create big data. All Nordic countries have strong historical traditions of documentation, beginning with medieval church records keeping track of births and deaths and followed up by eighteenth-century police registries and government statistics and early-twentieth-century population registries (Pálsson 2002; Lindenius 2009; Sætnan, Lommel, and Hammer 2011). Asdal and Gradmann (2014) talk about a Scandinavian political affinity for particular ways of building 'evidence' that interacts in reinforcing ways with infrastructures for data collection. The modern era of Danish registration began with the establishment of three base registries of identification in 1968: The Civil Registration System, which directly translated would be called the Central Person Registry (CPR), a registry of all property (BBR), and one for legal entities such as companies of various sorts (CVR). I use these abbreviations because they serve as terms in daily registry lingo, as when people suggest that you "check the size of your neighbor's property on BBR." The CPR identifies individuals by linking them to other individuals through kinship ties and to places of residence. It does *not* use biometric figures, unlike the world's largest, and much more recent, citizen database—namely, the Unique Identification Authority of India which has operated from 2009 onward (Nair 2021; Dagiral and Singh 2021). The Danish means of authentication is a network of data ensuring enough data to make up a consistent identity. Biometric evidence such as iris scans, facial recognition, and fingerprints are difficult to use in a database that follows people from cradle to grave. Bodies are too unstable.

The three Danish base registries were established for reasons of taxation—to know who is who, who works where, and who owns what. Once in place, however, the three registries delivered a neat way of keeping track of people, including for purposes other than taxation. The digital CPR replaced censuses in 1976 (A. Lange 2017). The three base registers of identification serve as the foundation for what is being registered in all other registries today. By means of the CPR number, health registries can be combined with data on schooling, employment, and social benefits. Registry data can be combined also with biological samples collected in the course of everyday care and screening activities (see figure 2.2). None of this was planned in 1968. Instead, layers of infrastructural integration have been added incrementally, and each registry has given rise to new ideas about use.

Since these data are permitted to be used for research, they constitute significant resources for epidemiology. Around the beginning of the new millennium, the prestigious scientific journal *Science* was publishing articles characterizing the whole of Denmark as "one big cohort study" (Frank 2000) and "an epidemiologist's dream" (Frank 2003). The Nordic data infrastructures share many traits (Sætnan et al., 2011; Tupasela 2017b; Tupasela, Snell, and Tarkkala 2020; Cool 2016),[7] but Denmark is the most research-radical country—a researcher's dream—because it is the most liberal in its regulations (Holm and Ploug 2017; Salokannel 2017; Nordic Committee on Bioethics 2014). In Denmark, there is an informed consent exemption for biobank and registry research (though since 2020, this is no longer the case for genomic data), and while biobank research presupposes research ethics approval, registry research is subject only to data protection rules, which include the European General Data Protection Regulation (GDPR). It is possible for citizens to opt out of biobank and genetic research, but not from registry-based research.[8] I have often spoken to researchers who view this type of research participation as an element of what Mette Svendsen (2022) has described as a "reciprocal relationship with the welfare state" (105): to receive good care, patients must accept donating their data to the common

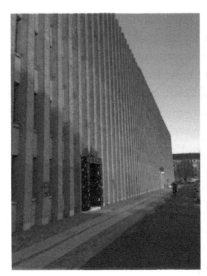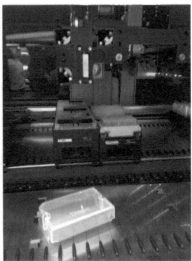

FIGURE 2.2

Statistics Denmark and the National Biobank. On the left, a picture of Statistics Denmark, serving as one of the key access points to the massive Danish registries. Note the numbers around the door. On the right, a robot works with genetic samples stored in the National Biobank. It uses a barcode that refers to the CPR number, which makes each sample traceable, as well as combinable with data from Statistics Denmark—throughout and beyond the lifetime of the individual in whom it originated. Photos by the author.

good (Pinel and Svendsen 2021). Patients, on the other hand, tend to resist discourses of obligation. Regardless of moral views, every single citizen is participating in research all the time.

It took a long afternoon in the company of a prominent British epidemiologist for me to understand the difference between what epidemiologists do in Denmark and in the United States and the United Kingdom. Typically, it seems as if they all make the same types of correlations among registries. Outside the Nordic countries, however, researchers need to infer the identity of the individual per proxy (using birthplace, birth date, and other information) and construe an algorithmic probability that different registries refer to the same person. Thanks to the CPR number, data refer directly to the same person (unless, of course, the person using this number borrowed someone else's identity, which the authorities responsible for the registries consider a rare event).[9]

I have recounted here a story of incremental construction of data infrastructures established to ensure fair taxation and to support the welfare state. The historical layers and the continuous fight for service entitlements provide a context for understanding how data integration emerged as a response to multiple requests. In the 1960s, countries elsewhere were also trying to harvest these new digital opportunities, but when, for example, a national data center was proposed in the United States, the federal ambition was turned down because it would involve too much centralization (Kraus 2011). In the 1980s, renewed federal attempts of data integration of criminal records in the United States were challenged for creating a "Dossier Society" (Laudon 1986). Jasanoff (2012b: 71) identifies

> a deep, and thoroughly American, suspicion of the state and its capacity to see, or know, for the people; in a culture committed to the discourse of transparency, the state arguably has no privileged position from which to see any differently than its individual members, who can see well enough for themselves.

In the United States and many other countries, most people have preferred to trust the market rather than the state. It was only after the 9/11 terrorist attacks that attitudes toward state surveillance seemed to change. In China, the social credit system has emerged to build trust by installing validation measures for individuals and companies, and this system has merged with a security agenda (Lengen 2017; Liang, Das, Kostyuk, and Hussain 2018). India has justified its mammoth biometric identification database as an aid in ensuring that the vulnerable can gain access to healthcare and other goods, but it is also known to serve as a source of surveillance (Dahdah and Mishra 2020; Nair 2021). The Nordic countries, in contrast, have mainly invested in data infrastructures to promote the administration and financing of welfare states. Gradually, the databases have come to serve more and more purposes. It is with this multiplication of purposes that data have come to both empower and disempower the citizens caught in their web.

A CENTRAL PERSON REGISTRY: BECOMING A PERSON IN A DATA-INTENSIVE COUNTRY

A fifth (and, in this chapter, final) way of providing a contextual understanding of data living is to provide narratives exemplifying what it can imply to live in a country with a civil registration system, typically referred to as the central person registry, the "CPR." Many Anglophone readers will associate the acronym CPR with cardiopulmonary resuscitation, and it does indeed represent life and death, albeit in a somewhat different sense: the type of life you can live depends on having a CPR number. Those who do not have that number encounter lives that are anything but seamless. For data-intensive government to work well for you, you need to conform to data standards and align with their prescribed norms. In Denmark, you cannot do any of the activities described here as leaving data traces without a CPR number. As commercial operators also depend on these data infrastructures, you cannot open a bank account, get employment, or rent an apartment without one. It is also necessary to have this number to get a phone number, or even just to sign up as member of a gym—and indeed, you cannot even be buried.[10] In a recent case, a local authority stored the corpse of an unidentified man for eighteen months before accepting that they had to construe an artificial CPR number so that an undertaker could bury him (Malacinski 2020).

For people working only temporarily in the country, the acquisition of a CPR number is like an initial rite of passage into the social texture of Danish society. The other Nordic countries also use civil registration systems. I remember the relief of getting my number when I was once living and working in Sweden. It was almost like getting a name or identity—to become a "person" (Bodenhorn and Bruck 2006). The CPR number becomes so crucial for the individual citizen partly because it is the entry point to a digital infrastructure used to assign rights and duties. Digital systems read data, not people, and therefore your CPR number is *you*, as it were, at least from a system perspective. It is your primary "data double" (Haggerty and Ericson 2000).

When living in the web of a centralized registry, even small mistakes can have serious ramifications, such as in the following case. On the morning of August 26, 2013, Sydvestjysk Hospital declared forty-seven-year-old Steen dead in its local electronic health record system. Steen, still very much alive, first noticed something unusual when some hours later, he discovered that his credit card was blocked. At the time, he was still an inpatient at Sydvestjysk Hospital, so he asked his girlfriend to check with the bank. As she was informed by the bank that Steen was "dead," Steen and his girlfriend began investigating and soon learned that this stemmed from an administrative error at the hospital—an erroneous data entry. Steen first thought of it as a joke worthy of a bad situation comedy. In a digitally integrated data infrastructure, however, it is not funny when an error makes its way into the Civil Registration System. Once "death" enters the integrated systems of the authorities, it is passed immediately on to other registries, and from there to companies and agencies hooked up to the Civil Registration System. Steen's bank account was closed (which explains the credit card), his insurance policies terminated, his passport and driver's license cancelled, and all planned bank payments stopped. The system is not set up for resuscitation: death is a one-way data entry. This meant that it took Steen four-and-a-half years to get his digital data-self up and running again (Jespersen and Hansen 2018). During the past ten years, seven persons have experienced a similar mistake at the same hospital.

Although the CPR number is essential to everyday living, there are people in Denmark without one.[11] There are illegal refugees and EU citizens without a job or an official purpose for staying in Denmark. Without a CPR number, they are living in a legal limbo, with no ways to own property, apply for welfare, or see a GP or any other doctor. There are also people who have been granted entry into the country for work but who are waiting for their number. Olsi Kusta, an Albanian PhD student of mine, learned upon arrival in Denmark that on certain Internet sites, you can "rent" somebody else's CPR number to establish yourself with rental contracts. It is illegal (and he did not pursue this solution), but for some people, it ends up being a necessary workaround.

The Civil Registration System providing people with CPR numbers holds such a central role in everyday data living that it became a major story in national newspapers when, at the turn of the millennium, a Danish-speaking man claimed to have forgotten his CPR number and identity. Journalists followed him around for weeks as he asked for help, but only encountered bureaucratic situations that would have made Franz Kafka green with envy. Without a CPR number, the welfare state could not offer any help, and only two homeless shelters in Copenhagen offered rooms to people without a number. In one newspaper article, a clerk explains why the authorities cannot help him: "The system cannot grant an expense when it doesn't know who the man is" (Beck-Nielsen 2003: 48). The journalist who had been following the man intervenes, saying: "But there is an evident need here. There is a man in need in front of you." The clerk replies that it is "administratively troublesome" without a number. To "know" who the man was implied knowing his number, not his suffering body. When the journalist later tries to file a complaint on behalf of the man, he is informed that in order to file complaints correctly with the responsible office, they also need a CPR number. An administrative manager later calls the journalist and explains the situation: "Look, we are living in a digital age. We do not have cool cash. If you do not have a CPR number [and a bank account], we cannot do anything. The system can't handle it" (Beck-Nielsen 2003: 50). As the man requests help from the police, a gracefully circular argument about his existence is presented by an officer: "He must have had a CPR number, and therefore he must exist" (47). Hence, the best way to help, the officer suggested, was to locate the number first. The CPR really is a number of life and death. It all turned out to be a stunt by an author who at the time called himself Claus Beck-Nielsen. Later, he called himself Helge Bille, Das Beckwerk, and Madam Nielsen. It is no coincidence, I guess, that an artist who enjoys exploring games of identity began with a CPR experiment. A selection of the articles and the man's personal narrative were later published as a book (Beck-Nielsen 2003).

Even when a person has a number, the number may constitute a prison rather than an option. In 1968, at the inception of the Civil Registration System, gender was considered a binary category. The CPR number is also binary. Still today, odd numbers are used for men, and even for women. Only in 2014 did Parliament enact the possibility of legal change of gender (from even to odd or vice versa), but only for people of legal age of majority (Folketinget 2014). To be a nonbinary person is not an option as a Danish data subject. Categorization can look as completely innocent as a ten-digit number, and yet it can reach into intimate aspects of identity. In an interview on national broadcasting (Norup 2019), a young man, Charlie, explained how it was to grow up within the web of the Civil Registration System. Charlie was categorized as female at birth and had to wait until turning eighteen to get a number that conformed to his identity. He explains:

> It is just important that the number corresponds [with who you are], because you would be surprised how often you use your CPR number, for everything, all the time. Just going to the doctor, to the bank, or logging into any system. (. . .) It's damaging to have to defend yourself, whether in the emergency room or in school. (Norup 2019: 1)

For years, Charlie had to respond to the name Anna in school during roll call because the lists get their data from the Civil Registration System giving people their CPR numbers.

Through the CPR, people come to exist in a manner that allows them to be seen by automated systems. That manner is, however, not always as they wish to be seen. The CPR makes visible, and it covers up. It empowers by making so many activities easy, and yet it disempowers when someone does not conform.

PARADOXES OF DATA LIVING

Data living has many surprises in store. You can only truly game a data system that you know how works (Henwood et al. 2003). The infrastructures described above are too complex for anyone to claim full overview. Data uses keep growing, as the previous chapter described, and with the new uses come new surprises. Some are empowering, others disempowering. Even a skilled patient like Lone, with whom I began this chapter, has had unpleasant surprises. Once, she thought she had cleverly protected herself by being selective about which data she shared with whom. Then, suddenly, she could not have her driver's license renewed:

> They constantly ask for informed consent for all kinds of people to have access to your medical record. I refused to sign that. Then I was told how I risk this and that. (. . .) Once I refused to report how many low blood sugar levels I had had in a given interval. I didn't want to (. . .). I couldn't see why it would be relevant. And then when I wanted to renew my driver's license, as you need to when you have diabetes, I received a letter that it was not possible because I had not reported blood sugar levels!

Lone's story exemplifies how data living in the web of the integrated infrastructures described above can have unexpected implications. As Lone had failed to document that her diabetes was under control, the systems automatically assumed her to have become a risky driver. She thought she was protecting her privacy and had not realized that the data she withheld were being used to prove her ability to control her disease—and therefore to drive a car. Attempts of empowering yourself can have disempowering effects. As Cheney-Lippold writes: "In the present day of ubiquitous surveillance, who we are is not only what we think we are. Who we are is what our data is made to say about us" (Cheney-Lippold 2017: xii). When data are repurposed they are also used to tell new stories, stories that might be counterproductive for the original purposes (a point I return to with additional examples in chapter five). Data-intensive healthcare systems therefore coproduce empowerment and disempowerment. The empowering and disempowering effects reflect the ways in which data both uncover and cover up particular stories about patients. Lone simultaneously aims to produce more data to direct clinical and research attention at what matters to her, but she also learns that data consume time, and data absences (her attempt of retaining privacy and control) become a ghost narrative that she cannot control about herself: a story about a disease out of control. These implications are paradoxical in the sense that they look like opposites, but they emerge in tandem with equal strength. As data living has both positive and negative effects, there is no easy way of choosing just one side of the story. The effects that people desire make it difficult to fight those they despise. Herein lies an important motor for data intensification.

In short, intensified data sourcing takes on local forms in response to what local infrastructures enable. The five types of context for the politics of data intensification explored in this chapter, each in their own way, tell stories about the infrastructures that the proponents of data promises now simultaneously wish to exploit and disrupt. I have alluded to the ways in which the technologically advanced integration often ends up with much more mundane implications than the promises suggest. In fact, most of what people do in response to disease remains pretty mundane, low-tech, and manual, even when mediated by data. This point about mundane, low-tech work will become very obvious as I now turn from data living to the *data work* unfolding in the clinic in the pursuit of data-intensive medicine.

3 DATA WORK

November 2016: "It was a big step for *me*, I thought, but I had never expected that type of public reaction," the chief gynecologist Morten Hedegaard[1] writes in a diary note about his resignation from his position as chief physician at the most prominent birth ward in Denmark. The resignation caused a big media stir, and the note was later printed in a magazine for doctors (Boysen 2016). For fourteen years, he had acted as a flagship of authority on matters of gynecology. He had been medically responsible for births in the royal family, and therefore also had experienced a certain amount of public interest before, but nothing like this. Every national newspaper covered the resignation. There were television interviews and massive social media reactions. It is rare to have the career choices of a doctor covered with such intensity, but the story was not so much *that* he resigned; it was *why* he resigned.

Hedegaard resigned, he said, because the ward had become too busy to ensure the safety and attentiveness that parents and newborns deserve. The working conditions had become intolerable. In the midst of the media hullabaloo around his resignation, the politician responsible, Head of the Capital Region Sophie Hæstorp Andersen, responded. Interestingly, she dismissed Hedegaard's professional concerns and stated as a matter of fact: "It is safe [to give birth at the hospital]!" She said so even though she was not a doctor and did not work on the ward. To support her claim, she argued: "No data indicate that we have more complications in relation to births taking place here. It is probably more a question of staff experiencing that they are running faster and faster, and many burn out. It is actually a serious problem, because we lack staff" (quoted in Maach 2016). In this way, she acknowledged a problem of human resources, which could be supported by data, but dismissed the doctor's concerns about the implications of this problem for safety. Her disregard of this senior clinician's disquiet was, ironically, based on data produced by the very doctors and nurses raising these concerns.

I followed this story with interest. At the time, I had already interviewed two data analysts servicing politicians and administrative management, who had proudly explained to me how, typically, they could document that levels of activity were absolutely normal when clinicians said they were too busy. I kept wondering: Who is right? What counts as knowledge about work? My sense of curiosity was stimulated further by the debate taking place in the ensuing months. In response to Hedegaard's exit, the political management defended itself by stating that the ward had received an extraordinary budget expansion of four million DKK. The staff had no reason to complain. However, the so-called reprioritization contribution, mentioned in chapter 1 (where operational expenses on hospital budgets have been reduced based on an expectation of 2 percent increased efficiency every year), happens to imply reductions of, yes, also four million DKK. Hedegaard explained to the media that the annual 2 percent reduction was, for him, the straw that broke the camel's back (Redaktionen 2016). In the following months, the picture became even muddier. When the minister of health, Ellen Nørby, was asked by political opponents to do something for prospective parents, she presented new data: from 2001 to 2015, the number of doctors and nurses had gone up 44 percent and 20 percent, respectively. In 2001, a midwife assisted delivery of sixty-five children on average, and in 2015, that number had fallen to thirty-eight. Nørby firmly stated: "There have been no cutbacks. Resources have been added" (quoted in Dørge 2017). Did Hedegaard then resign for no reason? Are healthcare professionals not busy at all? Or are they busy doing something else instead of taking care of babies and their parents? What counts as knowledge about clinical work?

Subsequently, numerous other stories have appeared in the media about doctors resigning in protest. Initially, these stories all referred back to Hedegaard. Then these accounts almost created a subgenre with its own narrative arc, with a new, increasingly prominent antagonist: *data work*. Many doctors now explicitly point to the time spent producing data when explaining their decision to leave the health services. Further, the digital tools offered for data work attract unprecedented public attention. In particular, in two of the five administrative Regions in Denmark, clinicians complain about a new information technology (IT) system (mentioned in chapter 1). Launched in 2016, it is delivered by the American company Epic and in Denmark it is known under the name *Sundhedsplatformen* (The Health Platform).[2] While the digital record systems used in the other Regions live relatively dull and unremarkable social lives, the Health Platform begins being featured heavily in news headlines with stories about clinical staff "who break down and cry" when having to work in the new system and who ask for (and receive) "psychological crisis assistance" (Heick 2016). One physician published a book in which he blamed his resignation from the post of chief physician on the current "yoke of Kafkaesque idiocy, grotesque over-administration, Health Platforms, crazy demands of documentation, [and] marginalization of medical competence and care" (Jacobsen 2018: 31). Another physician claims that as the health services are now "drowning in data work," health professionals are losing the motivation that used to be essential for them. He adds: "You have to survive, and you can cope only by letting a sense of indifference take over" (Olesen 2018: 84).

Also, in interviews with my colleagues and me, clinicians speak matter-of-factly about "meaningless work" as an integral part of clinical work. It is a startling observation. A recent Danish bestseller even describes meaningless "pseudo work" as a characteristic of modern organizations across all sectors in Denmark (Nørmark and Jensen 2019). Pseudo work can be considered a Danish version of what anthropologist David Graeber made internationally famous as "bullshit jobs"—jobs that make no difference and are meaningless even for those making a substantial income from them (Graeber 2018). According to Graeber, such work constitutes a form of "spiritual violence" that crunches the soul of the employee (67). When clinicians speak to me about the tasks that they think of as "meaningless," they often refer to something they also call "data massage" or "data fiddling." Data massage is typically related to what in organizational theory is known as "gaming"—to produce data in order to appear in a particular manner rather than simply as a procedure of clinical documentation. Their comments about data massage are typically followed by ironic gestures, jeers, and raised eyebrows. One general practitioner, Bente, who I interviewed together with my colleague Sarah Wadmann, used the phrase "it makes no sense" no less than forty-six times in the course of an interview, during which she said that the data tasks required by the regional authorities were "just plain idiocy, gosh, it's these kinds of absolutely foolish things (. . .) it's without meaning or purpose."

What is going on? Healthcare workers resigning. Complaints about meaningless work. Dull administrative matters such as IT systems suddenly making it to the news headlines. And politicians and administrators confidently asserting that there is no reason to worry. If Denmark really is at the forefront of digital healthcare, as the rankings presented in chapter 2 suggest, then it appears that there are some worrisome elements associated with this data-intensive mode of working. The pursuit of data promises seems to involve some unintended consequences. Once translated into everyday work, data-intensive healthcare is apparently not progressing as smoothly as the high-flying gospel from Silicon Valley would suggest.

In this chapter, I focus on *data work*. Data work is a key battleground for data politics. Again, I will suggest that the politics of intensified data sourcing involves paradoxes: apparently contradictory claims, yet both sides of the contradiction carry elements of truth. Data create less work *and* more work. Datafication both tightens organizational control *and* facilitates organizational disintegration. Data work involves tasks experienced by some as meaningless, and yet at the same time, data have become a prime source of meaning. Different versions of truth are presented on the one hand by clinicians and on the other by administrators (and politicians). Doctors and policymakers seem to live in separate realities, although they refer to similar data and ostensibly talk about the same clinical and organizational phenomena. Instead of opting for one or the other version as the "real" truth, the point is to approach these opposing stories as paradoxes and see what the coexistence of multiple truths allows people to do.

I begin the chapter with a discussion of the term *data work* and situate this discussion in wider, and indeed classic, discussions of organizational work and the role of technology. I then turn to the scandal surrounding The Health Platform as an interesting example of what happens when dreams of superior American IT tools meet everyday life in an e-health context, which is arguably more advanced in terms of data integration than the American healthcare system. Building on the purposes outlined in chapter 1, I then give examples of the data work that is supposed to underpin the goals of research, clinical performance, administration, and governance. Based on these examples, I suggest a rethink about why the data mill keeps grinding and what the implications might be for patients and health professionals alike.[3]

WORK: PRODUCTION, ANALYSIS, INSTRUCTION, AND USE

"Nice work if you can get it," Frank Sinatra sang about love. Data work does not seem to carry the same appeal. Still, in recent years, scholars have begun paying more attention to data work and to the clinicians, patients, or documentary specialists who deliver it (Morrison, Jones, Jones, and Vuylsteke 2013; Bossen, Chen, and Pine 2019; Bossen, Pine, Cabitza, et al. 2019; Pine 2019; Pine, Wolf, and Mazmanian 2016; Møller, Holten, Bossen et al. 2020; Fiske, Prainsack, and Buyx 2019; Pinel, Prainsack, and McKevitt 2020; Walford 2021; Petersson and Backman 2021). I described in the previous chapter how patients are doing increasing amounts of data work as a result of the shift in medical paradigms and organizational structures (Langstrup 2018; Torenholt, Saltbæk, and Langstrup 2020). In this chapter, I explore the data work undertaken by people employed in health services. So, what does data work involve, who does it, and why does it proliferate?

In the introduction, I referenced Berg and Goorman's *law of medical information*, which famously states, "The further information has to be able to circulate (. . .) the more work is required to disentangle the information from the context of its production." Berg and Goorman (1999) specifically pointed to a key question: "Who has to do this work and who reaps the benefits?" (52). They focused on the kind of work going into *producing* data: namely, clinical documentation. I think that intensified data sourcing generates other types of data work that also need consideration. Data work is carried out by people with a wide range of job titles and professional backgrounds situated in different parts of the healthcare system.

Consider again table 1.1 in chapter 1 and the many stakeholders interested in data. They all do some kind of data work. Just in the clinic, there are, in addition to doctors, nurses, and other clinicians, secretaries and information specialists working with data. Many people who work with healthcare data full time rarely visit the clinic. Some of them prepare data for quality databases. Some produce reports to management. Others assist politicians as described previously. Yet others work with how data can be used to intervene in and optimize work at all levels of the healthcare system, such as local "lean" consultants who work with management to optimize the efficiency

of clinical work by means of data analysis. There are also software program-
mers who work with data to design interfaces aimed at nudging clinical staff
into following particular guidelines or adhere to certain standards. There are
also all the public and private researchers who work with data derived from
the clinic to produce new insights or products aimed at goals such as prevention. Finally, data-intensive organizations impose an obligation on employees to know about the data analyses produced. Even when not producing,
analyzing, or managing data, most people have to spend time reading and
discussing reports and findings. While Berg and Goorman (1999) rightfully
asked who does the work, they focused only on the work associated with
producing data. I believe that to understand the dynamics of intensified
data sourcing, it is necessary to consider the other types of data work—and
thereby data workers other than those working in the clinic—as well. When
taking them into account, it is easier to understand how different groups
come to hold such divergent conceptions of the impact of data intensification on everyday work.

I suggest thinking of data work as four types of activity that partly overlap and feed into each other: production, analysis, instruction, and use
(see table 3.1). The distinction between these four types revolves around
how the worker is positioned in relation to the purpose of the data work.
When *producing* data, you are delivering data but do not necessarily enjoy
the thrill of doing the analysis. When *analyzing* data, you are engaged
in deciding what the data mean. When *instructing* people with, or being
instructed by, data work, the epistemological purpose gives precedence to
the political purpose: the meaning-making process is reduced to the effect

Table 3.1
The four main types of work associated with data-intensive healthcare

Data production	The work going into making data through actual documen-tation (e.g., application of a diagnostic code)
Data analysis	The work that transforms data sets into messages about what they mean (e.g., the making of a table, graph, dashboard or a narrative)
Data instruction	The work involved in governing others with, or being governed by, data
Data use	The work associated with understanding data or data analyses produced by others

on what people do and how they view each other. It subordinates validity to recognition and thereby positions people differently, as subjects of
governance. All these three types of data work, of course, involve some
form of use, but when I point to *use* as a distinct category, it is because
data-intensive organizations circulate so many data and so many analyses
that the use of data has become a precondition for retaining a right to
voice one's opinion. When *using* data and data analyses, the work revolves
around what it takes to make sense of the data analyses produced by others. You do not produce the data, you have not done the analysis, and
the data practices are not aimed at controlling your work: you are just
a user. It is a residual category aimed at capturing the fact that in data-
intensive environments, it can take a particular kind of data work to create
legitimacy around your person. When everybody refers to data, the right
to speak one's opinion can depend on the ability to cite relevant analyses
and to use analyses to make sense of the problems in front of you. It can be
time-consuming to find the right data and to locate the analyses that you
think you can trust. It takes work to disseminate what you have found. As
I could see people in the clinic spending time looking into all sort of data
analyses, reports, and rankings, I included it as a category of data work. It
struck me as one of those types of work that is not counted and is not featured in the data sets that administrators and politicians use when claiming that health professionals are not busy. Clearly, in practical situations,
all four can overlap, just as one type of data work can stimulate people to
engage another.

Intensified data sourcing affects what counts as knowledge about the
organization and intervenes in negotiations between professional groups
about who needs to know what. Questions about what counts as knowledge about work (and who needs to know what) have invigorated sociology
and organization theory for more than a century. In the current situation,
where data promises sweep across healthcare systems around the globe,
these questions are more relevant than ever. I now turn to these questions
and show how they can inform our understanding of the implications of
the four types of data work.

Historically, questions about work have stimulated controversies between
positivist approaches, such as Frederick Taylor's scientific management school
(Taylor 1998), and hermeneutic approaches, such as Elton Mayo's human

relations movement (Mayo 2003 [1933]). Arguably, Mayo used more numbers than Taylor in the actual writing, but he argued that workers need *meaning*. Mayo thereby developed Max Weber's hermeneutic approach to organizations and underlined the importance of Weber's warning against experiences of disenchantment and alienation in rational organizations—what Weber famously termed an "iron cage" (Weber 1947a).

At the time when Weber wrote about the rise of a legal-rational bureaucracy, records were kept on paper, in closed filing cabinets and archives. While professionals were expected to exert professional judgment and base decisions on their orientation toward organizational goals, they were also to be partly protected against political involvement when dealing with individual cases: "Every bureaucracy seeks to increase the superiority of the professionally informed by keeping their knowledge and intentions secret" (Weber, 1947a: 233). Max Weber identified a persistent longing for archival work in bureaucracies (Weber 1947a, 2003b). Professional data work (a term not used at the time) was aimed at supporting a professional role, much like clinical records used to serve primarily clinical goals (Bossen 2014). Today, however, there are many actors eager to use clinical documentation (again see table 1.1), and digitization has opened up many secret archives for inspection.

Management has long desired to "know" what employees are doing, as well as to optimize and control their performance. This urge was not born with digitization; digitization just provides additional tools. In 1911, when Taylor wrote his famous introduction to scientific management (laying out the seeds from which also Deloitte's mantra about "data and knowledge about what works" would later grow), he had already made it clear that he did not trust workers to understand or improve their own performance. He asserted that "the workman who is best suited to actually doing the work is incapable of fully understanding this science, without the guidance and help of those who are working with him or over him, either through lack of education or through insufficient mental capacity" (Taylor 1998: 9–10). An effective analysis of work, he asserted, should be based on numerical evidence and informed by statistics, not by the experience or opinion of the worker himself or herself. Today, digital technologies have propelled the pursuit of data-mediated optimization far beyond the factory floor and into professions that were previously more autonomous, including medicine (Moore 2018; Zuboff 1989; Rahman 2021).

Data on work still depends on data work. Management's knowledge typically builds on data that employees themselves produce. It is then not the same people doing the data work of production and the data work of analysis. Furthermore, digital tools are typically designed not only to *document* what people do, but also to shape *what* they do and *how* they do it (Amoore and Piotukh 2015; Moore 2018; Petersen 2019). Herein lies data work of instruction. The interfaces of electronic health records are designed to make them do the work in a particular order, but also to demand the documentation of particular tasks (Felt, Öchsner, and Rae 2020). Thereby, values and priorities become "inscribed" into the very tools offered for carrying out the clinical work (cf. Akrich 1992; Jensen 2021). Accordingly, Bovens and Zouridis (2022) claim that digitization has tightened the political control over public employees. The public servant used to have more room for professional discretion when meeting the citizen. There was what Lipsky (1980) called a street-level bureaucracy softening up the effect of new rules by being at liberty to exert judgment.

Bovens and Zouridis (2022) argue that it is now more appropriate to talk about screen- or system-level bureaucracy because frontline staff have to work in interfaces (screens) that steer and monitor their decisions. They cannot do their work without documenting it in data formats facilitating surveillance of compliance with organizational goals. They are under instruction. In some cases, performance management relies on criteria of measurement that remain opaque to the knowledge workers who increasingly find themselves under surveillance through their very tools of daily work (Rahman 2021). They sometimes need to hide what they are actually doing (Petersson and Backman 2021). Breit, Egeland, and Loberg (2019) suggest using the term "cyborg bureaucracy" to refer to a form of governance that is a mix of human and nonhuman forces. Cyborg-bureaucracy has coemerged with the new forms of "wired medicine" that patients meet when seeking care, as described in chapter 2.

Some forms of data work of production are aimed directly at facilitating the analysis of other actors or at tightening organizational control (in line with what I call instruction). Frontline staff, for example, are increasingly asked to "measure" the needs of citizens before attending to their care (Hoeyer and Bødker 2020; Lyneborg 2019). I gave an example in chapter 1 having to do with eldercare, but this trend cuts across areas and sectors, from education to social services and disability (Høybye-Mortensen 2015;

Fernandez and Lutz 2019; Shaw, Bell, Sinclair et al. 2009; Langstrup and Moreira 2021). In wired medicine, the problem has to be datafied before it can be solved. Parton (2008) has described how such documentation tools interact with and change the professional ethos and sense of purpose also among social workers. Parton points to datafication as one of the dynamics fueling this transformation: when asking for *data* on *what* citizens do, say, or want, rather than asking for a *narrative* about *why* they want it, professionals no longer provide an interpretation of the individual citizen. Through data points, citizens are monitored as a population. Datafication brings about a transformative process where interpretation is increasingly something that people can do elsewhere, based not on interactions *with* the citizen but on information *about* the citizen. It involves a separation of data-work-of-production and data-work-of-analysis, and it shifts decision making about individual patients toward seeing them as they are positioned in a population rather than as having a unique trajectory (Nordfalk, Olejaz, and Hoeyer 2022).

Work on instruction also goes into designing, implementing, and monitoring digital tools that can shape what people do. It can be with pop-up windows or interfaces that allow only certain options. In healthcare, it can take the shape of decision trees or alerts on risks, such as rare disorders, or polypharmacy (Wachter 2017).[4] I interviewed one data analyst who had designed a data tool reducing general practitioner (GP) prescriptions of dangerous drugs by 20 percent simply by giving the GPs automated feedback benchmarking their prescriptions against those of colleagues. What was interesting about this form of instruction was that it did not add data-work-of-production to GPs but stimulated data-work-of-analysis among the GPs: they now wanted to understand their own prescription patterns.

However, not all tools of instruction operate as subtly as this. Some attempts to affect clinical decisions focus on achieving particular political goals, such as reducing the use of physical force in psychiatry, shorter waiting lists, and the shift from eldercare to rehabilitation training discussed in chapter 1. In these cases, data work aimed at *instruction* can encroach on the professional sense of judgment and, in some cases, make health professionals feel that their work becomes less meaningful. To lose influence can give rise to feelings of meaninglessness, whether understood as alienation (Blocker 1974), moral disorientation (Oakley 2010) or powerlessness (Seeman 1975).

Before I turn to more examples of the data work aimed at supporting the clinical, research, administrative, and political purposes laid out in chapter 1, I will tell the story of the very expensive medical record system known as The Health Platform, which two of the five Danish administrative regions purchased from the American supplier Epic. This software exemplifies the type of reactions that an interference in data work can spur. It also illustrates how some of the high-flying data promises that fascinate administrators and politicians can crash when they hit the ground.

OPTIMAL DIGITAL TOOLS FOR DATA WORK: BUYING AN AMERICAN LIMOUSINE

Despite the Nordic countries' long tradition for integrated digital e-health, it should come as no surprise in the current climate of admiration for US IT that the biggest IT investment in Danish healthcare history had to be an American system. The medical record system called The Health Platform was implemented in 2016. As should be obvious by now, no other health IT system has received similar media attention. Unfortunately, the attention has been almost exclusively negative (Røhl and Nielsen 2019). I initially tried to interview people in key positions about The Health Platform, but I quickly realized that I had to rely mostly on media reports. People still in office would agree to an interview only if I promised not to ask about this purchase. It was "too political," I was told. Though key actors declined, I could hardly meet any clinician working in one of the two Regions—whether by chance on commuter trains or at dinner parties or in more professional settings at seminars or conferences—without hearing them talk about the system. Still, anonymity remained important. It is a system that raises emotions and strong opinions.

One of the doctors to resign while blaming this system, the surgeon Ulf Helgstrand states:

> The Health Platform steals your time. I am no longer in a position to provide the guidance and treatment that I believe patients deserve. (. . .) I am constantly sitting with my back to the patients because I have to look at the screen. (Baun 2017)

Another chief surgeon, Michael Halder, explains his resignation like this:

> It is a terrible system. It has drained all joy from work and from caring for patients and their relatives. (. . .) I will never work again in a hospital using The Health Platform. (Mortensen and Dencher 2018)

Like many of the people confiding in me off the record, Halder says that he very often had to stay behind after work to do his documentation. Apparently, Epic has not managed to fulfill the hopes nurtured by health professionals of a seamless, efficient, and safe e-health system. Instead the system has increased their data-work-of-production.

When Danish politicians and civil servants decided to buy the e-health record, they said that it would replace "thirty systems with one." Clinicians were working in a patchwork of systems, arguably not thirty for each individual doctor (more like six or seven), but there were around thirty systems from which some administrative workers needed to retrieve data. Better integration would be welcome, not least from the perspective of those doing the data-work-of-analysis: one tool rather than many. Epic was, at conferences, spoken about as an American limousine. "Limos" are rare in Denmark and associated with extravagant luxury. In line with this sense of indulgence, I remember the optimistic atmosphere before the launch, and how clinicians would talk about their hopes for more seamless interfaces facilitating their clinical work.

I first suspected in 2015 that some clinicians would be disappointed. It was when I heard a talk by a woman in a leading position in the implementation of the Epic system. She stated that codes were to completely replace narrative elements (free text) in the patient record because codes are easier to search and compute. They can be used for more purposes. I feared I had misheard her presentation and wrote her an e-mail. She kindly replied:

> It is correct that narrative elements shall be minimized and gradually be superseded. Epic facilitates monitoring of data fields so that a decision on when to terminate narrative elements will be based on actual data analysis. The first version of the Health Platform is not complete, hence this postponement.

It seemed that data codes indeed really were to replace narratives! The administration was inspired by the consultancy group Gartner talking about a five-step model of electronic health records, going from perceiving the health record as The Collector, The Documenter, The Helper, The Colleague, to, finally, The Mentor (Krogh 2016: 99). They thought it was time for the clinicians to get a mentor. The administration apparently felt confident that with enough data, they would be able to optimize clinical work—in line with Taylor's attitude.

To act as a mentor, the record system really had to be good. Being good, however, always begs the question: good for whom, and according to which criteria? Epic is constructed for American healthcare. It is built to support particular workflows, cultures, and purposes that are very different from those characterizing Danish healthcare (Allen 2019; Koopman, Jones, Simon et al. 2021). In American healthcare, each patient sees fewer doctors than in Denmark. When Danish doctors build a narrative, they write a short history, which is meant to help other doctors who are treating the same patient understand that patient's situation. Traditionally, Danish nurses have had more leeway to exert clinical judgment than do nurses working in American healthcare. Danish doctors and nurses also share tasks, but Epic is not built for that. Epic is excellent for billing purposes. Yet Danish healthcare is tax-financed: the economy of each hospital depends on sending data to national registries rather than on billing. In a number of major ways, therefore, the Epic system did not translate well into Danish practices (Bansler 2021).

There were also other elements lost in translation—and not only metaphorically. The builders of the system had relied partly on automated language translation with results that would have been laughable had they not been, potentially, so deeply serious (Allen 2019). "Right," for example, as in the *right* leg in contrast to the *left* leg, would sometimes appear as the "correct" leg, and "left" was occasionally translated into the Danish word for "abandoned," as in "left behind." The Latin word *cave*, meaning "watch out," which is used for highlighting drugs that risk giving a patient an allergic reaction, had been translated as "grotto" (Bentzon and Rosenberg 2021). Examples proliferated as health professionals agitatedly collected proof of their disappointment with the American limousine (Gadsbøll 2017). Doctors found themselves using interfaces that were described to me as "a dinosaur," "from the darkness of the past century," or "something you'd have expected to encounter in the 1970s, not in 2020." Also, American clinicians complain about counterintuitive and cumbersome data work when working in Epic systems (Schulte and Fortune 2019). A Danish doctor remarked to me once: "If this is a limo, I think a family car would have been a better match." In a sense, he acknowledged that the Epic system might provide new opportunities, but they were just not particularly relevant for the clinical tasks at hand. Some optimistic managers, in contrast, have shown me fascinating examples of what the system allows them to monitor, and they hope that their own enthusiasm eventually spreads to the clinical staff.

The integration element fared even worse than the initial translation problems. "Everything in one system" turned out to be a misnomer. Most clinicians continue to work in several systems. Doctors have to communicate with health professionals outside the hospital, but The Health Platform is a closed system, designed for the American healthcare system where data are proprietary assets. As the platform was not set up for integration with outside systems, there were now gaps in the data sent to the national quality databases, as well as to the otherwise famously complete registries. As I discussed this with two consultants servicing the system, they winced, and one said: "I basically think Epic had no clue what a national registry is or why central reporting would be important." Indeed, Epic has been criticized for lacking commitment to data sharing in other contexts too, including in the United States (Sheikh, Sood, and Bates 2015; Jones, Laurie, Stevens et al. 2017). In Denmark, however, the problems stretched beyond the clinic because Epic lacked the ability to integrate with existing infrastructures. After fifty years with outstanding registries known for their completeness, frustrated researchers spoke informally and at conferences about "data gaps." Considering that the biggest IT investment in Danish healthcare history was supposed to deliver more data, with better quality and in a more integrated manner, such breaches are astounding. A healthcare system known as having one of the most integrated data infrastructures in the world was now disintegrating. The American limousine was not made for public transportation.

The price was exorbitant. The two regions paid 2.8 billion DKK for the system. It was the same amount that the biggest health insurance company in Denmark paid in subsidies to all of its 2.3 million members the same year. On top of that, productivity went down considerably (Højer 2016). Or, at least, the registered productivity went down. Data gaps make it difficult to verify the exact drop. Data gaps partly reflect the problems of integration described previously, but probably also changed registration practices. With the arrival of The Health Platform, secretaries were fired and doctors told to document their own work. It was said to increase patient involvement with doctors by including patients in the record keeping. Laying off the secretaries also featured in budgets as a cost-saving measure. As data work turned out to be more demanding than expected, many secretaries had to be hired again (Ritzau 2017). Paper also saw a renaissance, as nurses and doctors began taking notes on paper, sticky notes, and napkins (Hecklen 2017). In short, it turned out to be surprisingly difficult to get data *into* the system (the data-work-of-production) as well as *out* of it (the data-work-of-analysis).

On top of the economic setback and the sense of burnout, health professionals have complained about the safety of the system. The dispensing of pharmaceuticals, for example, continues to be an area of concern (Sørensen 2016; Mirzaei-Fard and Baun 2019). Clinicians must choose from predefined options for prescriptions, which do not always fit their plans. Furthermore, the system has not always integrated well with the otherwise acclaimed national system of pharmaceutical dispensing. When outpatients and people in eldercare visited a hospital, their prescriptions in the centralized system were not always up to date. Overall, the number and range of clinical complaints have been massive, but some clinicians are tired of all the grumbling—they do not see the reason for all the fuss. One nurse said to me: "The old systems were bad. The new system is bad. Why complain?" Furthermore, there are people who enjoy playing around with the new features (see chapter 4). Even difficult systems can be fun, if you are so attuned. One civil servant, who actually had asked not to be interviewed about The Health Platform, decided, unprompted, to convey her impression to me while leaning in over the table, confiding "I think the clinicians have just forgotten how much they hated the old systems. The problem is they were told they would get a limousine, and they were disappointed."

She might be right. Clinicians thought they would get a system aimed at their own clinical objectives. What they got was a system helping the data work of the administrators. With its smart text and codes, it seems to be designed for easing the data-work-of-analysis, not the data-work-of-production. When the system was to be updated, clinicians again expressed hopes of more seamless interfaces. They were disappointed (Kristensen 2019). A representative for the management, Pia Kopke, responded to their disappointment as follows:

> It seems like we have not aligned the expectations properly at all levels of the organization (. . .). The primary reason for updating [The Health Platform] was to prepare it for integration with The National Patient Register. (Mirzaei-Fard and Korsgaard 2019)

The updates were not aimed at dealing with the problems faced by the clinical staff. They were aimed at servicing the data needs of administrators and researchers.[5]

In short, the Epic system redistributed work rather than eliminating it. It was said to deliver optimal integration, but this ambition relied on the idea of having "everything in one system." No single system can do the job when data are to flow between many actors, performing very diverse tasks. Denmark's colonial heritage, for example, entails that the main hospital in Copenhagen also provides specialized care to citizens from the Faroe Islands and Greenland—that is, from different countries, outside the European Union, and with their own record systems. Having one system as an ideal for integration is, perhaps, just silly.

When moving beyond the specific Epic system, how do people engaged in data work aimed at promoting clinical, research, and political-administrative purposes make sense of their tasks? How does data work interact with the way that priorities are decided? In pursuit of answers, Sarah Wadmann and I interviewed a wide range of clinicians, researchers, and administrators about data work. One could easily have imagined that the data-work-of-production would be carried out by clinicians, the data-work-of-analysis by researchers, the data-work-of-instruction was initiated by administrators, and the data-work-of-use by politicians. It is not the case. Clinicians, researchers, and administrators do all four types of data work—but in various degrees, in different forms and sequences, and with different senses of purpose and pleasure. I will not discuss politicians and industry, even though they are featured in table 1.1, because I have not been close enough to their actual practices. When data are used for multiple purposes, it can be difficult to discern which type of work goes into achieving what. This floating nature of data work is important, I suggest, because it gives rise to silent shifts in prioritization (see also Pine and Bossen 2020).

DATA WORK FOR RESEARCH, CLINICAL, ADMINISTRATIVE, AND POLITICAL PURPOSES

Data can be used to reach many laudable objectives. The list in table 1.1 is long but not exhaustive. Most of the data must be produced in the clinic. In general, in our interviews, clinicians are positive about data work when they are convinced that it serves the interests of the patient. They accept data-work-of-production when data serve a clinical purpose and the work takes as little time as possible. It is important for them to work in digital interfaces fitted to their tasks. It should be obvious from the description of The Health Platform that it is not always seen as an optimal tool, but there are other excellent digital tools—tools that are intuitive and easy to use, and therefore make data-work-of-production manageable.

Clinicians do not only *produce* data. Many clinicians do data-work-of-analysis to gain an overview of patients and patient flows, as well as to plan and optimize their work. Sometimes they get assistance from "lean" consultants and administrative data specialists. It is also part of the clinical routine to instruct each other with data. In a healthcare system communicating through data, there is no way to avoid data-work-of-instruction. The national pharmaceutical platform that I have mentioned is, in a sense, a data tool for instruction. It helps the doctor responsible to assign tasks to other health professionals. The tools for data-work-of-instruction for clinical purposes must first and foremost be stable and safe. Finally, clinicians are also users of the analyses produced by others. Data-work-of-use, therefore, also consumes their time. In short, data are essential for clinical work, and clinicians engage in all four types of data work. Yet many complain about drowning in data work. Clinicians are, of course, as varied a population as any other, and what some dislike, others enjoy. It is also possible to dislike producing data on a particular topic and still appreciate the analytical results arising from those data—just as many of us appreciate a clean home without enjoying the act of cleaning as such. Still, clinical complaints seem to be increasing. Why?

Clinicians do a lot of data work serving purposes defined outside the clinic. As also described by Winthereik, van der Ploeg, and Berg (2007), some types of data work are aimed at *both* clinical *and* political-administrative purposes. The National Quality Databases provide an example. Clinicians want to ensure—and document—high clinical quality, but the quality databases and their particular formats are partly an administrative invention aimed at governing performance. While the old-fashioned registries build on singular pieces of information about patients, such as a diagnostic code, the quality databases monitor entire stays in hospitals. There can be hundreds of data points a day on a patient, ranging from blood pressure and temperature to patient-rated outcome measures. The quality databases necessitate a lot of data-work-of-production. The systems that clinicians work in, such as The Health Platform, are set up in a manner ensuring that the everyday clinical documentation gathers these data in predefined formats. The data are then automatically transferred to the central quality databases (it was this feature that partly failed in The Health Platform). Although data collection operates through the interface that clinicians meet, clinicians are not always aware of why certain data have to be collected or where the data go. I have spoken to nurses who did not know that they were producing data for the quality databases. With the quality databases, information specialists analyze the data and send reports to local and central management through the management information system. The data-work-of-analysis is then no longer done by the clinical staff. Many clinical managers use these data in their daily running of the clinics. In such cases, the same nurse who produced some of the data may then come under instruction through the decisions made or become a user of the analysis when presented with comparisons among the local performance and that of other wards. Data work can act as a boomerang when you work at the front lines, as memories that you cannot control.

Many clinicians are also researchers. Doctors at specialized hospitals are expected to do at least some research. As researchers, they do data-work-of-analysis and depend on clinical data for this research. Several quality monitors pointed out to me that when the quality databases ask for so many data, this partly reflects research interests. The doctors on the database reference panels, who define which data to collect, are clinicians, yes, but their careers depend on the research they publish. By defining which data must be collected for quality assurance (an ostensibly clinical purpose), they can make nurses and junior doctors produce data for their own research. Both the documentation and the research take place in the clinic. It is, however, not necessarily the same people who do the data-work-of-production who then reap the benefits through data-work-of-analysis.

University researchers also benefit from massive amounts of data. Integrated digital infrastructures and intensified data sourcing have made doing research—especially epidemiological studies—easier. An experienced epidemiologist, who is a colleague of mine, once described to me how back in the 1970s, epidemiologists had to do a lot of manual work to prepare data for analysis. Data came in formats that were not interoperable. Today, complex data sets can be accessed on a virtual private network connection through Statistics Denmark. Although clinicians have ended up with more data-work-of-production, researchers have reaped some of the benefits. They can, whether for academic or commercial purposes, access data much more easily (though rarely easily enough, some maintain).

When more time goes into data-work-of-production to facilitate research, this indicates a shift between how the purposes in table 1.1 are prioritized. Francisca Nordfalk, a PhD student of mine, did some research with the

statistician Claus Ekstrøm documenting a shift in the use of blood samples
in the Danish Neonatal Screening Biobank, a part of the Danish National
Biobank. All newborn babies participate in a screening program where
dried blood spot samples are collected. Since 1982, the samples have been
stored in the biobank after screening. To see when and for what purposes
the samples were reused, the two identified all published articles listing the
neonatal biobank as a source (a total of 104 articles). Based on this, they
were able to document a clear increase in use of the screening samples for
research purposes over time. They also found a shift from use in research
projects close to the clinical screening purpose to more general research
questions, such as genetic disposition for psychiatric disease. An estimated
total of 794,157 individual newborn samples had been used for research
purposes, and an estimated 91,162 of them were used to study mental
illness—though psychiatric disease is not part of the screening program
(Nordfalk and Ekstrøm 2018). In the clinic, however, Nordfalk could also
observe how health professionals used the resources allocated to collection
of samples from newborns to pursue clinical goals. They used the task of
sample collection to actively make time for parents and discuss issues that
do not figure in evaluations of quality in official databases, but still matter
for many clinicians and patients (Nordfalk 2021a, 2021b).

If research affects data work, how does data work aimed at administrative and political purposes affect priorities in healthcare? In many ways,
the purchase of The Health Platform can be seen as a story about prioritizing data for administration and governance over clinical utility. Ironically,
however, because of the lack of integration with the central registries, the
investment ended up introducing data gaps that *undermined* the governance
objectives. It is a more general experience, indeed, that strong governance
is not always the effect of intensified data sourcing. When some years ago,
the former head of the Danish Health Authority, Else Smith, stepped down
to take a job at a hospital, she realized that she had been working "decou-
pled from reality." In a published interview, she said: "In the Danish Health
Authority we (. . .) had not realized how far the ideals were from practice.
(. . .) Seen from where I am now, it was too easy to "just" write instructions
and pass them on" (quoted in Steen-Andersen 2017: 4).

Datafication is a technology of distance. Distances can be productive. They allow what I discussed in chapter 1 as "functional stupidity" in

organizations (Alvesson and Spicer 2012). It can be expedient for people with overall responsibility *not* to know certain things happening at lower levels (Geissler 2013)—especially when they do not know what to do about them.

Most doctors actually agree with many of the goals set by central authorities, at least in the abstract. They agree with politicians that waiting time is a problem in cancer treatment. They mostly agree with politicians that the use of physical force in psychiatry ought to be minimized. They worry about the side effects of polypharmacy and agree with politicians and administrators that tools are needed to monitor these goals (Mainz and Bartels 2014). When clinicians across specialties and localities need to report in the same centralized systems, however, they often find that they need to do the data-work-of-production and -instruction, while others do the data-work-of-analysis. This distance and disconnection—decoupling—mean that clinicians sometimes cannot recognize their local clinical reality in the data. The data work then feels meaningless.

This is far from news to healthcare managers. Clinical department managers are aware that many clinicians find many data tasks meaningless. It is a challenge for managers to retain authority among clinical staff when also having to ask for data that are not essential to clinical work. One clinical department manager explained to Sarah Wadmann: "Of course, it's a little absurd. But it's a consequence of being measured in a particular way. It makes it important to tick the right boxes." I interviewed a quality coordinator who explained how she was spending a lot of time (data-work-of-instruction) making clinicians deliver "complete data" (data-work-of-production), not because it was clinically important but because "it did not count as quality" if there were gaps in data. What were considered meaningless data at the ward level made sense at the administrative level.

Jens, the strategy developer, gave an example of what he thought was a really successful use of data for governance: whiteboard meetings. There are now boards in all wards in the Capital Region where the staff are exposed to data on performance in relation to politically defined goals:

> Every week, new data gush out on the boards, and then clinicians say, "I don't agree with this; it must be a mistake." They engage with the data in a totally different way than I've seen before. It is extremely valuable. It is splendid!

Note how Jens is fully aware that clinicians think that data misrepresent their reality. It is not particularly important to him, however, because they are at least discussing the goals set by administrators and politicians. Their attention has been refocused: "It is splendid!" Jens disagrees with those saying that data need to be valid and correct: "God damn it, no! Data shall make people have a dialogue about how we can achieve the goal." Not all clinicians find these dialogues as stimulating as Jens suggests.[6] When questioning the validity of data representations, however, they sometimes feel inclined to begin collecting their own data to better represent the clinic as they know it (Wadmann, Holm-Petersen, and Levay 2018; Winthereik 2003). The grinding data mill accelerates.

THE GRINDING DATA MILL: WHY IS IT ACCELERATING?

There is indeed an odd thing about the complaints about data work: even clinical staff become hesitant when asked to name data tasks that they would like to see terminated. In interviews, I have several times heard full-time data analysts working in administration explain how they see themselves as the ones trying to reduce the "documentation burden" for the clinical staff. However, even when they set up meetings with clinicians on how to reduce registrations, they encounter requests for *more* data. One experienced quality monitor, Mona, gave this account of how such meetings typically proceed:

> They say, "we want something evidence-based," "we want to know what we are doing," "we want to have some ammunition if anybody says, we are really under great pressure," and really, it's the way you build an argument. You can't say "my gut feeling is that we are running very fast." Well, it might be right, but over there on the other ward they can manage and that is how it is. [Data collection] is *the way we build arguments;* it's the way we work (my emphasis).

Liselotte, the data analyst from the regional level, similarly said:

> I don't think anybody would sincerely say they saw a need for additional registrations. Absolutely no! Everybody thinks they produce data to the point of vomiting. It is crazy what needs to be registered. On the other hand, they also want the documentation. For instance, in cases of mistakes. What happened to the patient?

I think the point is that work needs to leave a data trace in order to *count as work* in the systems. Sarah Wadmann and I were struck by the way in which nearly all our interviewees presented themselves as merely responding to "meaningless" demands imposed by external actors or IT systems. In one of the hospital departments, the clinical staff complained that their ward management insisted they should document that they had examined and approved all prescriptions for all patients—even when no medication had been administered, as in cases with healthy relatives registered as "patients" because they were staying in the hospital to accompany sick children. When Sarah mentioned the frustration among the clinicians to the ward manager, it turned out he was frustrated too. He said it made no sense to count patients who received no pharmaceuticals as "not monitored," but unfortunately the IT systems had been set up to facilitate counting of how many who were "not monitored" because this was defined as deviations from the standard of good care, as "bad quality." The ward manager had the ward generate its own supplementary statistics to prove the centralized monitoring system wrong. Nevertheless, the ward manager routinely had to present at the hospital management's office and explain the supposed "quality breach." The ward managers would then be asked to audit their clinical records on the following day to compensate for this "lack"—a procedure he described with irony and references to Kafka's bureaucracy. When Sarah later asked one of the hospital managers about the standard that caused the clinicians' frustration, he also agreed that it did not make sense to demand pharmaceutical monitoring of *all* patients and added: "Sometimes it is so bureaucratic that it is almost unbearable." He proceeded to convey his frustrations with the officials at the regional administrative level who demanded explanations of deviation from the standard.

When I was trying to understand why the Regions would enforce these standards, several people at the regional level said that it was because the Regions needed to document their performance to the national authorities. Because cessation of regional self-rule has been on the political agenda for some years, the Regions have been under great political pressure. Moving a step up the hierarchy, I asked a representative from the state level about the pressures connected with data collection. She gave a really interesting insight into this sense of responding to data requests posed by others, even at the highest level of government:

> My experience is that a lot of people want more data, [and] it's also the clinical research staff that request more data. And a lot of patients cannot understand why they cannot get an answer on this or that, and there's a whole parliament also asking, "Why can't you tell us this or that?" And when we say, "No, we can't because we don't have the data," they say, "Well, then you've got to get them." So it's kind of funny (. . .) I think (. . .) it's not necessarily the ministry and the civil servants requesting more data. I experience it more as a response to needs articulated in various environments.

So even when we reach the highest administrative levels, staff see themselves as responding to demands raised elsewhere.

Data-intensive healthcare creates a form of bureaucracy-on-steroids where arguments only count when they are based on data. Administrators only seem to acknowledge the tasks that are documented. They have no data on the time spent on data work. The work related to data production remains invisible. It is not enough for doctors like Hedegaard to state that they are busy, when they do not have data to back their claim. To legitimately argue your case, you need backing by data. This is also what generates what I call data-work-of-use. It is by means of data that the staff pursue meaningful action even when this implies doing "meaningless work" in a strictly clinical sense. Here, we are seeing the accelerating motor of the data mill: an organizational environment creating interconnectedness through data—where being seen and recognized as doing important work of sufficient quality implies the use of standardized data that can travel across contexts. Well-known dilemmas of standardization (Brunsson 1999; Busch 2011; Hogle 1995; Timmermans and Berg 1998; Winthereik and Vikkelsø 2005) thereby generate the dual pressures of more locally initiated data collection (to be seen for what you do) and "meaningless work" in centralized systems (to respond to what the external parties want to see). While "building arguments" with data, clinicians still seek to produce patient-focused results. To some extent, the frustration they associate with meaninglessness might reflect their increased work pressure. Data work keeps them busy.

The trend toward "defensive medicine" discussed in chapter 1 also accelerates the data mill. The multiplication of data uses then again involves a shift in the priorities in the clinic. In an attempt to explain how data work has created a change in the "work culture," Mona (the quality monitor) laughed timidly as she said: "In the old days, we used to call it Cover My Ass [Da; Dæk Din Røv], DDR." With DDR, the Danish abbreviation, she made a pun on the former East German regime Deutsche Demokratische Republik (known in English as the German Democratic Republic, or GDR). The GDR is also widely associated with its use of surveillance. She said, "in the old days," but she also talked about a recent change, thereby illustrating how practices which used to be looked down upon have become normalized. Similarly, a leading quality program developer was recently cited in a medical newspaper for her warning against a changing hospital culture experienced as "an inferno of documentation" that "risks creating a Cover My Ass culture, where the physician's attention shifts from what is good for the patient to the physician's own ass" (L. Lange 2017, pp. 13).[7] Organizations eager to "punish" deviance stimulates peoples' urge to defend themselves (Fassin 2018).

In an organization where data means visibility, it can be dangerous to rely on "invisible work" (Star 1991). To have efforts acknowledged by superiors, work needs to be visible in a format that the organization values. As Zuboff (1989) argued, in computer-saturated workplaces, many tasks come to revolve around the "manipulation of symbols" rather than physical execution (23). It is by becoming visible to others, as data, that tasks come to count as working with (and for) other humans. Visibility is part of making the work meaningful. However, when meaning becomes a matter of communication and recognition within and among organizations, data work can become detached from the clinical goal orientation.

Could technology solve the problem of "meaningless" data work? It is certainly possible to build systems with more intuitive interfaces and seamless integration than those in place, which would reduce the number of complaints. However, automation will not halt the data mill. Automation cannot settle which purposes to pursue. It shifts data work around, but in the health services, it does not eliminate it (Vikkelsø 2005). When automation creates less work, it is mostly for those requesting data (doing data-work-of-analysis). Those in the clinic who have to respond to the requests get more work because many forms of data entry remain manual (Boyce 2016; Morrison et al. 2013). With automation, requests for data become easy to execute, and the tasks of responding become invisible to those setting up the system. Furthermore, automation can make data collection continue in perpetuity. Automation in this way adds fuel to the motor of the grinding data mill, but it is the pursuit of meaning through data that keeps the mill grinding. If the data mill is grinding with growing intensity, what does it produce?

PATIENT FLOUR: THE EFFECT ON RESEARCH, CLINIC, AND GOVERNANCE

Data work is meant to serve a range of laudable goals. However, when the data mill grinds, some of the objectives work against each other. The friction generates heat (Edwards et al. 2011; Tsing 2015), but it does not stop the grinding. It accelerates it. While I have shown that the result can be a loss of meaning, the motor of the mill also can ironically be located in the pursuit of meaning through data. In the examples discussed here, disagreement with data generates a longing for more, for better, data—data that can tell stories that people are eager to purport.

Datafication means that information about the patient is disentangled into small data elements. It is like wheat broken down into flour in a flour mill. My use of the term "patient flour" might seem to carry unnecessary violent connotations, but I refer here just to the informational representation of the patient. Datafication makes the small bits of information available for more users than the old clinical narrative. Flour, similarly, is a product with much higher utility than whole wheat. It can be used to make many things, from cake and bread to sauces. Information in the form of diagnostic codes, precoded "smart text" phrases, or searchable digital narratives can be employed for far more analyses than the old paper-based narratives in clinical records stored in closed archives. It can, however, be difficult to reassemble an understanding of the full situation of the patient from the flour produced by the data mill. A sense of the person does not always emerge from the individual data points just as the sense of wheat plants in the field is hard to generate from a package of flour. The patient as a person with a history can dissolve. This effect of datafication has been found in other contexts as well (Hunt, Bell, Baker, and Howard 2017; Hutchinson, Nayiga, Nabirye et al. 2018; Olesen 2018; Taylor-Alexander 2016; Verghese 2008). This is, however, not the only implication of the pursuit of meaning through data. In the following discussion, I wish to suggest that intensified data sourcing makes people relate to and use data in new ways. Data can come to operate as symbols rather than as references to patients. This has ramifications beyond the care for the individual patient. It introduces a profound epistemic doubt—doubt about what is going on in healthcare. Like flour thrown up in the air, data can become a haze impairing visibility.

The epistemic doubt relates first and foremost to "data massage," and then from an inability to understand data at a distance. The tendency to have more data-work-of-analysis carried out, detached from the data-work-of-production, leads to mistaken conclusions. When clinical data furthermore become the primary tools for governance, they gradually change in character for those who are simultaneously producing data and instructed by analyses made with the very same data. Some people are very frank about manipulation, as when a hospital manager said to Sarah Wadmann: "One thing is certain: you become very creative. If you are pressured on something that you can't possibly deliver, you cheat." Margit, a quality coordinator I interviewed, preferred not to call it "cheating." Instead, she explained the ambiguous nature of data validity in the current system in this way:

> Times are changing. People are getting more used to having everything out in the open, so if you haven't documented it, somebody will be chasing you down asking for it. I actually think you can hide as many things today as you used to be able to, because you can just produce bad data, invalid data, then the documentation is there. It's just as if a slippery slope has been opened somehow.

It is an interesting observation: "you can just produce bad data." Such data massaging is equally well known elsewhere. In the United States, one observer notes how Medicare "pressures hospitals to cheat, saps doctors' and nurses' intrinsic motivation to do good work even when no one is looking, and corrupts the data" (Himmelstein and Woolhandler 2015: 5).

Liselotte, the data analyst from the regional level, was very aware of data manipulation practices among clinicians, but she decided to use data anyway "as if" they were valid. She saw no alternative. She also admitted that data manipulation took place not only in relation to data production. Her own data work related to analysis was not all that different; she said, "You can manipulate data endlessly, and you can get practically any result that you'd like. You can clean the data so much that you get rid of anything that contradicts your point." She felt confident that she knew when to trust her own results, but she also admitted that she was under increasing pressure to get particular results desired by the administrative management or at the political level. The pharmaceutical industry has long been accused of manipulative data practices (McGoey 2010; Creager 2021), and it is worrisome to hear public data analysts articulating these pressures (Knudsen 2011). Jonna, a data analyst working in one of the big municipalities, explained that "you sometimes just have to do the dirty work." She referred to cases where top management needs "a particular number" for a purpose like legitimizing letting off particular people. It is always possible to find something in the data to support the story they want to tell, she explained. For some, validity problems represent opportunities.

Taken together, these reflections point to a very profound effect of intensified data sourcing: an experience of referentiality as an illusion that can be departed from. Data need not refer to—or pretend to refer to—something "real" to have effects. French postmodernists such as Lyotard and Baudrillard awaited and embraced such a moment (Baudrillard 2021 [1994]; Lyotard 1984). Baudrillard spoke of a culture of signs operating as simulacrum: copies with no originals. Drawing on this tradition, Mark Poster (1990) argued that the "database" transforms data into a *self-referential* sign. Data serve as signs *without* any connection to an external "reality." What is real to the organization is what is in the data—what can be found in the database.

Liselotte, Mona, and the other people who do data analytical work in Danish healthcare would not agree with the postmodern interpretation. They insist that some analyses are better than others. They mostly dislike pressures, biases, registration errors, and corrupted practices. Still, they have come to accept working with data as signs that are desired as much for their performative effects as their epistemic veracity. Data lie at the heart of their meaning-making practices. They need data to feel that what they do is meaningful, even when the data act partly as self-referential signs.

In addition, a sense of epistemic doubt creeps into research uses of data. The epidemiological literature explicitly discusses data validity problems arising from reuse (Chan, Fowles, and Weiner 2010; Pedersen, Klarlund, Jacobsen et al. 2004; Severinsen, Kristensen, Overvad et al. 2010). From these quarters, the proposed solution is, like the response from politicians, to collect *more* data to make up for data omissions and errors. The result is a self-enforcing epistemological kaleidoscope relying on data that need verification by other forms of data, which are then in need of verification from yet other data in a potentially endless regression loop.

Industry researchers, or at least the lobbyists working to ensure access to data, seem a lot less worried about validity. I have pondered this point a lot. How come people like Bent, the lobbyist cited in the introduction, do not fear data validity problems? Is it because they do not know the registries well enough to have the data analytical skills needed to make sense of them? Or might it be that industrial research has gone further down the postmodern lane and acknowledged "dissolving referentiality" as an opportunity? Epistemic doubt creates space for the most powerful actors to promote the narratives they see fit (Oreskes 2019; McGoey 2010). It is well known that some industrial actors have used data access for years to debunk claims made by public researchers about topics such as risk stemming from tobacco use, environmental pollution, and climate change (Angell and Relman 2002; Sismondo 2008; Egilman 2005). While epistemic doubt can be favorable for certain interests, it is important not to overemphasize suspicion. I do not even think of the embrace of data massaging as driven (primarily) by corruption or greed.[8] It is not useful to give in to one's paranoia (Sedgwick 2003). Paranoia derails the understanding of intensified data sourcing. Instead, I see a key driver in the pursuit of meaning through data.

I opened this chapter by describing a particular conflict between clinical and administrative perceptions. When Hedegaard resigned in 2016, he claimed that patient safety was at risk because the staff were too busy, but the politicians said that no data supported his claim. Indeed, Hedegaard and colleagues had just published a research study about the falling risk of stillbirth as a consequence of a more proactive approach where all prolonged pregnancies were acted upon earlier than previously (Hedegaard, Lidegaard, Wessel Skovlund et al. 2014). In 2020, the hospital released new figures showing that stillbirths had doubled in the preceding five years (Lidegaard, Krebs, Petersen et al. 2020). The primary explanation was that due to high work pressure, births were no longer initiated in time in cases of prolonged pregnancy (Munk 2020; Knudsen 2020). Perhaps the staff were right when they said, back in 2016, that the work pressure had reached a level where it affected safety. At the time, however, data did not yet support their everyday experience. Instead, their experience was overruled by data.

PARADOXES OF DATA WORK

This chapter has shown how intensified data sourcing has changed the conditions for professional work—as well as what counts as valid knowledge about this work. The imposition of data work for objectives other than clinical purposes influences the moral landscape of the clinic by changing the work culture and priorities of clinical attention. Digital tools now structure work practices, and the documentation formerly kept in closed cabinets is made available for continued monitoring and reuse. In the course of that process, the epistemic status of data has changed. The attraction of data no longer hinges on the belief that data refer to an external "reality" or serve a "rational" clinical goal. What is real to the organization can be simply (and only) what is in the data. Data are multiple, and people in different places with different agendas may use the same data with very different interpretations, drawing conspicuously dissimilar conclusions. A radical implication of this is that the pursuit of meaning no longer is determined by clinical goal orientation. Health professionals, however, continue to see patients. They care about patient outcomes. This is, perhaps, why they find themselves so busy. They encounter actual people and cannot work only with symbols.

With this in mind, the paradoxes outlined in the opening of the chapter are no longer logically inconsistent. Intensified data sourcing produces both less and more work. Work, however, is redistributed (see also Svenningsen 2004; Vikkelsø 2005). The very concrete experience of less work (for some) legitimizes more work for others. In this sense, the paradox is productive: it does something for some of the stakeholders. Ironically, the increasing amounts of data seem to legitimize new recruitments among the administrative data users who get easier access to data. There has been a consistent growth in administrative staff relative to frontline staff at least since the 1930s—and it does not seem to be about to stop (Østrup, Jørgensen, and Zwisler 2020; Vallgårda 1992).

The second paradox is similarly productive. Data intensification tightens organizational control and facilitates organizational disintegration. With data, the political and administrative layers have better options for controlling the narratives that are told, as in the conflict between Hedegaard and the politicians, while being comfortably unaware of what is going on in the clinic. Organizational disintegration, however, can also be beneficial for clinicians and other frontline staff. Data can serve as shields deflecting further interest. But such data massage practices propagate a sense of epistemic doubt. Epistemic doubt informs the productivity of the third paradox. Data create meaningless tasks, and yet they still are used as meaning-making tools. As data purposes mingle in multiple ways, the same data can be seen as meaningless in one context and yet meaningful in another. Meaningful and meaningless are not two distinct classes of data. Epistemic doubt provides room for multiple stories. It allows them to coexist. Thereby, people can work alongside each other with an equal sense of conviction, though with different perceptions of the problems they confront. Still, they seem to agree that they need data to tell their stories.

The French postmodernists happily embraced the dissolving referentiality. They considered references to the "real" as tools of power. Lyotard (1984) associated claims of truth with totalitarian ambitions and said: "In the computer age, the question of knowledge is now more than ever a question of government" (pp. 8–9). His ambition was to open up access to data and "give the public free access to the memory and the data banks" (67). For him, open access to all data was the way to ensure a plurality of voices.

Baudrillard (2021 [1994]) similarly detested the longing for the real and concluded: "There is no hope for meaning. And without doubt this is a good thing: meaning is mortal" (164).

Be careful what you wish for, some might say. Opening up for the reuse of data indeed created a plurality of voices, but also a loss of meaning (Rahman 2021). Dissolving referentiality is a double-edged sword. In 2020, American voters were told by their president, Donald J. Trump, that they did not have to believe in election results if they did not agree with them. Today, after having seen the success of Trump at promoting "alternative facts" (Fuchs 2018), the postmodernist attraction has faded. There is reason instead to sustain and speak to the sense of integrity that makes clinicians and data analysts most proud.

For patients, dedication to "truth" has a particular and very personal urgency: What helps their fight against suffering? For their sake, there is a need to embrace the search for robust knowledge. Chapter 5 explores the role of data in generating robust knowledge. First, however, I believe that there is a point to paying much more serious attention to how data form part of meaning-making practices. I am thinking here of how people experience data. There is an experiential dimension to data that has not yet been explored adequately. I suggest paying attention to how people engage data work as sensing bodies, not just analytical beings. Chapter 4 is therefore about *data experiences*.

4 DATA EXPERIENCES

February 25, 2017: I have joined Jesper, my husband, at the optician's to check out some glasses that he had had put aside a couple of days earlier. At the counter, a friendly optician's assistant asks for his "CPR" – his personal identity number from the Civil Registration System. Happening to glance at the screen, I cannot help noticing the number of the previous customer. With the CPR number, she quickly retrieves my husband's record, where they have noted not only his optometric measures and previous purchases, but also the numbers of the spectacle frames that he found interesting on a previous visit. He could walk into any shop in this chain, Jesper tells me, and they would be able to look all of it up in seconds. The CPR number also links his purchases to his health insurance and bank, and can automatically allocate subsidies for any purchase even if he changes his address or moves to another bank. The Civil Registration System facilitates automatic updating (see chapter 2). Jesper loves the efficiency of it.

The woman quickly finds the frames and we step aside, discussing how he looks. They are not quite right for him. As we return the spectacle frames, I ask why they connect this commercial information to his state-sanctioned CPR number. It strikes me as a very centralized way of keeping track of people . . . for a shop on the high street. The optician explains that they are legally obliged to keep "patient records"[1]—and then adds that it is very important to log out of the system so that nobody sees the CPR number of the previous customer. I point out that they apparently forgot to do that when we arrived. She smiles gently and thanks me for alerting them.

Meanwhile, Jesper is stepping on his own toes, so eager is he to leave the shop. He practically pulls me out into the bright February sunlight, where he explains how embarrassing that was. Why did I have to question the use of the CPR number? Why did I mention that I could see the number of the previous customer? I stare at him, surprised, and just as I am about to defend myself, I realize how I am in the middle of an ethnomethodological moment. In his introduction to ethnomethodology, Garfinkel (1984) spoke about experiencing tacit cultural rules by breaking them. Without deliberately deciding to do so, I have begun breaking rules about data practices—rules I did not even know existed. Having at this point worked for about a year trying to understand the politics of intensified data sourcing, I am now more and more often asking questions that make people feel uncomfortable. Jesper is not easily embarrassed: I think this is the main reason why I went home and immediately described the episode in my field notes. I was beginning to realize that the invisible data infrastructures that often make life in Denmark so seamless and "integrated" involve a particular social texture—a set of tacit assumptions—that demand attention if I am to understand the politics of intensified data sourcing. Assumptions about data are nested in intersubjective relations between the users of data, and they catch people's attention only when somebody transgresses the social rules—as I did on this occasion. Data infrastructures thrive on seamlessness, on a sort of invisibility. While they cannot be observed as objects, we still feel what they do. We encounter them through interfaces. In these encounters, an analytical potential resides. This potential can be actuated when we think of data and data infrastructures as producing a bodily experience.

In this chapter, I argue my point about data experiences by presenting my own methodological engagement with Danish data infrastructures—that is, my own data experiences. I thereby discuss a number of my methodological choices, but the point of focusing on data experiences is not limited to methods. My discussion of methods serves as an entry point to understanding how the politics of intensified data sourcing reaches into intimate aspects of how humans understand the world around them.

Data infrastructures are not places you can visit, nor objects you can hold. They are inapproachable, or transient, field sites. Still, they work on us. They inform the sensory anticipation of data promises. They shape data living. They permeate data work. However, we see *how* they do so only when we are able to translate our personal experiences into tools of observation (Verran 2021). Academics like me, who study healthcare organizations and data infrastructures, as well as people working in the healthcare services with data tools, have to embrace their own sensory experience to assess how those tools work. It is necessary to make well-informed decisions.

It is not easy to study data experiences. First, where are the data? At the optician's, I realized that features of my everyday mode of data living were opaque even to me. Service providers can access and use data about Jesper and me, but I do not know how, when, or for what purpose they do so. In what I called "wired medicine" in chapter 2, healthcare providers often see data instead of patients—data that can be read, stored, and exchanged by computers without the patient being present. Data work is thereby embedded in a basic paradox: data dematerialize interactions whereby data can be in many places at the same time and connect people and systems *at a distance,* while data simultaneously rematerialize interactions because they connect to people through *physical interfaces* (like data dashboards) and *embodied experiences* (like the one at the optician's). Data are used by people to affect other people, but this mostly happens through wires and computer interfaces. Datafication relies on interactions mediated by materiality. Experiences with hardware and software shape what people do and know. This mutual dematerialization and rematerialization constitute the first paradox that this chapter deals with, and this is important because the paradox involves methodological challenges relating to where to go and what to do when studying data.

There is a second paradox I will discuss in this chapter. It revolves around standardization. Data become successful through standardization, and yet they are never able to fully standardize human experience. The seamlessness that Jesper enjoys rests on standards. Standards are a prerequisite for systems to become integrated so that computers can communicate effortlessly with computers. Standards for integration are the reason why Jesper does not even have to inform his health insurance if he opens a new bank account: his identity number is linked to a primary bank account and automatically updated in all systems drawing on information from the Civil Registration System, the CPR. Yet standardization affects people differently. Each person experiences and reacts to data and digital interfaces in her or his own way. What stimulates curiosity for some creates embarrassment for others, as when I violated tacit rules at the optician's out of curiosity and embarrassed Jesper (and possibly the woman behind the counter). By talking about data experiences, I want to create greater awareness of the variation in how each of us engages with data in the course of everyday life.

Equipped with this awareness, it is possible to look for the experiential dimensions of data work in healthcare organizations. There is every reason for acknowledging data experiences, and yet it is as if there is no vocabulary for talking about them. I therefore begin with a discussion of what I mean by the term "data experience," and then turn to examples of experiences emerging in relation to the types of data work discussed in chapter 3 (production, analysis, instruction, and use), each time beginning with reflections on my own data work—my methods—and then relating them to examples from the health services.

EXPERIENCE: BEYOND EPISTEMIC CONCERNS AND POWER CRITIQUE

Data are typically approached as epistemic objects (conveyers of information) or political objects (shaping relations of power and resource allocation). Consider, for example, the important work in anthropology, science and technology studies (STS), and critical data studies, where scholars question the *epistemic* assumptions found in policy discourses (Borgman 2015; boyd and Crawford 2012; Busch 2017), or criticize the *power effects* of data (Iliadis and Russo 2016), including power understood as pertaining to inequity (van Dijk 2020), infrastructural and cultural change (van Dijck, Poell, and De Wall 2018; van Dijck 2013), economic disruption (Hoffman 2018; Zuboff 2019), or the impact of data on issues like privacy (Taylor 2017; Obar 2017). I discussed this body of literature in the introduction. Although delivering fascinating insights, these approaches nevertheless pay limited attention to *direct experiences* with data. For these scholars, data experiences means the type of lives people live—their data living—as a consequence of data infrastructures (Ebeling 2016; Cheney-Lippold 2017; Kitchin 2021), not *how they experience data*. Even though these are important issues, the direct engagement with data and data infrastructures is black-boxed: data remain epistemic, political, or economic rather than *experiential* objects.

A few scholars have begun paying more attention to the way that data and data infrastructures can be experienced as beautiful (Halpern 2014), and how data aesthetics (color coding, graphs, interactive maps) mediate power effects by privileging particular representations and silencing others (Ratner and Ruppert 2019). They study how the beauty that data visualization experts like Edward Tufte strive for works on people (Tufte 2020). Others note how data provoke feelings such as "data anxiety" (Crawford 2014;

Pink, Lanzeni, and Horst 2018; Cool 2019) or "enchantment" (Smith 2018). Studies of self-trackers and patients who use various wearables and data tools illustrate how people respond emotionally to "seeing" their own data (Kristensen and Prigge 2018; Lomborg, Langstrup, and Andersen 2020; Oxlund 2012). Kristensen and colleagues, in particular, has emphasized how people relate to data goals, such as walking 10,000 steps a day or eating a certain amount of fruits and vegetables, without engaging with the scientific evidence supposedly guiding these goals (Kristensen, Jacobsen, and Pihl-Thingvad 2017; Kristensen and Ruckenstein 2018). Data work on the users, not as conveyers of truth but as partners they can interact with. Immaterial and diffuse goals become material when, for example, red turns to green in an app on your cell phone or when a pedometer makes a sound. Lupton (2020) similarly suggests that the study of self-tracking should be about "paying attention to practices, affects and sensory and other embodied experiences" (6), and she has also suggested that such affective dimensions might be relevant for health professionals (Lupton 2017; Lupton and Maslen 2017). I think these lessons about embodied experiences gathered from studies of self-trackers should indeed be used also to study data experiences among clinical staff—as well as among policymakers, administrators, researchers, and patients.

"Experience" is, I admit, a troubled and ambiguous word (Asad 1994). I use it to build a bridge to the phenomenological dimensions that are easily forgotten in epistemological and political debates about data. The phenomenological turn in anthropology and STS has already sought to attune us to the experiential aspects of technology (Gunnarson 2016; Jackson 1996, 2002b; Mattingly 2010). It draws on Merleau-Ponty's phenomenology, which explored how people make sense of the world around them in a bodily conscious way (e.g., Merleau-Ponty 2002). People are not computers. They engage information as embodied beings, not just through logocentric analytical computations (Hastrup 1994, 1995).

As noted by Mauss (2007), the body is the primary instrument of any human being. Although emphasizing the body as the locus of experience, Merleau-Ponty (2002) also acknowledged the role of technology, noting how people can learn to experience through, for example, a stick as an extension of the body (175). Appreciation of technology as an embodied way of experiencing the world has been developed further in postphenomenology (Ihde 2002; Verbeek 2011; Olsen, Selinger, and Riis 2008; Selinger 2006). Today, it is through data—processed and accessed through digital technology—that people engage many aspects of the world (de Boer 2020; Schwennesen 2019). With data, people learn to sense themselves and the world around them in particular ways (Torenholt, Saltbæk, and Langstrup 2020; Kragh-Furbo, Wilkinson, Mort et al. 2018). Digital data infrastructures not only convey information about the world, but they also make particular worlds emerge as experiential phenomena.

From a philosophical perspective, Sokolowski (2000) has argued the need for appreciating phenomenological experience also when exploring aspects of the world otherwise left to science (consider, for example, climate change) (see also Knox 2022). His point is that we cannot evade or circumvent the phenomenological dimension, even when wishing that people could analyze data as dispassionately as computers:

> We could not live in the world projected by science; we can only live in the life world, and this basic world has its own forms of truth and verification that are not displaced but only complemented by the truth and verification introduced by modern science. (148)

I take this point as an invitation to explore how data feature in life-worlds. How do people as embodied beings experience data?

Data are always experienced through a medium (O'Riordan 2017), as also pointed out in the introduction. The medium materializes the data. Today, the medium is typically a digital interface. Also, the form—graphs, tables, spreadsheets, and so on—matters. The social nature of the encounter with data similarly shapes data experiences: With whom do people experience data? At work, in the clinic, or at home, for example? In the course of doing what? I contend that data experiences in healthcare primarily play out in relation to the four types of activity outlined in chapter 3 as data work: *production* (the work going into data production), *analysis* (the work related to data analysis), *instruction* (to govern with, or be governed by, data), and *use* (to access and utilize data products). I have outlined these with examples of potentially important parameters of variance in table 4.1.

The categorization is not exhaustive. Some types overlap. There is, for example, no absolute distinction between analysis and use, as any use will involve an element of interpretation. Accordingly, my examples in this chapter will illustrate overlaps. The table primarily means to illustrate the diversity of data encounters. We should not expect data to awaken similar reactions even in the same person when situations are so diverse. Also, in

Table 4.1

Four types of activity that give rise to data experiences

Data production	At own will with your own purpose (e.g., doctors trying to systematize their work, a researcher or administrator wanting data to answer a question, or a self-tracking citizen)
	When asked to make data for others and for purposes defined by others (e.g., a nurse asked to fill in quality data to document performance or activity, or a patient filling in questionnaires)
	When (consciously or unconsciously) leaving data traces in the course of doing something else that can be used by others (e.g., digital surveillance through monitoring tools)
Data analysis	When initiating your own analysis on your own data (e.g., citizens using self-trackers, or researchers pursuing research questions, or general practitioners [GPs] seeking to identify patients with special needs)
	When initiating your own analysis using data produced by others (e.g., administrators using clinical data, or epidemiologists using registry data for research)
	When performing analysis for others on demand (e.g., data analytical teams asked to support particular political projects with "facts")
Data instruction	When governed by data analyses produced by others (e.g., performance-based management)
	When working in or designing digital interfaces that use input to modify behavior (e.g., decision-support tools, reminder systems, algorithmic feedback)
	When granted or denied a privilege based on a data profile (e.g., patients' access to treatment or experience of prejudice based on diagnostic profile) or designing programs for such decisions
Data use	When accessing data on yourself (e.g., patients logging on to see their health records or use data such as ancestry testing for educational or entertainment purposes)
	When accessing data on others—legitimately or illegitimately (e.g., health professionals using data produced by other entities as part of care—or to spy on, e.g., an ex-partner)
	When reading data analyses (e.g., as when policymakers receive input to decision-making, or as when staff, patients and citizens read data products that claim to represent them)

relation to what might be considered *one* data practice, there might still be *multiple* sites for data experiences, each with their own implications (Moerenhout, Fischer, and Decvisch 2020). Consider again table 1.1 in chapter 1 on the many purposes with data, and it becomes obvious that even though policy discourses talk about for example a diagnostic code in the singular as *a* piece of data, this code is produced in one practice, analyzed in others, and used for governance and remuneration purposes in yet others. The doctor producing the code in a medical record system such as The Health Platform can have an experience which is very different from, for example, the epidemiological researcher analyzing this code on the servers of Statistics Denmark. The "same" data give rise to different data experiences as part of different types of data work, through different interfaces, in different social situations. Just as Merleau-Ponty (2002) pointed to the fundamental situatedness of all experience, any analysis of data politics must accept this basic awareness of the situatedness of data experiences.

The concept of experience remains, of course, anthropocentric. It directs attention toward the human side of the human-technology equation. This is not to say that data experiences are created by humans alone: materiality matters—hence my point about rematerialization. Still, a focus on human engagement is crucial because this inevitably varies even when technology seeks to standardize. There is no end to human variation, as Mills (2000 [1959]) insisted. Data politics unfolds and has implications in the tumult of multiple actors, each one differently situated and variously disposed toward data, and working toward different ends. Awareness of such variances can help raise useful questions about the complexity of data-political effects, while simultaneously providing new methodological angles from which to examine data infrastructures.

Once you acknowledge your own emotional reactions to data, you can begin observing them in others. First, it can make you think: "Why should the others be altogether different from me?" If I myself am not as cool and rational as a computer, for example, I should probably not expect others to use data as if they were computers. Second, the next thought should be: "Some of these other people probably *are* very different from me! They are definitely not as cool as computers, but what do *they* feel? How do *they* react?"

With these theoretical reflections aimed at mobilizing data experiences as an analytical term, I can now turn to the four types of activity: production, analysis, instruction, and use. I begin in each case with my own methodological experiences and choices, and then relate them to observations in the health services. I use my own engagement with data because it illustrates the challenges associated with the paradox of dematerialization and rematerialization, but also because I think awareness of one's phenomenological experience can be helpful whether done during academic analysis or working with data in healthcare.

PRODUCTION: DATA WORK GENERATES EMOTIONS

It gradually dawned on me that it would be useful to theorize data experiences as I acknowledged (I should perhaps say admitted to myself) that I was having emotional reactions to my own data production. These reactions were not particularly flattering. I sometimes experienced a form of exhaustion. One day in October 2017, I added a reflective note about my own data production in my field notes:

> I've been out of office a few days, and opening my email it is as if I am drowning. I feel dizzy. I'm flooded by data. I am now fully dependent on digital tools to keep track of the constant stream of news, reports, papers, and press releases. These sources of information probably sometimes become research data partly as a consequence of their digital format and availability through the technological infrastructures I'm embedded in. (. . .) Thanks to my phone, this flow of data hits me constantly and everywhere—when queuing for an airplane or in the [coffee] break at a conference. I transfer links to emails and send them to myself to have them waiting in my inbox when I am back in office. I get too many data and have to make them searchable with keywords. I then transform them into an archive, just like other data sets that need rinsing and preparation. Constantly dreading to lose track or forget something. But I can't help asking: Why does it exhaust me in this way?

What I am admitting to myself here is not just a lack of control and direction. I am admitting to a set of emotions. I had begun wondering why my documentary data practices *felt* so different from my memory of the joyous task of writing notes during earlier fieldwork in Tanzania and Sweden. When doing fieldwork in those places, I used to fill books with handwritten notes and later index them. The very act of writing gave a sense of orientation, as if I gradually mastered the complexity in the course of narrating my experiences. Subconscious omissions probably helped me select among memories and add a sense of clarity, but if that was the case, then the comforting sense of understanding overrode my doubts.

People use narratives to orient themselves (Frank 2012). In the field note, I describe a data production that has become disentangled from analysis. It might be why it was disorienting and exhausting. The note also reveals another source of exhaustion: the technological mediation of my notetaking. Today, it is always on a computer, if not at the time of the initial notetaking, then later (see also Gehl [2019] on the emotional engagement with digital tools). Digital pervasiveness also means that data are potentially everywhere and can be anything (although anything already in a digital format has a greater chance of making it into data archives, as I write in the note with a hint of bad conscience). The Internet has changed my research practices (Meyer and Schroeder 2015). My notes have begun to overflow with hyperlinks and pictures. The notetaking is easier with links. Ease overrides the sense of analytical reward. Digitalization does change "memory practices" (Bowker 2005), but it does so through our emotional reactions—joy, shame, ease, exhaustion—as much as anything else.

If emotional aspects of my data production inform my research choices, why would they not inform organizational and clinical actions? Of course, people in the health services also feel joy, shame, ease, and exhaustion. They do not, however, necessarily react in similar ways to the same tasks. Today, I have come to think that my lurking sense of shame partly reflects an awareness that by admitting to a lack of digital thrill, I have relegated myself to a group of people with limited standing in a world dominated by data promises. It is embarrassing even to talk about handwritten notes to young people who can barely write properly by hand anymore. You feel like the dinosaur who forgot to die.

But my point here is not to defend myself. I wish instead to argue the relevance of acknowledging how emotional reactions to data production shape what we produce, as well as which lives we live in data-intensive organizations. Once you dare to admit your own emotions related to data work (including the not-so-favorable emotions proving that you are not as systematic as a computer or as thrilled about digital interfaces as data promises suggest you ought to be), you begin to see the emotional reactions of others everywhere. Emotions shape what we do, not as some form of primary state of affect (Martin 2013), but as elements of the social texture of being human (Hochschild 1979). Of course—and inevitably—they are important for data politics.

The complaints among health professionals about "meaningless work," as discussed in chapter 3, are emotional reactions. When clinicians complain about data production as meaningless work, it might very well be related to the shift from producing narratives (the old means of record-keeping) to producing scattered pieces of information (data entries, smart texts, or codes in response to pop-up windows) (Parton 2008). This type of data work no longer gives the gratifying sense of orientation that narratives do—something I had also lost as I shifted from making handwritten notes to digital recording of links, reports, pictures, and press releases.

Once I had begun thinking analytically about my own data experiences, I was able to notice how clinicians seemed to have a range of reactions. As I pointed out in chapter 3, most clinicians dislike data work without clear clinical relevance. However, their responses to "meaningless" data production come in a range of emotional registers. While some feel ridiculed, others talk about being drained of energy, and still others do not really mind. A nurse, for example, spoke endlessly—while treating me as a patient—about the "ludicrous" Epic system, The Health Platform, "It makes no sense, of course," and then surprisingly she added: "But actually I don't mind it that much. It's kinda like having a break, just filling in stupid numbers." Apparently, it is possible to experience data work as "a break" even while finding them "ludicrous" at an analytical level. Yet others seem to experience an actual thrill of excitement when confronted with a new digital interface.

Excitement appears not to be as common in relation to data production as it is with data work relating to analysis. I noticed how the face of a psychologist at a seminar lit up when telling me how she would spend hours after work exploring what the Epic system could do. Although she had not yet found anything of particular clinical applicability, she found the "opportunities" fascinating. For her, the system was like a puzzle, inviting curiosity. I have also noticed such enthusiasm with new software among my colleagues. They have sparkling eyes and move their heads forward, looking at the screen, in ways that tell me that they react in emotionally more compelling ways to new data interfaces than I, the dinosaur, tend to do.

Acknowledgment of emotional reactions to data production can also add to the understanding of the implications of dissolving referentiality presented in the previous chapter. Those clinicians where the imposition of data work potentially undermines their professional motivation have to find pride in their work, as well as motivation, in new ways. Pride in producing good data is one such strategy. Lars may serve as an example. I interviewed Lars, an anesthetic nurse, a couple of times. He explained how he personally had come to like some of the features of The Health Platform because he could do his documentation while the patient was anesthetized. Thereby, his data production did not compromise patient safety, he explained, but he obtained significantly better data:

> The product that I deliver is better. The way I anesthetize the patient has not changed. It is no better and no worse. But I can document it better. The quality of the document I hand over afterwards has improved.

What he refers to here as the "product" of his work is the data he produces, not the treatment of the patient.

In the national quality organization, where I conducted a number of interviews, the data analysts similarly spoke about "good data" as having value independent of the actual use. Taking pride in good data is an obvious outcome of an organizational culture that distributes praise and blame based on that data. To find pride in data with limited clinical value is a coping mechanism as well as an effect: it helps to reenchant otherwise meaningless data work, though the patient fares "no better and no worse." My point is that data work generates and operates through such emotions. Data failures can give rise to shame; data confidence can inspire pride. Emotions therefore run through not just data production, but also the other three types of data work: analysis, instruction, and use.

The field note mentioned previously suggests that there is reason to question whether I chose the data or they chose me. Of course, serendipity has always characterized ethnographic methods, but I have no way of understanding the algorithmic forms of selection that shape what I encounter. Of course, I have kept doing what I can. I sign up for press releases and listservs, I follow relevant lobbying organizations, and I do systematic searches on selected topics such as The Health Platform.[2] A lot of it is fun. Production without analysis, however, is not that stimulating for me. I cannot, like the nurse above, consider it "a break." My sense of exhaustion might reflect how my data production had become increasingly disconnected from analysis. The informational overload makes the thought of subsequent analysis appear overwhelming. If digital infrastructures were part of creating the information overload, it is striking how this overload in turn inspires the use of digital tools to make sense of the "infoglut" (Andrejevic 2013). Thinking becomes a cyborg act. I am well aware that the feeling of information overload is not new. As historian Ann Blair (2010) remarks:

> We describe ourselves as living in an information age as if this were something completely new. In fact, many of our current ways of thinking about and handling information descend from patterns of thought and practices that extend back for centuries. (1)

Blair points out that even Immanuel Kant complained about exhaustion in his attempt to keep up to date. Still, the ongoing datafication of our documentary practices sustains the feeling of disorientation. Disconnected, scattered pieces of information, kept in databases that are to be analyzed later, imply postponement: the pile in front of you keeps growing, and it does not yet make sense. Postponement is at the heart of data politics, as I argued in chapter 1, but people relate to it in different emotional registers.

ANALYSIS: PEOPLE LEARN FROM PEOPLE, NOT JUST DATA

I have just described how the speed of communication and overload of information can provoke feelings of inadequacy. Yet observing close colleagues, I see how they can appear empowered and invigorated by the very same elements. For example, during a workshop where we discussed software that analyzed texts by counting "positive" or "negative" expressions in enormous digital data sets, some participants delighted in the ease and sense of quantitative certainty. I focused on algorithmic obfuscation: not knowing what the software does, how it deals with irony, and other such aspects. Conversely, I can observe the sense of unease when quantitatively trained colleagues or students feel uncertain about their own analytical choices when involved in qualitative analysis. I am well aware that some would argue that the workings of the human mind are no less obscure than algorithms (Kahneman and Klein 2009). We are, at least on the surface, remarkably different in this respect as well: some people tend to trust computers more than the minds of humans, and others trust human judgments more than digital calculations.

The point is that the data experiences of analysis are not epistemological alone. They are embodied. Embodiment is social. It emerges through interaction with other people. How we feel affects our analytical decisions and which analytical products we trust. Once we acknowledge the inevitable human variations, we can avoid seeing the choices of others through a deficit model compared to our own,[3] and instead rethink our reasons for trusting an analysis, case by case. This goes for research as well as organizational decisions and clinical work. If data experiences shape the dimensions of reality that researchers decide to include in their analysis, why should policymakers, administrators, and clinicians be any different?

Even those people who prefer calculations to human judgments still have to make judgments themselves. These judgments are inherently social. Even people who are the most digitally invigorated and enthusiastic also orient themselves toward fellow humans. Chapter 3 described the rising authority of data ("we build arguments with data"). As Charles Taylor (1994) avows, people want the recognition of other people. Therefore, people feel attracted to the types of analysis that are acknowledged by people around them. When I have participated in meetings, I have begun noticing that they are full of references to relations, experiences, and personal impressions. Which *data* are allowed to count—that is, to be considered significant—depend on *whose* opinions and experiences likewise count in that given meeting. Data as such rarely dictate decisions among people. The politics of recognition guides data selection in any given organization. In a healthcare system permeated by data promises, quantitative data tend to provide speakers with more recognition and authority. It is to gain recognition from others that clinicians "build arguments with data," not out of mere epistemic curiosity.

We are all influenced by the thoughts of others, but we each react very differently to the various *forms* in which we encounter them. For me, interviewing is engaging in ways textual analysis is not. Others feel exactly the opposite (Žižek 2020). In participant observation, we take clues from people in an embodied way. Some researchers feel comfortable, even enlivened, by that form of intersubjectivity, while others feel uncomfortable or exhausted. Similarly, classic studies of organizational managers showed how some prefer taking clues for action from people, and others from written sources, when forming opinions (Stewart 1967).

To provide an example of how interviews work on me with more strength than documents, I return to Mona (discussed in chapter 3), the experienced data analyst who had worked with the integration of data at the regional level for years. I was struggling to understand why quality databases previously kept by the regional level had to begin sending backup files to the Danish Health Data Authority. According to the written documents, the board was not supposed to use the data as such, so why did they have to be pooled? In the course of an interview, Mona then explained:

> Yes. Now they want to pool the data, and then you've suddenly got, so to say, a *hell of a lot of* information about all citizens in Denmark. There might be ten [citizens] who are not registered somewhere, but then they must have been born abroad, really. . . . Then combining all these data sources we can actually have sort of a constant state-of-health register, which provides us with a real-time picture of the state of health in the population: How many smoke, what do people weigh, how much do they exercise? (her emphasis)

There was something about the sparkle in her eyes and her gesticulating hands as she conveyed her sense of pervasive overview that worked on me very differently from the various reports making similar claims about data power. She was bolder. It was obvious that she believed in the power of data; it was not just a strategic discourse to her. What is more, Mona went behind the polished statements in the reports. She conveyed her doubts. It turned out that Mona was not 100 percent comfortable with the compilation of data at the state level. Referencing George Orwell's novel *Nineteen Eighty-Four*, she says it makes her think of "Big Brother." She then goes on to refer to this "Brother" as an unspecified plural "they": "The reason I am a tiny bit worried is that they can't say why they want all these data. They just want them (. . .) I guess it provokes some form of anxiety; that they will be abused."

Although Mona is proud of what she thinks data can do, the conversation allows her to communicate doubts of a different order. Again, bodies read bodies in ways that affect them personally. I feel worried, not because of any specific information provided, but because *Mona* is worried. The change in her mood, the way she was trying out the thought, affect me in ways that documents cannot. I had previously interviewed Teis, who also used the image of Big Brother, as he said:

> Really, George Orwell, *Nineteen Eighty-Four*, he only touched the surface of what we store on citizens today. If Denmark was to become a dictatorship—it's difficult to imagine, but if—it would be GDR [the former East Germany] on speed. We could keep everything under relentless surveillance and constantly know everything about the citizens. It really could be abused, if anybody wanted to.

The difference between interviewing him and interviewing Mona is that Teis expressed no worry. It was Mona's lack of comfort with data pooling that made me bolder. After several such encounters, I dared questioning the logics of data accumulation more openly. If emotional clues from people affect me, why would others be altogether different?

Knowing is socially embedded all the way through (Mauss 2007; Hastrup 1995). Not only are our thought styles shaped by communities of practice, as observed already by Fleck (1979), but we also glean much more than information from the people we work with. When we have repeated meetings with people, for example, we learn to respect (or sometimes disrespect) the opinion of others. They become a filter through which we take in new information. We orient ourselves through the values and beliefs of the people we respect. Sometimes emotions probably shape what count as facts rather than the other way around (Durnová 2019), even among anthropologists (Horowitz, Yaworsky, and Kickham 2019).

The ability to orient myself through others has been a very concrete experience for me in the project that led to this book. As described in the preface, I have had the privilege of working closely with a group of excellent scholars. They have conducted fieldwork in various clinical environments, and it is by collaborating with them that I have been able to engage everyday practices across many clinical specialties. I could never have gained intimate familiarity with so many clinical settings on my own. Working with other people entails a methodology of traveling experiences, as it were, where the experiences and interests of others become part of my thinking (see also Korsby and Stavrianakis 2021). I have often found myself pondering, "What would this-or-that colleague say?" when considering an idea. Relations direct curiosities and shape judgment.

Continued collaborations are therefore much more than data exchanges: they shape which data to look for and how to make sense of them. When we reflect on our own data experiences in this way, we can begin to recognize how the people we study also take clues from other people, not just from data. If I learn something about data infrastructures from interacting with Mona—something that I cannot discern from documents—then the people building these infrastructures probably also use multiple forms of impressions when doing their work. They do not just compute information; they learn from other people. In line with this, Jensen (2022) shows in her work on organ transplant coordinators how it often takes social skills and diplomacy to make health professionals produce and use data. What data do depends on the social networks in which they operate.

Finally, the way that people take clues from people, not just from data, relates to the need for context. When discussing organizational questions, we academics do not just throw data at each other: people expect context. If scholars do this when comparing research sites, why do organizational policy papers today increasingly disregard these classic forms of knowing the organizational context and claim a need for data instead (Pedersen 2019a)?

In organizational matters, people always learn from people, not just data: analyzing is a social act. Clever organizational decision makers know that organizational issues vary according to so many parameters that they need to discuss ideas that were developed or tested in other organizations with local teams before they can assess their feasibility in their own case. Still, data promises are marked by a consistent longing for standardization and transferability. Strategies aim for forms of analysis that can be streamlined, applied to all organizations, and scaled up, and give the same result each time. They aim for predictability. At the heart of predictability lies standardization. In order for data promises to fully materialize, people would have to become more standardized and predictable—that is, more like computers.

INSTRUCTION: PEOPLE ARE NOT COMPUTERS

People are not computers—or even like them. It is as embodied beings that humans experience data. Just like it is an embodied experience to produce and analyze data, it is an embodied experience to be governed by data tools. I think all academics feel the yoke of data instruction crunching in on them. We feel the increasing weight of tasks that we are asked to do so the administration can monitor, in particular ways, our academic performance, our teaching, and our financial expenditures. In this regard, academics experience demands akin to those faced by health professionals (Biagioli and Lippman 2020). What may we learn from our own complaints about "meaningless work" when governed through data tools?

I admit to feeling an irrational resentment of having to use a *particular* accounting system for reimbursement of travel expenses. I can hear myself complaining about the time it consumes and how I am certain that it makes traveling more expensive. Actually, I know that these reactions are also a consequence of my dislike of working with the system, not just the potential costs associated with it. My dislike preceded my analysis of the system. Had it been smooth and fun, I might not have bothered to analyze the financial cost. In contrast, consider the delight of a Google search. It is so easy and efficient—at least if you do not bother to read the terms of agreement policy. The accounting system that I dislike has a counterintuitive interface and yet I have no free choice. I must use it. Counterintuitive computer interfaces eat motivation for breakfast. Conversely, seamless and engaging interfaces like Google and Facebook eat data-security awareness for breakfast. They leave you feeling good, with no urge to analyze their implications.

The use of data governance in academia is about more than bad information and communications technology (ICT) design. It changes priorities. Just like clinicians, academics respond to measurements (Shore and Wright 1999, 2001). A colleague of mine at another university told me that he could see the rush of adrenalin when people looked up their own citation numbers. I have rarely observed other academics looking up such numbers. It is a private practice in my institution. Still, it is obvious that academics respond emotionally to data representations that pertain to themselves. Like the clinicians described in chapter 3, studies show that they also begin gaming the system to get better scores (Power 2020). Wounters (2020) argues that academic gaming is not even really cheating; it means to respond to signals in the system—delivering what you are asked to deliver. I cannot count the number of times that I have been called naive when arguing that we need to think about the *goals* of the university, not just its *measurements* when assessing performance. Gradually, I have come to acknowledge that perceptions of academic performance are now inseparable from measurements of academic performance.

When acknowledging that academics respond to data instruction in embodied and emotional ways, it becomes obvious how data politics in healthcare is full of such data experiences. Clinicians can be proud and happy when reaching a goal, even while questioning its clinical relevance. Administrators *feel* data achievements, they do not just work to achieve them. My notes are full of scribbles about people referring to "green" numbers (goal reached) with satisfaction, and to "red" numbers (suboptimal performance) with distress or shame—even while calling into question both the validity and the relevance of the measurement in question.

How about the data experiences of patients? Patients increasingly receive instruction through more or less automated systems. Automated systems are also used for data collection. As the people creating the system and those summoning the patient to an examination often do not themselves see the patients, they do not always realize that the data are never used. A physician told me that often patients would be "furious because they fill in all of this and then I never comment on it. But I simply haven't got the time!" Langstrup (2018) has shown that the people who design these questionnaires are very aware that they need to be used in a clinically relevant manner, but they cannot control how they are distributed and used.

In 2020, for the first time in many years, I had a number of medical appointments for what turned out to be innocent ailments, although they—due to my age, as I was repeatedly told—prompted standard examinations to rule out cancer as the cause. These examinations allowed me to experiment a bit with the role of the patient. Sometimes, for example, I would fill in the questionnaires that popped up automatically on platforms on which I was informed I needed to check in before an appointment. Sometimes I decided not to fill them in. It did not seem to make any difference. I also received an automated instruction to print a questionnaire and bring it along, but when I tried to hand it in, they said they did not want anything on paper. The nurse welcoming me said, "I really don't know who sends out those letters." It was something "that came with this Epic system," I was told. Others asked me to fill in the questionnaire a second time because they could not access my answers in the system, again blaming Epic. It feels slightly odd and rather unsettling to have just filled in a questionnaire and then be told that the data are already "lost" in the system. For another appointment, a nurse called me on the phone, saying I would get a letter in my electronic mailbox that I should not read—she just did not know how to stop it from being sent. It was an automated function in the Epic system. I could not help myself—I read the letter. It began with "This letter contains very important information. You must read it carefully." The whole episode made me laugh, though it was of course very sad.

As with my distaste for the accounting system that I am obliged to use at work, I noticed how being obliged to use particular data-gathering tools as a patient affects the experience. When some apps suddenly become very popular on the global market, it is because they are picked up by users wanting to experiment with them. Often they abandon them later (Finkelstein, Haaland, Bilger et al. 2016). The availability of options can make a world of difference for the data experience, but it is rarely taken into account when the health services seek to find, for example, the best monitoring tool for all patients associated with a given ward or clinical specialty: healthcare systems tend to depend on one size fitting all. The chosen tool, however, will give rise to different experiences for different patients. No size is best for *all*.

Most people, whether working in academia or in the health services, like rewards and dislike punishments. In that sense, they are like computers—they are just not as easily standardized. People evade, omit, and transgress systems because they—as individuals—are working toward slightly different ends. They remain unpredictable. Furthermore, for most organizational decisions, data are not used in a truly automated way, but selectively. The selective use of evidence (discussed in chapter 1) makes more sense when we accept that people are not computers. The cases that caused the most distress in the data analysts that I have interviewed were those where the analysts had to deliver data to legitimize planned redundancies, cutbacks, and firings of unpopular employees: these were decisions made by humans on grounds that were anything but data-driven; data were just the fig leaf covering up the real reason behind the act. Humans react differently from computers when confronted with such decisions. Decisions like these matter to humans on an emotional level on which computers, as far as we know, do not operate.

USE: DATA EXPERIENCES INFORM THE PATH OF ACTION

How do people, as embodied beings, use data products? How does a person *experience* seeing a graph, a heat map, a list of red-yellow-green statuses? How do they experience an interview quote or clinical narrative? Through which medium, and in whose company, do they engage these data representations? To appreciate this dimension, I again have had to reflect on my own methodology. How do *I* engage with data representations, and how do *my* methodological choices reflect what I consider good data? Which type of data user am I? Only then have I been able to look for differences in others. Users engage technological products in a range of different ways (Oudshoorn and Pinch 2003; Hyysalo, Jensen, and Oudshoorn 2016), and data technologies are no exception.

As embodied beings, we are all at the mercy of our own embodied being-in-the-world. It took some time before I realized that the discussion of "what data mean" (as presented in the introduction) involved this more phenomenological dimension too: what do we, as users of data, even recognize as data? In my initial anthropological training, I was always told that "everything is data." This was—of course—a lie (Brinkmann 2014). The constant encouragement to see everything as data was intended to persuade us, as students, to pay attention to that which other disciplines often neglect. Being *present* in the course of everyday life is supposed to allow anthropologists to go "beyond the words" (Wikan 1992). Instead of numerical clarity, the point is to create dense and thick descriptions. In that training, the word "data" clearly meant something very different from the general use of the term in the health services that I now study. Ethnographic data do not come in computational formats only.

Ethnographic presence gives access to types of knowledge that data science does not, exactly because it draws on bodily experiences and the ability to build a rapport with people. It is through this rapport—as when Mona conveys what she can hardly articulate—that interesting interview data are produced. The willingness to acknowledge the messy and intangible, the tacit (Polanyi 1966) and that which is difficult to record and document, also has proved itself useful when working with datafication processes, as demonstrated by Sally Merry Engle, Vicanne Adams, Cristal Biruk, and others (Hunt, Bell, Baker, and Howard 2017; Biruk 2018; Adams 2016a; Hutchinson, Nayiga, Nabirye et al. 2018; Merry 2016; Sullivan 2017). Not everything makes it to the field notes, however, and Jacques Derrida's point that the archive is characterized not only by what it contains but also by what it omits has enduring relevance for qualitative researchers (Derrida 1995). The anthropological ambition creates its own silences and omissions. The credo of ethnographic presence downplays the value of stories in television and in newspapers, such as the media reports on a man without a CPR number (chapter 2) and the public conflict about Morten Hedegaard (discussed in chapter 3). Still, I maintain that data politics is also what is happening in this type of public contestation. Although not ethnographically thick, it is "thick data" in a different sense when Hedegaard's resignation or a man without a CPR number attract massive attention. Journalistic framings say something about what is considered newsworthy in a given context, even though the individual story behind the news will have other facets. Any form of academic training establishes its own hierarchy of data, and in some cases it is important to rethink what might be data for the topic at hand rather than limiting yourself to what can be studied with what is usually considered good data in everyday organizational practice, as well as in research.

If I sometimes select data according to tacit disciplinary habits and fear negative reactions when I do not follow conventions, why should other people—researchers, administrators, or clinicians—be any different? When data users select which data to consider, I have come to think that they often do so partly in light of how they themselves experience data. Just as interviews invigorate me but are deeply uncomfortable for others, I have begun noticing the relief that colleagues express when finally presented with a graph or table after a discussion of quotes from interviews. Just as we approach the analytical tools with different dispositions (as in the case of algorithmic software counting negative and positive words that I have already mentioned), we consume data representations within various emotional registers. For some, a graph is alienating, but for others, it is a comforting reduction of complexity. Healthcare organizations employ people who feel differently about different data types and data representations. Each person gets a different energy from interacting with data representations, and each makes different selections and omissions. It might be dangerous, however, to ignore the competences of people in areas such as clinical care just because they are not particularly good with digital tools.

Without appreciating the variation in how patients engage data and data presentations, medical professionals cannot communicate treatment plans and monitoring goals effectively. Some patients find graphs comforting, but their interest in being comforted can also make them pay attention to only those data that provide such gratification (Weiner, Will, Henwood, and Williams 2020). Selective attention and registration is similar to gaming the system, but with the aim of achieving a particular data experience. Some patients feel vexed when realizing that they have moved without their pedometer and lost the data (Wienroth, Thomsen, and Høstgaard 2020). Emotional reactions to data practices make us into different types of data users. They shape the paths taken in research, organizational practice, and everyday life.

PUTTING DATA EXPERIENCES TO WORK: THE CASE FOR SELF-EXPERIMENTATION

What began at the optician's as an ethnomethodological moment, by sheer coincidence, has for me become a stable ingredient in my methodological toolbox. As human beings, we have to use ourselves to grasp the phenomenological experience of data. Now I take this point a step further and argue the value of self-experimentation by design, not just by accident or necessity. Self-experimentation involves working reflexively with yourself as a sensing tool. I have illustrated each of the four types of encounters with data with reflections on my own methods. Reflexivity may sound like something an individual builds in an armchair in solitude. It is not. It emerges through social practices. By acting in the world and getting reactions, you learn from those reactions. To do so, you do not necessarily have to be an embarrassment to your fellow human beings—or an obtrusive patient experimenting with questionnaire compliance. You can self-experiment in less intrusive ways. I will provide a few examples (and let readers judge the level of embarrassment I should feel).

When reading a paper stating that back in 2008 that it would take on average 201 hours a year to read the terms of agreement needed to access the number of digital services a typical citizen uses (McDonald and Cranor 2008), I decided to try it out myself. For a year, I would read all new terms of agreement before clicking "Accept," and I would on each occasion record the time it took. I wanted to see how it would be to actually do what most agreements write at the top of each document: "Read these terms carefully." Admittedly, I could not carry this task through. First, I gave up recording the time. Measuring time was in itself time consuming . . . and—for me—it was too boring. Boredom is a feeling that (unfortunately) influences many choices of data production, as noted previously. Second, sometimes it was just too grueling to figure out whether I had followed all the links in the agreement. I simply could not figure out what the terms of agreement even were. Third, some weeks were too busy, and I had to employ an assistant to read the agreements (typically between 5,000 and 9,000 words) and send me a short summary so that I could at least categorize the type of agreement.

Nevertheless, by reading several hundreds of terms of agreements, I did learn a lot about the conditions of capturing data from citizens (Larsson 2017). Just as important, I learned a lot from experiencing the feelings of apathy and disempowerment involved in trying to understand what I was agreeing to (Obar 2017). Sometimes I had to click "Accept" no matter how unreasonable the agreements were because of relations of power. For example, I ended up accepting data sourcing in a case where an internationally publisher of high standing had made an online portal mandatory for authors to sign contracts. As I complained about how the conditions for using the portal included offering my data for sale to third parties, it turned out that the contact at the publisher had not himself read the terms of agreement—and could not locate anyone who had. In the course of the year of enduring this self-experiment, I understood the absurdity of presenting terms of agreement as a contract protecting the rights of users, and at the end of the year, a childish joy—a form of conscious cheating—could erupt when I again was at liberty to click "Agree" without even trying to read the terms. Yet there is no way back to innocent clicking once you have seen enough of the often absurd terms.

Another form of self-experimentation is to throw yourself and your ideas into the arena you study. That is, you can turn your thinking into data representations that you can then observe being processed by others. For me, this has involved engaging in discussions about data politics in Denmark as well as abroad. As part of this engagement, I published a book in Danish about health data designed in a short and popular format to stimulate debate (Hoeyer 2019). It did the trick. I was invited to speak at numerous meetings and conferences, as well as in informal meetings with policymakers who were preparing new initiatives and looking for feedback on the feasibility of the proposed ideas. Some of these events were high-profile ones with leading figures such as the prime minister, cabinet ministers, and key industry representatives. Others were low-key, for the people engaged in the everyday work of maintaining a data-intensive healthcare sector. During these seminars and in the course of conversations with the organizers, I made observations on their reactions: What works on people in these organizations? What do they recognize as data? Audiences became sounding boards for the ideas presented in this book, and informal chatter with organizers and participants generated new data for me. Reactions from people are more than data, though; they have come to shape my concepts and thinking as I searched for a vocabulary that made sense also to them (Marcus 2021). I also saw that even when people claimed to "build arguments with data" and aimed for a "data-driven organization," I needed to speak to the *emotions* that data work entailed for them—for example, to speak to the pride evoked by careful data analysis and point out how much work it takes to deliver that type of analysis. Speaking to the sense of pride works much better than warning against hype.

In general, I also respond to hearings on new legal proposals and ethical reports. In this way, I take on the role of political actor and not just an observer of data politics (see also Sharp 2019). Working as I do in a medical faculty, several of my colleagues are involved in planning and executing data-intensive initiatives for health sector research. As a "data expert," I am regularly seconded to committees and advisory panels of various kinds and attend seminars, inaugurations, and management meetings where I hear colleagues discuss the types of work that I study. Meetings are intriguing, at least methodologically speaking. However, when anthropologists write about meetings, they generally approach meeting participants as "study objects" (Brown, Reed, and Yarrow 2017). I talk about attending meetings because I had to, as one of the participants. I was not doing participant observation; rather, I was an observing participant. Some of the examples given in this chapter come from notes taken during or after these meetings.[4] In the meetings, people informally articulate their fears, their pride, and their longing—sometimes even their shame—relating to data in ways that they would never publish or concede to in an interview. These meetings have confirmed that data are indeed experiential objects that work on people as people work with them. By bringing attention to data experiences, I want to encourage those working with data and infrastructures to begin using *what we know as human beings*—not just what happens to feature in the data sets that our disciplines or organizations make us think of as paths to "real" knowledge.

PARADOXES OF DATAFICATION

The kind of politics that revolve around data is coproduced with the experiences that people have when engaging with the data. By becoming aware of our bodily data experiences, and of how we engage the simultaneous dematerialization and rematerialization, we stand a better chance of seeing when emotional and embodied reactions matter for others. This awareness is a bridge to understanding data politics, but also to building more inclusive data infrastructures. Human beings differ in infinite ways. The infrastructures in which their lives unfold must provide space for all this variation. Datafication depends on and becomes successful through standardization, but humans are never fully standardized (Büchner 2018). At the heart of this paradox lies a reason for continued curiosity: nobody should expect data tools to do only what they expect of them.

Which type of politics do these paradoxes propagate? Why do the paradoxes persist? If everybody knows that people differ, why would somebody insist on the ultimate power of standardization? This is similar to the paradox of dematerialization and rematerialization: If everybody is an embodied being and every being can work with data only through material interfaces that generate emotional reactions, why would anybody insist on thinking of data in a purely dematerialized way? Perhaps the reason is that many things are easier with selective knowing, in the short run at least. A policy focus on *one* side of the story, dematerialization or standardization, redistributes and focuses epistemic authority. When Negroponte (1995) suggested that bits would take over from atoms (as mentioned in the introduction), he was writing on a computer made of atoms. He did not produce atoms, but he was a master of bits, and his narrative form privileged his own kingdom.

Loukissas (2019) suggests that Negroponte's dogma about dematerialization is facilitative for governance at a distance in a more general sense. If we relate it to the organizations described in chapter 3, it means that those who use data for instruction are not confronted with how other people—as atoms—are affected by their decisions. Some of these effects are planned, others unexpected. The two paradoxes allow people to use standards and see the inevitable variation as "human error"; coexisting narratives allow them to exert power as information and to ignore the diverse material effects. Those making the decisions can focus on the aspects they wish to govern and ignore the others, whether they relate to race, age, sexuality, or anything else reflecting the endless variation in human lives. Through awareness of the paradoxes, conversely, the effect of data on everyday living becomes thinkable—and thereby actionable—in new ways.

I have written this chapter to create an awareness of data experiences as being the embodied way in which every human must deal with data. My interest in data experiences began with the challenges associated with the second paradox that has been weaving through this chapter: data dematerialize and rematerialize interactions. I was studying ephemeral data infrastructures that I could not localize. My problems reflected the multiplicity of data: data were many things and in many places at the same time, as when a CPR number could at once be at the optician's, in an insurance agency, and in a bank—and simultaneously be used for very different things, such as record keeping, marketing, calculation of remuneration, and money transfers. While data dematerialize interactions and create connections between people who do not themselves know how they connect (or even that they are connected), data also rematerialize. They appear on computer screens—through material interfaces. Through such interfaces, people experience shame, joy, and pride—sometimes provoked by clumsy questions. Data have material effects. These wider and socially engrained experiences are *part of* the infrastructure, and when acknowledged as such, they are options for understanding important dimensions of what data do.

The points I have made here can be summarized as five lessons about data experiences: (1) data work generates emotions; (2) people learn from people, not just data; (3) people are not computers; (4) data experiences inform actions; and (5) the primary tool for understanding data experiences is self-experimentation. The fifth lesson suggests that both researchers and organizational actors should reflect on their own experiences to understand what data tools do in practice. Self-experimentation is the bridge to the other four. In our own reflections, there is no point in limiting what counts as data to that which can be processed by a computer. It is better to let computers do what they do well, and let human understanding draw on as broad a set of experiences as possible. We are our own primary research instruments. When we reflect upon our own reactions, without prejudice about what counts as good data, our understanding expands. Often, we become better at seeing even those around us who are clearly very different from us.

Awareness of data experiences also provides new avenues for exploring other abstract phenomena known only through data, such as population politics (Grommé and Ruppert 2020), climate change (Edwards 2010), and the COVID-19 pandemic (Caduff 2020). These phenomena all depend on data to emerge as political entities. Data also make them subject to experience. It is through experiential appropriation—*data experiences*—that datafied entities become subject to action. To know how and why some people react to datafied phenomena (such as a pandemic threat) as they do, it is unwise to ignore how they experience data and representations of data such as graphs, tables, and heat maps. When scholarly work and policy papers refer to data as only epistemic or governmental objects—as carriers of information with purpose rather than objects for emotional and bodily engagement—this reduces disagreements about these topics to questions of misunderstandings or "fake news." Contemporary political struggles, therefore, might find new paths out of the deadlock of "truth wars" if scholars are willing to explore the experiences through which disagreements emerge.

Computers are good at computing. Humans, however, possess a reflective capacity for thinking about *how* they know something. This capacity is central for making judgments. Many policymakers—and some computer scientists—nevertheless seem to wish that humans would be more like computers—that they would simply *compute*. Wisdom does not arise from data without judgment; however, and therefore, chapter 5 explores what it takes to exert judgment and use data *wisely*.

5 DATA WISDOM

May 2019: "We make trends in data visible," Torben says when I ask him what he does. Torben is a civil servant working at the national level figuring out how to use data to optimize clinical performance. He spends a good deal of his time facilitating informed debates among politicians on which areas of concern to prioritize. To do so, he works with finding ways of turning data into something visual, such as graphs, maps, or color-coded tables: "It's so that you can say, 'Oh, there was something interesting here. It's going down, and it's been going downwards for years. Why is it doing that? Why is this Region red?'"

A curve or a color coding inspires change, Torben says. He first mentions problematic areas, the "red" ones, as examples, but later he talks about using measurements to celebrate achievements and learn from best practice. All his examples revolve around learning through comparisons: over time, as curves are going up or down, or geographically and organizationally, through revelation of differences between Regions and Municipalities, or units. The graphic visualizations build on data from clinical reporting systems, administrative systems, or both. For Torben, the key point is that interventions should be "based on facts rather than opinion." Considering how I have shown throughout the preceding chapters that people in paradoxical ways produce very different facts with similar data, it is time to examine in more depth such claims about factuality. It is time to explore the relationship between data and wise decisions.

Torben wants to be clear about the nature of the governmental aim: the point is *not* to set standards derived from evidence-based medicine (EBM).

"What is the right level?" he asks rhetorically, "Really, often we don't know." The point is to set a *direction*. He mentions the use of physical force in psychiatry as an example. Everybody agrees that use of physical force should be avoided when treating psychiatric patients, but despite doctors' best efforts, force cannot be completely ruled out. There is no "right level," but less force is most preferred. The politicians, therefore, want data to document that the use of physical force in psychiatry really is going down.

In my interview with Torben, he speaks mostly about a form of quality monitoring called "National Goals" (Sundheds-og Ældreministeriet, KL, and Danske Regioner 2018). This has replaced earlier forms of quality assurance such as accreditation, which included experiments with standards from the American Joint Commission. The Danish Ministry of Health works with the ninety-eight municipalities and the five administrative Regions to compile data on performance according to eight overall goals, and the performance measurement in relation to each depends on hundreds of indicators, each drawing on multiple data sources.[1] Examples of some of the data representations can be found in figure 5.1. Currently, the monitoring mostly uses data already collected in the health services. Torben imagines a near-future, however, where the effect of the health services can be measured directly by measuring the well-being of patients: "Hopefully, sometime soon, data will be generated automatically, I mean, something like citizens wearing watches with in-built sensors." It sounds like a grand vision. Still, I have some nagging doubts, and they are not just related to privacy issues. I wonder: Is it really possible? How would data from wearables become useful for healthcare governance, remuneration models, and monitoring of the quality of service delivery?

Torben is not naive in any way. He knows how difficult it is to make sense of data. He provides several examples of inaccurate data analyses featured in the governmental report on National Goals. For example, it annoys Torben when comparisons between years are sometimes said to illustrate a trend even though they are made with indicators where the sources have changed the data formats during the period measured. A couple of weeks later, on Torben's recommendation, I am interviewing Flemming, who has constructed a number of the indicators for the National Goals measurements. Like Torben, he is aware of trends documented in National Goals that do not reflect the actual organizational performance. In some instances, Flemming remarks that this is just because clinicians have changed their

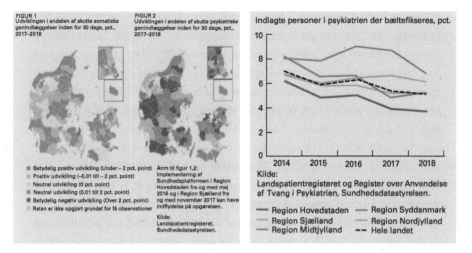

FIGURE 5.1
Examples of visualizations from National Goals, 2019. To the left there are two maps of Denmark where unplanned readmissions to hospitals for somatic (left) and psychiatric (right) disorders are indicated in different municipalities as degrees of positive and negative developments (percentages compared to the previous year). To the right there is an example of a graph that illustrates the number of persons who have been restrained with belts in psychiatric care over time and in the five administrative Regions (shaded lines) and the country as a whole (broken line). (Credit: The Danish Ministry of Health).

registration practices, akin to what I described in chapter 3 as "data massage" and "gaming." Also, Flemming explains, there are in some units significant data gaps and missing values, not least after the introduction of the Epic system described in chapter 3. He mentions how people at his section at one point realized that for a particular indicator, they had data on the same thing from three different sources showing three different results.[2] At least two of the data sources had to be wrong (and perhaps all three were), but they could not know which was most accurate. The central authorities decided to use data from just one of the sources, not because it was definitely right but because they needed to have just one value for the report. In short, the data visualizations in the report do not correspond in any straightforward way to a particular "reality" outside the data. They are not so "factual" after all.

I keep having this feeling that there is something I do not understand—that there is a link or an argument that I have missed. In the course of the interview with Flemming, I hear myself asking again and again in different ways: Do the numbers and visualizations in National Goals convey the performance that they are said to measure? Do they give an accurate impression of the quality of the service delivered by the respective units in each area? At one point, Flemming looks at me with the forbearing gaze of an indulgent father ready to explain the most elementary stuff a hundred times to a slightly dimwitted child. He takes a deep breath and then carefully explains that (1) the reports are no better than the data on which they are built; (2) it is not possible from these data to determine who reaches the "right level" of whatever they measure, whether it is use of force or unplanned readmissions (see figure 5.1); and (3) based on data of this type, one cannot conclude whether measured differences reflect the performance of the respective health services in those areas, divergent registration practices, or differences in background population. When Flemming mentions background populations, it is because the ninety-eight municipalities are composed of citizens with varying health profiles and socioeconomic backgrounds, as well as differing levels of exposure to environmental risks. Such variations—rather than the performance of the healthcare offered—could be the cause of any measured variation.

I already know this. What confuses me is why people working with the governance of the health services—who also know this—nevertheless insist on acting on data as if this uncertainty did not exist. Why do National Goals not draw on any of the established research methods for investigating the data and see whether it might be, for example, variances in the background population that give rise to differences? Case-mix is one such method for controlling for differences in background population.[3] Why suggest adding wearable data—something so complicated—when *existing* research standards are not being implemented? Why suggest massive data tracking on the well-being of all citizens when we already know that it will not reveal what the authorities need to know about organizational performance? Reflecting on the current practice with National Goals, Flemming admits that "from a strictly disciplinary perspective, these analyses make no sense. It's more like a political maneuver." Still, he maintains that they are useful. They help to create that sense of *direction* also highlighted by Torben. They are tools for governance, not research. Still, I keep asking: Is the epistemic difference between governance and research not supposed to relate to novelty rather than accuracy and validity? Flemming and Torben then both explain that

there are so many users of the data presented in the National Goal dashboards that it simply does not make sense to talk about what constitutes the
right, the accurate, the valid analysis. The different users want to know different things. I cannot help thinking: But is it *knowing*? What do they "know"
in this way?

Torben and Flemming point to an interesting paradox: data gain power
by appearing as tools of knowledge in a positivistic sense ("fact, not opinion"), and yet organizational actors find them useful even when fully aware
that these data are not especially representative of the world these actors
wish to govern. People readily admit that data can give rise to erroneous and
invalid claims, and yet they maintain that having no data, or too few data,
makes things even worse. Contemplation of this paradox, I suggest, adds
again to our understanding of data politics because it invites us to understand the appeal of data even when those data do not deliver the insights
that data promises announce.

The question of how data relate to knowledge has been running as an
undercurrent to the previous chapters. When do data give rise to knowledge? What type(s) of knowledge? What further types of knowledge might
the health services need when caring for patients? It is, however, difficult
to contemplate "knowledge": for consciousness to understand itself is like
asking a man or a woman to carry himself or herself. Ideas about what counts
as knowledge have thousands of years of philosophical baggage, and those
suitcases can hardly be lifted by a single chapter of a single book. Still, it is
also dangerous to avoid the topic altogether because data promises thrive
on fuzzy ideas about knowledge—a fuzziness that opens up a space for
powerful commercial and political actors. Remember how, in the introduction, I cited civil servants and industrial lobbyists who conflated data and
knowledge. When claims about data *as* knowledge become more and more
authoritative and aimed at control (Cheney-Lippold 2017; Poster 1990;
Zuboff 2019), it is time to discuss knowledge claims in a candid and direct
manner.

Nevertheless, I will go light on the classic epistemological canon. I am
avoiding established dichotomies such as idealism and realism, constructiv-
ism and positivism, as I have nothing much to add to those debates. By talking about data as *ontologically* multiple objects, I have already shifted the
focus from what data mean to what they do. As a consequence of integration and reuse, the same data are involved in very different practices,

engaged by different networks, and have effects in several different places. They have become like cogs operating in several machines at once. Still, it is too easy to simply replace the epistemic question about knowledge with an ontological claim about data being multiple, when data in all the various practices in which they operate continue to be thought of in an epistemic register. If I wish to claim that data do *not* equal knowledge, I must be able to say something about what *does* constitute knowledge—in what sense, for which purposes—in each of the many practices where data operate.

In this chapter, I am proposing the concept of data wisdom as a form of practical ability to use data well. The use of the term "well" begs consideration of the questions "Well for whom?" "Well according to which criteria?" Normativity is built into the ambition of knowing. The pragmatist John Dewey famously evaded what he called the "problem of truth" by focusing on what knowledge claims do for people in the pursuit of something. He spoke about how knowledge claims take the form of an "inquiry for it" (Dewey 1998). For Dewey, knowledge was always inherently normative and guided by aspirations. The anthropologist Fredrik Barth (2002) similarly emphasizes the link between understanding and motivated action and even defines knowledge as "what a person employs to interpret and act upon the world" (1).

Analyses always bring norms with them (Callon and Law 2005). With *data wisdom,* I wish to integrate the analysis of knowledge claims with the ability to think about whose interests they serve. It is necessary because the same data serve so many purposes. With additional data reuse comes an increased risk of misunderstanding what the data signified and were meant to do when they were first produced. With data reuse come new forms of data error. I long thought about calling this chapter "Data Error" rather than "Data Wisdom." This was because I was struck by the many obviously erroneous claims that are made with data. I became almost obsessed by error and compiled an archive full of examples. I even tried to categorize these examples into error types before I gradually realized how fruitless that was. There can be no exhaustive list of errors (Thylstryp 2021), not least because errors have as many dimensions as the people they affect. In the following discussion, I therefore cover examples of error without setting them up as if they could have had an imaginary twin of "Data Truth."

To reflect on how data can be used wisely, I first address the relationships among data, knowledge, and wisdom. I then reflect on data challenges in medical research and clinical practice before I turn to how new algorithmic inventions interfere with those established ideas about knowledge. After that, I consider citizen and patient experiences of data errors. My point is that to care for patients, both scholars and policymakers need to reflect on how to use data wisely, and I end the chapter on that note.

WISDOM: HOW TO USE DATA WELL

Data wisdom, as I suggest, is the ability to produce and apply "robust knowledge" with beneficial outcomes for those affected. It also implies consideration of how the reuse of data can interfere with several practices at once, thereby having both positive and negative implications for different people, or for the same people over time. Data wisdom means understanding both *how* and *when* to use data—and also when *not* to use them. In addition, it involves the willingness to consider what data do for those patients (and staff) who fit neatly into established norms, as well as those who deviate from them. In chapter 4, I highlighted the tension between endless human variation and data-imposed standardization. Prompted by my observations of people evading standards, I agree with the anthropologist Tim Ingold (2018) when he suggests thinking of wisdom as a willingness to embrace the unexpected: "Knowledge fixes and puts our minds at rest; wisdom unfixes and unsettles. Knowledge arms and controls; wisdom disarms and surrenders" (9). Data promises propagate the power of prediction, but healthcare systems must be able to care for those with unexpected problems as well. Unfortunately, as Ingold (2018) dryly observes: "At no previous time in history . . . has so much knowledge been married to so little wisdom" (10).

Knowledge, particularly the sort of knowledge that is generated with data, is increasingly treated as an asset that can be traded (Pinel 2021; Geiger and Gross 2019; Sadowski 2019a). Wisdom, in contrast, is a gift passed from generation to generation. It stems from processes of maturation. It is relational, created at the moment of gifting, not an object of barter. Wisdom is nurtured by strong institutions. In these institutions, wisdom is reinvented by each expert, but no expert can arrive at it by "mining" knowledge alone. It stems from socially sustained nurture and care. It takes wisdom to produce useful knowledge.

Kitchin (2014) suggests, in his acclaimed book *The Data Revolution*, that we should think of data as presenting aspects of the world that can be turned into information, which can then be used to produce knowledge that might (but only *might*) be used wisely. He uses a triangular figure to illustrate his point—building on similar figures from Ackoff and other esteemed scholars (see Beaulieu and Leonelli 2022: 60). Figure 5.2 shows an adaptation of Kitchin's version of the figure (though it leaves out "information" because this word is so often used interchangeably with both data and knowledge and therefore tends to create more confusion).

The figure is helpful because it reminds readers that not all aspects of the world can become data, not all data become knowledge, and not all knowledge is used wisely. However, I do have some reservations. It conveys an impression of higher levels being subsets of lower levels. In figure 5.2, all types of knowledge seem to build on data, and all wisdom seems to build on knowledge. I, conversely, think that there are types of knowledge needed in healthcare that do not derive from data. Furthermore, what might be right for one purpose can be wrong, or unsuitable, for another. The triangle also gives a temporally unidirectional impression—a path upward from world to data to knowledge to wisdom. This unidirectionality is also problematic. Leonelli (2012a) has reminded us that it takes knowledge to create good data, just as I suggest that it takes wisdom to create useful knowledge.

If I am complicating what counts as knowledge, why even use the word "knowledge"? Would it not be easier just to depart from this word altogether and simply focus on what people do with data and whether they like the results? It might, but I believe that it is important to hold on to "knowledge"—not only because policymakers insist on using this term, but

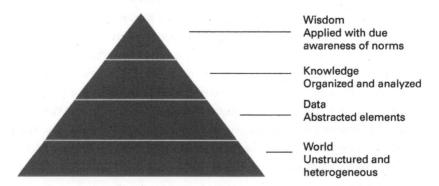

FIGURE 5.2
Data, knowledge, wisdom. Adaptation of the model of the path from world to wisdom presented by Kitchin, Ackoff, and others.

also because it speaks to something important and motivating for people, not least the ones working with data. Most of us have a phenomenological experience of knowledge as a moment of understanding something: the beauty, the contentment, and sometimes the dread and fear that arise when realizing something and comprehending a situation in a new way. I would like to keep an awareness of this experience of "getting to know" as part of our thinking about data. "Understanding," or "knowledge," is one of very few phenomena carrying intrinsic value. That places it in the company of, for example, "love" and "beauty." The sense of understanding can make a person feel at home in the world. To be without it can be disempowering (as described in chapter 2), lead to feelings of meaninglessness (as described in chapter 3), and evoke disorientation and exhaustion (as described in chapter 4). Its value is instantiated right at the moment of comprehension. It is a practice, not a thing. This experience lies at the heart of what many researchers love. When Weber (1947b) spoke of science as a vocation, he articulated such love. The word "philosophy" is derived the Greek words for "love" (*philo*) and "knowledge" (*sophia*), which also suggests a deep devotion to insight among the earliest scholars in Western history. Learning something new is also at the heart of debates about confidentiality (Grossman 1977; Fainzang 2002), and very important for the politics of data: who gets to know what about whom? For these reasons, I am not willing to give up on "knowledge."

Rather than abandoning knowledge, it is more useful to think about it as coming in many forms. I therefore wish to suggest a vocabulary that can foster reflections on the various types of knowledge already used in healthcare. As I shied away from the philosophical canon and contemplated how people *experience* knowledge, I was drawn to psychology and found a vocabulary in the work of the American pragmatist and psychologist William James. In his seminal book *Principles of Psychology*, which came to form a foundation for modern psychology, he approached "truth" as those beliefs that are useful for the believer (James 1950 [1890]). Not surprisingly, he here aligns with Dewey. But James did something more. He spoke of a human capacity for different types of knowledge. He conceived of these forms of knowing in a developmental and hierarchical way, but when the hierarchy is disregarded, elements of his thinking can be useful even today—at least if you accept twisting and tweaking it a bit.

James claimed that human babies, as with nonhuman animals, begin in pure *sensation*. Humans only gradually develop the ability of *perception*. Sensation is a bodily engagement with the world. The baby does not see light; it *is* light, as it were (James 1950 [1890]: 4). The world is sensed in its totality. Perception, in contrast, is a conceptually mediated experience of the world, where categories of thinking shape objects of experience and make light into an object that can be recorded (76ff). In growing up, James suggested, humans lose the ability of pure sensation, but not sensation altogether. What they retain comes across as something that James terms "associative thinking." Associative thinking is what happens when people sense a situation as a whole and compare it with previous experience. Associative thinking can imply an empathic understanding of the pain, anger, and fear that others feel, but it is first and foremost about drawing upon experience with "wholes"—similar situations—rather than delineated objects.

For me, associative thinking resonates with phenomena that others have spoken about as, for example, experience-based knowledge, bodily knowledge, and action skills (Zuboff 1989; Mauss 2007; Connerton 1989). I am grouping together vastly different traditions here, but my point is to say that a lot of work has identified bodily ways of knowing that do *not* stem from analysis of data and yet remain key to clinical work (Goodwin 2010; Gardner and Williams 2015; Moreira 2004; Friis 2021). These forms of knowledge shape what is known as clinical judgment, as well as the tactile skills needed for good clinical care. Experienced nurses do not analyze data when holding the suffering body of a patient, nor should they. Surgeons do not depend on analysis alone to become skilled. They draw on a range of tactile types of knowing. In her seminal work on the digitization of the workplace in the 1980s, Zuboff (1989) described tacit bodily knowledge as a form of "action skill" where hands "know" how to treat materials in ways that are not easily turned into data: "Some forms of meaning are comprehensible only as a whole and can be destroyed when objectified and analyzed," she observed (186). Even though I am perhaps a little "hard-handed" with the term "associative thinking"—adapting the term to suit my own purposes—I hope James would forgive me for borrowing it to describe a type of knowing that does not stem from analysis of parts, but rather from experience with similar wholes.

James maintained that to identify causal factors, there was a need for "reasoning" instead of associative thinking. Reasoning, he said, builds on perception rather than sensation. By taming perception, particular *aspects* of a situation are turned into data and related to other similar aspects of comparable situations. Each situation, however, remains unique (Verran 2021). Any situation can give rise to infinite aspects, including smell, visual impressions, humidity, and others. James (1950 [1890]) writes:

> Every reality has an infinity of aspects or properties. Even so simple a fact as a line which you trace in the air may be considered in respect to its form, its length, its distinction, and its location. When we reach more complex facts, the number of ways in which we may regard them is literally endless. Vermilion is not only a mercury-compound, it is vividly red, heavy, and expensive, it comes from China, and so on, *in infinitum*. All objects are well-springs of properties, which are only little by little developed to our knowledge, and it is truly said that to know one thing thoroughly would be to know the whole universe. (332; italics in original)

In order to reason on something, in James's sense of the word, it is necessary to choose an aspect of the unique and momentary whole and focus on that to build an abstract phenomenon. As a product of his time, James believed that women, children, and the uneducated classes were more disposed toward associative thinking, while well-educated men like himself were better at rational reasoning. This dichotomous hierarchy between these groups appears ludicrous today. For people working in the health services, the point is to find the right places for different types of knowledge.

James was writing at a time when respect for *numbers*—and the authority they represented—was mounting. Science was aspiring to fulfill a new role in society. His British contemporary, Lord Kelvin, famously asserted (just one year after James published *The Principles of Psychology*):

> I often say that when you can measure what you are speaking about and express it in numbers you know something about it; but when you cannot measure it, when you cannot express it in numbers, your knowledge is of a meagre and unsatisfactory kind: it may be the beginning of knowledge, but you have scarcely, in your thoughts, advanced to the stage of *science*, whatever the matter may be. (Thompson (Lord Kelvin) 1891: 73, italics in original)

It is a bold claim, "whatever the matter may be," but the strident and slightly pompous tone may reflect how Lord Kelvin, along with others, saw themselves as engaged in an important struggle. They were building secular alternatives to the authority associated with religion and class (Hecht 2003). Today, however, this valuation of "reasoning" and its association with numbers is no longer in *opposition* to regimes of power. It is integral to how modern organizations work.

The type of numbers that Lord Kelvin was longing for depends on data-fication, and this datafication involves categorization. Categorization has long occupied anthropology and science and technology studies (STS), but it was Immanuel Kant who several hundred years earlier had turned categories into central issues for modern philosophy. It was at the height of the Enlightenment period. He asserted that it is necessary to reflect on the relationship between one's categories of thought and the phenomena in the world which one is contemplating. In *Critique of Pure Reason*, Kant (2017 [1787]) stipulated that things cannot be perceived as they are, in and of themselves. He thereby thoroughly established how analytical knowledge (of the type that James would later relate to reasoning) must build on a reflec-tive engagement with the involved categories of thought. The world does not just magically turn into data. My critique of the unidirectional assumptions conveyed by the triangle in figure 5.2 stems from this long tradition of work demonstrating that data do not precede knowledge. As stated previously, the converse is true: it takes knowledge to create good data.

A reflective engagement with categories also is the basis for counting. Counting may sound simple. It is not. It takes thorough disciplinary training to learn to delineate objects of counting (Martin and Lynch 2009; Deville, Guggenheim, and Hrdlicková 2016). In laboratory science, counting also involves relatively practical tasks, such as how to document what happens in a test tube. Latour (2014) talks about this as "inscriptions" where aspects of the world are "flattened" and turned into "immutable mobiles." Inscrip-tions generate a form of flat ontology, where data regardless of provenance and type can be used in the same analysis (Stark 2018; Andrejevic, Hearn, and Kennedy 2015).

In her work on data practices, Borgman (2015) observes: "Every category, and name of category, is the result of decisions about criteria and naming. Even the most concrete metrics, such as temperature, height, and geo-spatial location, are human inventions" (26). Data wisdom involves investigating these inventions. It means looking *at* data and not only *with* or *through* data. In her important book about data-intensive research, *Data-Centric Biology*, the philosopher Sabina Leonelli (2016) similarly encourages

> philosophers, historians, and science scholars to take data seriously as research outputs and think of them not as inert objects with intrinsic representational powers but as entities who acquire evidential value through mobilization, and may undergo significant changes as they travel (198).

In a similar way, the data analyst and media scholar Yanni Loukissas (2019) urges practitioners and scholars to pay attention to data as objects of knowledge in their own right, not just as means for acquiring knowledge: "You must learn to look *at data*, to investigate how they are made and embedded in the world, before you can look *through data*" (xv–xvi; emphasis in original). For Loukissas, it involves investigating what data mean in local contexts: "Do not mistake availability of data as permission to remain at a distance" (196). Still, this is exactly how data are often used politically: to govern at a distance. Chapters 1 and 3 are full of examples of this phenomenon, and the international rankings discussed in chapter 2 often exhibit a similar lack of care for the local meaning of data.

To use data wisely, it is important to care about knowledge, but also to remain aware that data can be involved in several knowledge projects at once and have different implications in each. What appears to be a solution for one problem may carry the seeds of a new problem. Foucault (1997) once said: "My point is not that everything is bad, but that everything is dangerous, which is not exactly the same as bad" (231). I take this as an invitation to look into the interconnection between problems and solutions and to explore how "solutions" build on forms of knowing that are coproduced with specific forms of blindness or "unknowing" (Proctor 2008; Geissler 2013; Gross 2010; Michael 2015). It makes it possible to consider whether the most exciting forms of "new" knowledge might sometimes lie in recovering lost knowledge, a form of reknowing, where silenced voice are rearticulated (Hoeyer and Winthereik 2022). There is no perfect way to use data that works for all, but conversely, we should not think that no data or no attempt to generate knowledge would be a viable solution.

MEDICAL EVIDENCE AND CLINICAL JUDGMENT: TACTILE SKILL AND INFERENCE ERRORS

When, after World War II, Archie Cochrane and other founding figures of what later became known as evidence-based medicine (EBM) began developing new ways of testing the effect of treatments, they were also solving one problem while inadvertently sowing the seeds of the next. They wanted statistical treatment of data to take precedence over clinical experience, or—in James's terms—to let perception and reasoning replace sensation and associative thinking. EBM continues to be a "malleable range of techniques and practices" (Ecks 2008: 2639) and its exact definition remains subject to contestation (Kemm 2006; Stegenga 2018). Still, it is fair to say that EBM seeks to isolate aspects of complex wholes to determine their "independent" effect, and also that this approach has been central for the development of regulatory efforts aimed at ensuring the safety and efficacy of pharmaceutical treatments (Daemmrich 2004; Faulkner 2009).

A key feature of EBM has been the randomized clinical trial (RCT) (Bohlin 2011; Lambert 2006) and development of evaluation standards such as the GRADE (Grading of Assessment, Recommendations, Development, and Evaluations) guidelines. As the RCT seeks to isolate effects, it necessitates limiting the factors that can influence the result. Herein lies the potential for what I would call "inference errors": trials are based on narrow groups, and inferences are made about a lot of other people who have not been studied (Langstrup and Winthereik 2010; Kaufman 2015; Stegenga 2018). Drug testing is carried out on particular groups, typically white adult men, so the results from the trial might not be representative for people of color, women, and children (Epstein 2007). As Armstrong (2007) observes, EBM cannot erase uncertainty. Still, the use of drugs without any testing is not particularly appealing either. In short, RCTs can give rise to error as a result of the simplifications built into the method, but it can be worse for patients if the alternative is no testing of drugs at all. To mitigate inference error, medical researchers typically request more data. If this is how medical research typically works, at least ideally, then how do the probabilities of medical science translate into clinical practice?

What might be true on average—for the population—might not be true for the individual (Henderson and Keiding 2005). EBM is a study of the generalized body, but a generalized body is a data invention. In real life, all bodies vary on an infinite number of parameters, like James's line in the air. Epidemiologists talk about an "ecological fallacy" when doctors mistake knowledge about generalized bodies with predictions for individuals (Piantadosi, Byar, and Green 1988). Nevertheless, clinicians must treat individuals, not "generalized bodies." They must find ways to translate EBM into practice. How do they do that? Clinicians employ a range of strategies, and data play a role in many—but not all—of them. I even wish to make a daring suggestion: clinicians sometimes use forms of associative thinking when trying to fit EBM guidelines to individual patients.

I first came to think about this as I interviewed Lars, a very experienced anesthesiology nurse also mentioned in chapter 4. When I asked Lars about his data needs in clinical care, he responded in this way:

Lars: Most of the data I get stems from the moment I walk up to the patient and do this [*he grabbed my hand, gave me a firm handshake, and looked me right in the eye*]

Klaus [*affected by the handshake and the intensity of the gaze*]: A firm handshake?

Lars: A firm handshake, yes, but more than that . . . how is the physiological tone [*Da: tonus*], is he warm, dry, cold, humid, and what kind of contact do I get? Physically as well as intellectually. I've worked with this for so many years, so I have learned to take in so many data in that moment.

Klaus: Do these data have any clinical implications?

Lars: Definitely! Absolutely! And I really make a point of this when I am teaching younger nurses . . . but I don't write it down. It just contributes to my *sense of the situation as a whole* [*Da: helhedsfornemmelse*, my emphasis]: what needs to be done in this specific case.

He later explained that although he was calling it "data" here, he did not regard this information as "real" data. To become that, his impressions would have to be entered into the electronic record, which he would not do. Lars tries to teach young nurses how the state of the patient—including fear and exhaustion—affects the metabolism, and it is necessary to adjust the dose of the anesthetic accordingly. He thereby seems to combine sensation with reasoning, if we use James's terms as I have suggested.

Lars in this way points to a fundamental clinical skill: the ability to "read" a patient's body. This is what I wanted to capture with my use of James's term "associative thinking"—the ability to draw on experience with other persons ("I've worked with this for so many years"). Lars uses a wide range of impressions, and with the handshake he actively engages his own body in collecting them (Gardner and Williams 2015; Goodwin 2010). In recent years, it has become common for older doctors and nurses to complain about the younger generation having lost the "clinical gaze" (Olesen 2018). A loss of clinical competence is also widely criticized in the international literature, which, in chapter 3, I discussed in relation to the datafication of clinical work (Nettleton, Burrows, and Watt 2008; Adams 2016a; Hunt, Bell, Baker, and Howard 2017; Hutchinson, Nayiga, Nabirye et al. 2018; Prainsack 2017; Taylor-Alexander 2016). Perhaps more emphasis on associative thinking in clinical training, in line with Lars's approach, could address the problem and reintroduce the ability to read patients' bodies.

All the same, clinical work today *also* does involve reading data. With increased outpatient monitoring, many clinicians spend several days a week in office buildings looking at data rather than patients (Torenholt, Saltbæk, and Langstrup 2020). Clinical work depends on both associative thinking and data skills. Looking only at data is dangerous, but in a data-intensive healthcare system, the clinicians who cannot look at data at all are just as alarming. It can be incredibly difficult to make sense of data in clinical work. Thanks to the highly integrated data infrastructures, Danish clinicians have access to an abundance of data, but they often struggle to find and discern data, even on relatively simple matters.

Several clinicians have told me about their challenges. Take cholesterol levels, for example. It is not just difficult to find all the necessary measurements in a patient history: just figuring out where to look can be a challenge. Even when clinicians do know where to find all the relevant test results, reporting standards can change. Historically, some laboratories have reported cholesterol levels as above or below a threshold, and in these cases, clinicians must remember that clinical guidelines have changed over time. This could mean that although a value might first appear as "green" and later as "red," the patient might have had the same value throughout (Green, Carusi, and Hoeyer 2022). A medication's coding number also can change, and some patients buy medicine abroad, whereby it is not registered in the Danish databases (Frandsen 2019). How would the physician know about this? There are also plain data gaps, such as the ones from The Health Platform described in chapter 3.

In short, even with the best intentions, and even in relation to simple issues such cholesterol levels and prescriptions, it can be difficult for clinicians to find the answers they require just by having access to data. Giving clinicians access to more data on their patients is not the same as giving them more knowledge—and certainly not the same as training them to use data wisely. Conversely, denying clinicians access to data is not very helpful either.

ALGORITHMS, MACHINE LEARNING, AND AI: AUTOMATION AND PREEMPTION ERRORS

As it is time- and labor-consuming to produce valid claims with data, it is not surprising that many people hope to find a digital shortcut through computer automation. What do terms such as "algorithm," "machine learning," and "artificial intelligence (AI)" mean? In policy documents (Regeringen, Finansministeriet, Erhvervsministeriet 2019; Digital Vækstpanel 2017), they are often used interchangeably. For computer scientists, conversely, they can connote a range of significantly dissimilar approaches. There is no agreement on exact definitions, but for those doing the programming, there are profound differences between, for example, an algorithm treating data in specified ways and forms of machine learning where computers search for patterns in unstructured data. Alan Turing defined a classic measure of AI—namely, that humans experience an interaction with the computer as no different from an interaction with a person, what has become known as the Turing test. In principle, this definition of AI could both cover simple algorithmic chatbots and advanced machine learning products—at least if the test person interacting with the computer is gullible enough. Here, I will not seek to settle definitions. Instead, I wonder: how do such technologies of automation affect the points I have made about data, knowledge, and wisdom?

The simpler algorithms typically depend on established theory building (or, as it is often called, "model building") and validation of the categories in use. Some uses of machine learning, in contrast, depart from this type of analytical engagement with category formation and theory building. There are epidemiologists doing both types of research, but they typically remain engaged in a particular topic or area of health. Some data scientists, conversely, move relatively freely among subject areas and search for patterns in data without necessarily knowing existing theories of pathology, causation, and effect—and in some cases without caring about known validity problems with the data sources (if they subscribe to the belief that with enough data, bias and validity become irrelevant). In these cases, everything that Kant cared so much about and many of the methodological refinements from decades of medical research seem to be dissolving. Gone are careful conceptual reflections; what is left is a fascination with computational power attuned to pattern recognition. It was the perceived power of pattern recognition that led the editor of *Wired*, Chris Anderson (2008), to famously declare, in an article titled "The End of Theory": "Forget taxonomy, ontology, and psychology. Who knows why people do what they do? The point is they do it, and we can track and measure it with unprecedented fidelity. With enough data, the numbers speak for themselves" (2).

Researchers have challenged his assertion endlessly, but it is fair to say that Anderson did not propose it in a piece of serious research. Still, it continues to inspire developments associated with automated data processing. Whereas classic epidemiology tried to build models and make carefully balanced assessments to avoid jumping from mere correlation to assumptions about causation (Hill 1965; Rothman and Greenland 2005), the new, data-intensive technologies challenge these ideas about how to exert judgment. A review has shown that it is now increasingly common in the medical literature to present a mere association as a prediction (Varga, Bu, Dissing et al. 2020). Furthermore, some of the new technologies in effect black-box some of the steps of the analysis (Fedak, Bernal, Capshaw, and Gross 2015). Black-boxing can be augmented through a division of labor whereby programming is outsourced or delegated to others who do not discuss their choices with those knowing the substance area (Anthony 2021).

The potentials associated with algorithmic prediction and rapidly expanding computer power are at the heart of the powerful data promises with which I opened this book (Krumholz 2014), though they are, of course, also much older than the recent Silicon Valley iterations (Greene and Lea 2019). It is likely that some readers would have expected the whole book to be primarily about how machine learning is disrupting clinical practices. However, I have consciously downplayed the grand claims about doctors being replaced by Google's DeepMind or IBM Watson. In the clinic, data intensification mostly comes about as a continuation of existing regimes, incrementally transforming, first, clinical work, and second, what counts as evidence (Gjødsbøll, Winkel, and Bundgaard 2019; Torenholt and Langstrup 2021).

In a few cases, though, machine learning has changed clinical practice. A Danish example is an algorithm that was trained on recordings from Danish emergency call centers to identify signs of heart failure. It is now used as decision-support software to alert health professionals about the risk of heart failure while they are taking calls (Blomberg, Folke, Kjær Ersbøll et al. 2019). Computer scientists cannot say what the algorithm identifies, but they can prove a high predictive value, and it is claimed to help the human operators. Such tools are sometimes embedded within decision-support software and can potentially help raise awareness of rare diseases and broaden the scope of clinical thinking (Wachter 2017). In Denmark, some radiologists use automated image analysis as a backup to alert them of potential pathologies (Friis 2020), and since 2021, some hospitals have replaced one of two radiologists looking at each mammography image with AI (Albinus 2021). These applications depend on thorough data cleaning and years of development—they have not magically popped out of a computer. Still, they do represent important innovations, and it is fair to expect other similar innovations to gradually bring about important changes in healthcare.

Sometimes machine learning can help generate new hypotheses that can be tested with classic means for building evidence. Machine learning has, for example, been used to suggest potential changes to antibiotics to help counter antimicrobial resistance (König, Sokkar, Pryk et al. 2021). The exact value of these findings can then be determined in more classic laboratory experiments or RCTs. Still, we are *not* witnessing a healthcare system where digital monitoring of all citizens using wearables are about to facilitate automated administration of prevention and treatment as well as automated remuneration schemes, as Torben suggested.

Novelty goes hand in hand with continuity. While the current appetite for data and automation feeds on the eschatological sense of being on the brink of a new era, I think that this appetite gains voracity from the well-established culture of metrics that already has such a strong grip on medicine and healthcare organizations. As Lord Kelvin's blunt assertion about the ability to measure as a prerequisite for knowing has become how many policymakers and clinicians think (Mau 2019), investments come to focus on making data available. These investments are informed by old, but persistent, dreams of having access to all information in all places at all times (Poster 1990). Today, these dreams circulate in Silicon Valley (Wiener 2020), as exemplified by the quotation from Domingos in chapter 1 (Domingos 2015), but they can be traced right back to Laplace in early-nineteenth-century France (Busch 2017), Lovelace and Babbage as they invented the first "computer" in nineteenth-century Britain (Plant 1998), and Tesla's and Well's early-twentieth-century hopes for a "World Brain" of all available information (Wells 1938).

The thought of having all available information at hand permeates the open data movement that is seeking to make public data sources accessible in a machine-readable format, the work with the European Health Data Space, and the so-called FAIR data policies that seek to make research data "Findable, Accessible, Interoperable, and Reusable" (Jirotka, Lee, and Olson 2013). FAIR in reality means making it possible for *computers* to read the data! Open data policies downplay the problems that persist in finding the *right* data and *interpreting* what they mean (Denis and Goëta 2017; Gregory 2020; Gregory, Groth, Scharnhorst, and Wyatt 2020; Wyatt 2017). The trouble that a clinical doctor experiences when looking for information about a patient's cholesterol levels could be a useful reminder to proponents of open data about the difference between having *access* to data and being able to *find* what you need and *understanding* what you find.

Many proponents of open data also ignore the previous concerns about categorization. With pattern recognition, data are about whatever the analyst aims to predict. Every type of data can be health data if somebody can find a correlation with a health outcome (Schneble, Elger, and Shaw 2020). If a person's electricity use can be associated with heart attacks, then electricity data are also health data. Also the caution related to categorization and statistical probability, which I referred to as "ecological fallacy," is evaporating, and big data scholars matter-of-factly talk about predictions that operate at the "single-patient level" (Jørgensen and Brunak 2021, 7). In the pursuit of data for the old positivist dream, the very conception of knowledge is thereby tacitly reconfigured.

When Auguste Comte (1988 [1830–1842]) announced the birth of a positivist sociology in the middle of the nineteenth century, he proposed a clear distinction between premodern magical thinking and a new type of science to come. He was confident that through "reasoning and observation," it would be possible to arrive at "the actual laws of phenomena" (2). Does machine learning finally deliver on that ambition, then? Do open data finally generate a digital "world brain." I do not think so. In contrast to Comte, Claude Lévi-Strauss (1966 [1962]: 13) suggested that rather than "contrasting magic and science," it is better "to compare them as two parallel modes of acquiring knowledge." He pointed out that the "great arts of civilization—of pottery, weaving, agriculture and the domestication of animals" (13) could not be seen as "chance discoveries" (14); rather, they were the result of a determined search for meaning. Unlike in the trained scientific experiment, magical thinking takes everything available and tries it out until the solution is found. It is a dedicated process. The same may well apply to big data enthusiasts. They construct trials without the dogma of established science. It is a material form of magical thinking, working with whatever is available in a computer-readable format. If driven by genuine curiosity (and combined with other modes of knowing), there is no doubt that this explorative approach can generate brilliant new ideas. It is, however, not a path to establishing "the actual laws of phenomena" in a positivist sense.

There is something striking about comparing Neolithic pottery making with the brute usage of ontologically flat data in contemporary computer science. Besides seeing data science as a meaning-making practice like any other human endeavor dependent on experience, skill, and imaginative capability (Franklin 2006), the comparison is compelling because it points to the way that certain uses of big data methodologies can be seen as "bracketing" scientific theory building. It also suggests that it is not necessarily (or not always) a bad idea: important innovation can arise from brute experiments. Still, the "savage mind" described by Lévi-Strauss would not limit itself to what a computer can process. The Neolithic pottery maker would take in all aspects of the world and work by analogies and comparisons, again akin to James's associative thinking. She would insist on meaning. Indeed, the clever data scientists who produce the major breakthroughs in big data research probably do use associative thinking, bodily experience, and imaginative power. Perhaps greater awareness of this experimental "pottery mode" also could serve as an inspiration for computer scientists and big data proponents to broaden their argumentative style and repertoire when translating their findings to worlds inhabited by people.

Humans remain problematic to work with. They vary a lot. They are not consistent. They harbor prejudices. In a popular book about diagnostic uncertainty, Steven Hatch (2016) even calls his fellow physicians "error machines" (30). When humans rate each other, the rating often says as much about the rater as the rated (Scullen and Mount 2000). Deloitte also saw this in their own organization in relation to performance measurement: scores said more about the managers doing the scoring than the employees who were scored (Buckingham and Goodall 2015). Prejudice can generate a human form of what I call *preemption error*, where people preempt their own chances of realizing they were wrong because their decisions become self-affirmatory. A famous example is a group of research participants who had claimed to be mentally ill just to test the reliability of psychiatric assessment. Once inside the walls of the psychiatric institution, they could not convince the doctors that they had only faked their illness and should be allowed to leave the ward (Rosenhan 1973). Once a person was labeled as ill, this preempted reassessment.

It is in many ways justified, therefore, when many policymakers look for solutions to the persistent challenges with human prejudice, lack of consistency, and inattention (Kahneman and Klein 2009). With new solutions, however, come also new sources of error. Algorithms can also carry prejudice, and they also involve the risk of preemption error. They may replicate societal prejudices engrained in datasets and perpetuate racism, sexism, and other injustices (Lee and Larsen 2019; O'Neil 2016; Achiumi 2020). They are no better than the data on which they are trained (Jaton 2017, 2020). When implemented in healthcare, Henriksen and Bechmann (2020) suggest that AI "may prompt a world that is fit to algorithms rather than a world to which algorithms are fit" (813). To make patients fit into the algorithmic tools offered to clinicians, medical decision-making risks becoming "a matter of classification rather than judgment of individual cases" (Peeters and Schuilenburg 2021: 2). The clinical work becomes a matter of fitting patients to risk scores, and then algorithmic scoring tools determine which measures patients are offered (Amelang and Bauer 2019; Holmberg, Bischof, and Bauer 2013). Algorithms then preempt judgment.

Faced with digital interfaces, patients and staff cannot argue their case: "Algorithms do not argue. They present an outcome without an argument or reasoning. They present a truth without revealing sources or assumptions" (Schuilenburg and Peeters 2021: 198). With automation, therefore, the key point is to figure out whether reality has a chance of kicking back: do automated decision-making practices preempt the chance of realizing that the assumptions built into the system were wrong? Computers cannot get an epiphany or suddenly feel concern. It is therefore important to ensure that their applications are designed so that somebody can detect potential errors. This caution is missing when some Danish municipalities want to use big data to assess, for example, "parental preparedness" (Mortensen 2018). Predictions of this type risk becoming "self-fulfilling prophesies" (Merton 1968), with very important implications for those who are algorithmically assessed, as suggested by Mertens, King, van Putten, and Boenink (2021).

When algorithmic decisions preempt the discovery of mistakes, it can turn the paradox around: it can be dangerous without data, but it gets worse when decisions are made based solely on data. Automation, therefore, does not replace human folly with science; rather, it produces different sources of error in need of other tools of correction. In some cases, keeping "a human in the loop" can be source of error because of human inconsistency and prejudice, and yet in other cases a human in the loop will be the only way to detect error. Data wisdom therefore involves ensuring that different types of knowledge can complement each other and mitigate the risks involved (van der Niet and Bleakley 2020).

There is an ontological dimension of this argument that is rarely appreciated. AI builds on a unidimensional perception of phenomena—a flat ontology. Machines treat data as representative of wholes—a representational view. Data, however, represent only one dimension of situations and practices with many dimensions. When AI researchers such as Max Tegmark warns against a super-intelligent Master Algorithm that could potentially conquer the world (see chapter 1), he speaks of networks of machines optimizing everything toward a particular goal, such as economic value (Tegmark 2017). If powerful enough, such a network will dominate all other values thanks to its superior calculative ability. Associative thinking carries a form of intelligence that differs from calculation: because humans can experientially engage wholes rather than merely calculating datafied aspects of those wholes, they can balance different types of values against each other. This is a key reason for continuous training of associative thinking in clinical practice. Although human judgment often appears inconsistent, this inconsistency might partly reflect a key ontological resource for overcoming the preemption errors of automation: the ability to appreciate how every situation involves an infinite set of dimensions and a need to weigh them differently over time.

CITIZENS AND PATIENTS: EXPERIENCING DATA AND CODING ERRORS

How do citizens and patients experience the types of knowledge, and errors, that datafication produces? When posing this question, it is important to note first that for many patients, integrated data infrastructures do exactly what they are built to do: patients can expect healthcare professionals to have access to the information they need in order to deliver high-quality treatments. Still, as datafication implies that healthcare professionals communicate increasingly through codes, the potential for coding error—along with the failure to *decode*—perseveres. Coding errors can be when people like Steen are declared dead in the computer system even though he is very much alive (as I described in chapter 2). In most cases, however, the veracity (and falsity) of data cannot be as easily ascertained. Doctors and patients sometimes disagree about diagnoses; and general practitioners (GPs) have told me how some patients oppose simple diagnostic labels because the corresponding codes poorly represent complex social and medical problems. Again, data can never fully capture the multidimensionality of individual experience (Middleton 2022).

Here, I wish to focus on types of coding error that are generated specifically by data *reuse*. They are particularly relevant for intensified data sourcing because they stem from actors wanting more data while disagreeing about how they should be used. A telling example came about when in 2016, Søren Brostrøm, the director for the Danish Health Authority, stated matter-of-factly in an interview that psychiatric diagnostic codes were no longer medically valid among the young (Rasmussen 2016). His point was that municipalities (and with them, schools) had begun demanding a diagnostic code, such as the one used for depression or attention deficit hyperactivity disorder (ADHD), before they would provide special pedagogical support to children. It had put pressure on GPs and psychiatrists to provide diagnoses and thereby help families to get extra resources for the child. The diagnostic labels were stretched, as it were.

It turns out, however, that what a doctor does to help a ten-year-old can have unintended consequences when the child reaches adulthood. When people apply for a driver's license, for example, the Danish Patient Safety Authority checks with the registries. Just as Lone was surprised to find her driver's license cancelled when she had not reported her diabetes measurements (see chapter 2), there has been an increase in young people who have to wait for months to get a license, simply because the registries contain old diagnostic codes that trigger a warning of having the would-be drivers' psychological reliability assessed (Guerdali and Nielsen 2018). Similarly, from 2009 to 2017, Danish military authorities noted an increase of 72 percent of young men under nineteen years old who were not allowed to join the military because of psychiatric diagnostic codes acquired during childhood (Forsvaret 2018). Data that open doors to pedagogical support in childhood can in this way close other doors later in life. A diagnostic code is not necessarily right or wrong—but it can do things for persons that over time feel right or wrong.

Diagnostic codes can raise even more kaleidoscopic questions about veracity and error. Next, I will recount in some detail the story of a young man, Sebastian, to illustrate how coding errors become a lens through which a patient must experience subsequent encounters with healthcare. In his case, it was a psychiatric diagnosis that caused him problems. Sebastian was referred to me by a colleague who knew about my interest in data. I met him in my colleague's apartment in a town a few hours' drive from the capital. It was a warm and sunny afternoon, and the three of us first sat outside getting to know each other. After a while, Sebastian and I moved inside and logged on to his electronic health record through the online portal *sundhed.dk*. During the next couple of hours, he used the data on the screen as prompts to tell his story. We both struggled to understand the data, where they came from, and what they meant. For him, however, it was more than a puzzle. He has to live in the shadows of these data as they convey a story that he cannot control.

Sebastian grew up in a family where things had not always been easy: "I guess I didn't have the best childhood. It could have been better, well yes, but it's what lots of people experience." A troubled childhood in a small town was, he assumed, part of the reason why he, as a very young man, reacted strongly to getting type 1 diabetes. He was out of balance. At the time, he was also accused of a crime that he himself found hideous, and though later acquitted, he found it very challenging to see his name in the local news in relation to this case. He felt isolated and ostracized, and he thought that he really needed to talk to someone, preferably a psychologist. At that time in Denmark, however, people had to pay psychologists out of their own pocket, and Sebastian could not afford that. Psychiatry, conversely, was tax-financed, but when psychiatrists take on a patient, they usually need a diagnosis.[4] It is built into the remuneration system. Sebastian explains it like this:

> I ended up in the psychiatric system because that is where you are sent if you can't afford a psychologist. Psychiatry is the answer from the public system, when you ask for help. In the course of this treatment, they added this diagnosis, paranoid schizophrenia, or first "schizophrenia," and then later "paranoid" was added.

He could still have had the diagnosis even today had he not later been reassessed by the psychiatric system. The doctors wondered how he had acquired the previous diagnosis and declared it an "error." Paranoid schizophrenia is not something that comes and goes. He seemed to have been misdiagnosed, he was told.

Sebastian wanted to delete this code. However, from a system perspective, data are never supposed to be deleted. It is only possible to add corrections. Deletion would open up the possibility of covering up malpractice, so the system is carefully designed to retain everything. Data are multiple in this sense as well: data might be erroneous as diagnostic statements and still true as statements about what doctors have entered into the record in the course of treatment.

Looking at Sebastian's file on the online portal for health records, I could see how his insulin and other medications came in as "health record notes" [*Da; journalnotat*] under the diagnosis "paranoid schizophrenia." It kept moving this particular diagnosis to the top of the list of what you would see when looking at his records. Algorithmic ordering is supposed to help create a relevant overview, but here, it had come to misrepresent his pharmaceutical and medical history. He was worried about the implications for how health professionals would view him if they thought he was a paranoid schizophrenic.

> You can't help wondering whether it affects how people view you . . . For example, last year, I broke my wrist, and as I enter the emergency room I get this impression—I can't be sure that it's true—but the doctor [after having viewed the record] dismisses my case. The way I was treated, there was something, I couldn't work it out at the time, but it was as if I wasn't being treated objectively. . . . And there was this nurse, she was really rude. . . . I tried to get an X-ray, but the doctors just said [the wrist] wasn't broken and I was sent home. . . . It turned out it was broken, in two places actually, and it is a little annoying if they were somehow colored by the [psychiatric] diagnosis.

Sebastian does not know whether the health professionals were biased on account of the obsolete psychiatric diagnosis. He also admits that he is not even certain that the health professionals in question saw the diagnostic label. He did not see their screen. Still, he cannot help wondering whether they might have seen him through the lens of that label. It illustrates how coding errors are not limited to the pieces of information they pass on—whether correct or false. The errors also operate through the interpretations people make—and those that they in turn think other people make.

After spending the afternoon with Sebastian, I tried for a couple of months to figure out what had happened on the technical side: why were insulin prescriptions featured under a psychiatric code so that the code kept moving up to the top of his record? I called several people whom I had interviewed on other occasions or knew as experts. Sebastian had already asked multiple doctors who did not know what to do, and now the experts did not know either. With intensified data sourcing come very complex forms of integration, which make it increasingly difficult to find a responsible human being capable of mitigation. In the end, the hospital that entered the original diagnostic code figured out how to close the erroneous health record. It had taken years for Sebastian to achieve this outcome. He had acquired a data label that haunted him, and for which nobody felt responsible.

Sebastian could see his own data online because of a political commitment to patient empowerment. Online patient access to data also constitutes a form of data reuse—another purpose with data. Still, access is not always empowering. Patients have online access to all the specialized medical data serving to document their hospital trajectories and use of laboratory services. If we define it as a coding (or decoding) error when patients who are given access to data do not understand what they see, then there are certainly many coding and decoding errors as a result of the Danish system that gives immediate online access to laboratory results and health records. Even with my background, I have felt worried, confused, and in need of help when I have looked up my own laboratory results, brain scans, and other examination data. There used to be a time delay placed on cancer results to avoid worry and confusion, but this delay has been removed.

To learn more about this, I interviewed Jenny, a civil servant who had been working on the task of removing the time delay. At the time I interviewed her, however, she had also experienced seeing her own cancer diagnosis on a test result from a pathology laboratory. She thereby came to tell me the story from the perspective of a patient, not a civil servant. She told me how she began trembling as she looked at *sundhed.dk*:

> I could see it was a very long test result, masses of text. That was the first thing that struck me, "there's a lot here, that's not good." And then I read "malignant" and I thought, "Is that good or bad, is that good or bad, is that good or bad?" . . . and then I thought "Shit, I've got cancer. I've got cancer" . . . I started trembling all over.

Jenny explained how she found it provocative to think back on the small disclaimer she had had to click before accessing the results, which informed her that she might prefer to see a doctor before reading them: "What the f . . . is that? Such political cover-my-ass bullshit. . . . Of course, it won't stop me when I'm already logged on to *sundhed.dk*. (. . .). This is not protecting my interests."

Even a well-educated, competent woman with a great deal of knowledge about this area—and who, moreover, used to be inside the system—ended up feeling anxious when finding herself in the patient position. She emphasized that for data to make sense, they must be exchanged among people who understand what they mean. Today, however, data are not just conveyers of knowledge. They do many different things for different people and what they do can shift over time.

A different type of error comes about when some people use integrated data infrastructures to access information they should not see. Two interviewees have told me that on average, six health professionals are caught every year peeping into the medical records of lovers, ex-lovers, or others. In a few cases, medical secretaries have complained about their employer having looked at their data, as their labor union informed me. Patients can also be pressured into sharing their data once they have access. GPs have told me about young women who are forced by family members to share access to their medical records (which is used, for example, by parents to look into their daughters' means of contraception), and insurance companies that ask their client for a full printout instead of paying the physician for a statement, whereby the company also gains access to irrelevant—and private— pieces of information.

The authorities have tried to counter these pressures by offering citizens the opportunity of hiding data from view, including self-viewing, through something they call "privacy marking." It generates new sources of potential error when access to data might be selected in ways that the viewer does not realize. Conversely, patients have also used the log system on *sundhed.dk* to identify and threaten the doctors who have treated them. In a particularly tragic case in 2019, a doctor was killed by a former patient. The police found a printout from *sundhed.dk* where the patient had used the log to identify the doctor and six other health professionals involved in this patient's treatment (Dalsgaard 2019). The murder has generated anxiety, and some health professionals have mobilized to ensure their anonymity so they are featured only with numbers on the online portal and cannot be identified by patients (Clante and Allerslev Eriksen 2021). Such as solution, however, would make it difficult for patients to see whether somebody they know have peeped into their record. More commonly, of course, patients simply complain about elements in their health records that they dislike. This has caused doctors to change their documentation practices, omitting information or writing it in ways that they believe patients will not understand (Kristensen, Brodersen, and Jønsson 2022)—something that was also observed in Sweden when their health records went online (Petersson 2019; Petersson and Backman 2021). Viewed from a doctor's perspective, patients thereby instigate coding errors.

DATA ERROR REVISITED: QUALITY, MISCALCULATION, AND DEEPFAKE

The examples of "errors" presented in this chapter do not constitute an exhaustive list. As stated at the outset of this chapter, I do not think it is possible to produce such a list. Unintended errors can arise in relation to each of the four types of data work (production, analysis, instruction, and use), and for each of the four groups of purposes (research, clinic, governance, and industry). Errors are not just epistemological. They can happen simultaneously in several dimensions, as it were, affecting different aspects of people's lives, interacting with different interests and ambitions. Again, this is why I say that data are ontologically multiple—they are part of several practices at once.

There is a lot to learn from errors. I have highlighted inference error, preemption error, and coding error as types in need of more attention in organizations eager to become "data-driven," but these terms only add to the existing literature. They are not meant to stand alone. In the literature, there already are well-developed vocabularies for many other types of error, including types of missing data (Hand 2020) and types of error occurring when data are used for governance (Wadmann, Johansen, Lind et al. 2013), or what I have called data-work-of-instruction.[5] There are also terms for data quality and methods for assessing it,[6] and for data cleaning and curation (Plantin 2019; Gabrielsen 2020). Despite all of these well-established insights and their associated terminology, Deloitte and other consultancies insist on a simplifying positivist vocabulary about "data and knowledge about what works," without any serious acknowledgment of what it takes to produce knowledge out of data and how often error occurs. The European Union data strategy papers, the open data movement, and the Silicon Valley "gospel" make practically no mention of existing research into data errors and how to mitigate them. What is in fact so striking, so utterly fascinating, but also scary is the way in which the powerful data promises announcing a new era of data-driven healthcare have swept away old concerns about data error.

I have participated in numerous committee meetings where computer scientists and industry representatives have argued for their need for direct and unmediated access to Danish registries, and where they have not even been aware that most registries have documents describing how variables have changed over time. Although they thereby reveal themselves to be unaware of the simplest ways to detect and avoid a principal type of data error, they maintain that they only need *easy access* to data. Trained epidemiologists, conversely, maintain that often it is not even enough to read the documented coding histories stored with the registries. For instance, Schmidt, Schmidt, Sandegaard, and colleagues (2015) suggest discussing coding practices with clinicians before using new data derived from the clinic. In one article guiding newcomers to registry-based research, they write, "Before engaging in extensive retrieval and analysis of data, it is . . . important to consult clinicians from the relevant specialty to learn about current and previous coding practices" (462).

To consult with clinicians also can be considered a way of drawing on the resources associated with associative thinking and ontological multiplicity: it involves learning from the practices where clinicians code amid many values and interests. While many epidemiologists (including some of those who would also call themselves data scientists) continue to adhere to these norms, the effect of data promises has been that it has become legitimate in some communities of practice to sidestep this old care for understanding the data well.

Besides the mostly unintended errors that I have described, there are of course also *intentional* errors of various kinds. As I stated in chapter 1, some people want access to data to cover up, distort, manipulate, control, or misrepresent phenomena to suit their interests. Sometimes it can be difficult to tell the difference between intended and unintended errors. The clinicians doing "data massage," for example, may think of these "errors" as attempts to get remuneration or quality indicators right. Still, not even intentional cheating with data is given much attention in policy discourses and consultancy reports. This is surprising, especially considering that fake data is nothing new. Discussions of data cheating have a long intellectual history. In a famous essay, Charles Babbage (1830 [2018]) accuses his fellow English scientists of four "impositions": hoaxing, forging, trimming, and cooking (108–110). They are all forms of what today might be called "data manipulation."

Contemporary international research integrity manuals usually talk about falsification, fabrication, and plagiarism, where the former two again clearly revolve around data manipulation (Jensen, Whiteley, and Sandøe 2018). As already mentioned, commercial interests are also known to make companies sometimes pick data selectively or color their interpretations in conspicuous ways (Bekelman, Li, and Gross 2003; Barnes and Bero 1998; Sørensen 2013; Pisinger 2013). All of these examples of insights into intentional data error also seem to have been forgotten by the people now advising governments and authorities about how to become "data-driven." Years of accumulated insights into data difficulties also seem to evaporate when decision-makers contemplate automated algorithmic tools. In the words of the epidemiologist David Grimes (2010): "In recent decades, the computer science concept of 'GIGO' (garbage in, garbage out) has somehow come to mean 'garbage in, gospel out'" (1019). I do acknowledge that it is possible to combine suboptimal datasets carefully so they contain different types of error and thereby produce meaningful results even with somewhat problematic data—but still, if these technologies are to deliver the progress suggested by data promises, I maintain that care and caution need much more space in governmental and organizational practices than the current race for big data allows.

When approaching a future where AI is gaining increasing influence within healthcare systems, it is important to remember that it is not only a means of analyzing data. It has become a way of producing them (Peeters and Schuilenburg 2021). This point has gained new urgency with the rise of deepfake technology. Most people will know deepfakes from entertainment. They have, perhaps, seen a video with President Barack Obama saying things that are wildly out of character (Warzel 2019)—and learned that it was produced by AI. Or they have witnessed public debates about nude pictures and porn videos featuring people who never took part in those activities (Harwell 2018). The visual material was produced by a computer program. Deepfakes have moved into healthcare too. Pharmaceutical companies have been caught submitting protocols of RCTs that never took place (Hildebrandt 2017a). A computer generated the data. To combat deepfake technology in the pharmaceutical industry, authorities such as the US Food and Drug Administration (FDA) and European Medicines Agency (EMA), as well as major companies, are inventing AI so it can detect AI-generated fraudulent protocols (Hildebrandt 2017b). Healthcare is entering a race on fake data.

Ironically, in the midst of this deepfake race, artificially produced data (also known as "synthetic datasets") have also become an official way to circumvent privacy issues. Researchers and authorities produce virtual data sets generated by computers to facilitate *in silico* trials (Hogle 2018) and to create open-source data that do not reveal sensitive information derived from real patients (Carusi 2014, 2016). Such synthetic data can be used as "sandboxes" (see chapter 1), where companies can explore correlations without data protection violations. This blurs even further the notion of data as a reference to something outside the computer: data-derived knowledge can be produced in its own closed circuits.

PARADOXES OF KNOWLEDGE MAKING

Data are needed for generating robust knowledge about abstract phenomena. Many medical problems are knowable only through data. Research, therefore, depends on good data. Data is also of vital importance in clinical care when they help ensure consistency and symmetry where human judgment may suffer from inattention and prejudice. Furthermore, data can be important elements of ensuring accountability and transparent forms of governance. Data wisdom is therefore not to abandon data, but to use them with awareness of potential errors and to be able to assess whether the problem at hand can be solved with data or is in need of other types of knowledge. Big data methodologies are also potentially very useful. They can identify novel patterns that can inspire new theories, new questions, and new curiosities (Swierstra and Efstathiou 2020). They should, however, support—not replace—human judgment. Judgment presupposes training (Kahneman, Sibony, and Sunstein 2021), and I have suggested that judgment is helpfully guided by experience with other similar situations—that is, *associative thinking*. The five lessons summarized at the end of the previous chapter are also ways of sustaining judgment to support wise data use.

Not all decisions are necessarily improved by being based on reflection or data analysis. Mercier (2020) suggests that in relation to most of our daily tasks, experience-based habits provide a better protection against mistakes than a quick analysis. Data analysis can generate reflections, which disturb good habits without having established a firm and valid alternative. It usually takes multiple experiments to overthrow an old insight, but in those organizations that aim to become "data-driven," we see people suggesting that organizational changes should be based on a quick-and-dirty gaze at the latest data available in the organization. Quick-and-dirty analyses of data then risk becoming very dirty indeed. A decision does not become scientific by referring to data if scientific care has not informed the data analysis. If the available data are not sufficient for drawing any firm conclusions, or if they reflect a random variation or are used to transfer insights between incomparable organizational situations, decisions do not become better by being based on data. Furthermore, it is important to acknowledge that some problems do not even call for analysis as such. When caring for people who suffer, warm bodies can sometimes deliver more comfort that cool brains. The health services continue to need people who know how to meet other people with openness, dignity, and care. Human bodies learn to deliver comfort through guided experience and associative thinking, probably more than through analysis. It takes strong institutions to pass this type of experience from one generation to another.

In this chapter, I have pursued the paradox that though data might well be used for drawing invalid conclusions, the situation can be even worse without data. I have also suggested that this paradox occasionally has to be formulated in reverse: the problems faced are dangerous without data, but they are even worse if data take primacy. It all depends on who has what at stake in the given situation. Data are used to pursue very different goods—knowledge, health, governance, and wealth—and in some cases, they may be seen by some stakeholders as serving one goal perfectly well while working against the goals of other stakeholders. An example of this is when a child acquires a diagnostic code of ADHD as part of a data practice aimed at streamlining the allocation of resources in schools (a governance goal), but this use of diagnostic codes then undermines clinical communication (a health goal), as well as the validity of registries for research use (a knowledge goal). It can undermine even the opportunities for the child as a grown-up.

I believe that most of the people I have interviewed are working to improve healthcare. The errors they introduce emerge as they pursue solutions to earlier errors—and sometimes just from lack of experience. In most of the organizations I have visited, public *and* private, people complain about constant reorganization. They talk about being moved around and constantly given new tasks, their sections being closed and later reopened elsewhere; and they talk about a tier of managers who try to prove their worth with yet another reorganization as a step to their next promotion. This modus of constant reorganization is not how you nurture wisdom. This is not how to sustain and train judgment. What is politically expedient, therefore, is not necessarily the path to good governance. Data *create* a reality that makes political interventions possible. Perhaps this is why Torben and Flemming insist that data do not have to convey a representative impression to be useful. Political utility does not always equal "good politics," however, at least from the perspective of the affected staff, patients, and citizens.

The proper use of judgment presupposes the courage of delegation. Delegation of decisions implies giving up certain forms of political control. It takes judgment to figure out what to delegate, just as it takes judgment to determine which type of problem needs which type of knowledge. For democratically elected leaders to be able to govern, they need some form of data. Data are their primary means of control. However, I showed in chapter 3 that if data are overused for governance, they lose referentiality. Data become detached symbols of communication. Accountability, therefore, hinges on a balance between *delegation* of decisions to health professionals and *documentation* (in line with what I call data-work-of-instruction). A good place to begin when looking for that balance is to focus on using only data that are deemed clinically relevant for governance purposes—that is, to let clinicians design data practice and let administrators figure out how to carefully analyze the resulting data instead of asking health professionals to document what policymakers would like to see.

Data wisdom involves the willingness to ask questions such as: How can data inform judgment rather than replace it? Are data needed for tackling this problem? With COVID-19, such questions acquired an all-new sense of urgency—for politicians, researchers, clinicians, and citizens alike. It is to the data politics of the pandemic I turn in chapter 6.

6 DATA PANDEMIC

April 17, 2020: "The numbers speak for themselves!" Mathias exclaims, pausing briefly, as if he wants to let it sink in. Mathias, at eighty-three years old, has kindly offered himself for a telephone interview during Denmark's first national lockdown in the face of the COVID-19 pandemic. With a group of epidemiologists, I have initiated a project to document how people understand and cope with the lockdown, and Mathias has been recruited for the interview, as he had responded to a questionnaire we had developed. Reflecting on the severity of the viral threat and the need for concerted governmental efforts, he then continues: "Just look at the US. It's running totally wild over there!" Yet there is still something nagging him: "I can't help thinking . . . they say COVID-19 causes this and that, but many people die also of cardiovascular diseases, diabetes and so on. . . . How can you know that they die *because* of corona? . . . If you count 100, then 60 percent of them might have died anyway?" While trusting the Danish authorities, Mathias, an ordinary man with no specialist background in medicine or statistics, cannot help reflecting on the data and what they mean. He cannot help pondering how to interpret the data now ruling his world.

During 2020, as a consequence of the COVID-19 pandemic, citizens all over the world, much like Mathias, were beginning to follow and discuss health data on a daily basis. In some countries, people were flooded with daily numbers, graphs, and heat maps. In other countries, debates focused on missing data or data gaps. Some citizens used government sources; others began building networks for disseminating alternative information. In supermarkets and public squares, you could hear people discussing epidemiological questions relating to the reliability and validity of testing numbers, as if they had always had an opinion about these matters. People with no epidemiological training would casually use expressions such as "the R number" and consider how to interpret aggregate test results with an interest usually only granted to their favorite sports. COVID-19 brought citizens into the scientific conversation about health data in an altogether new way.

The historian of science Lorraine Daston comments on the pandemic that it is as if "we are back in the seventeenth century, the age of ground-zero empiricism, and observing as if our lives depended on it" (Daston 2020: 57). Ground-zero empiricism is when a community seeks to know about the world without a "settled script for how to go about knowing" (56). Another historian, my colleague Adam Bencard, said during a seminar that thanks to the pandemic, the wider public could suddenly "witness the scientific sausage as it was being made." I immediately liked the analogy. Sausage-making can be a pretty messy process, and yet sausages are consumed in large numbers by people who usually seem to agree on the benefits of ignoring what went into making them. Now they all had their hands in the filling.

COVID-19 is a *data pandemic*. I mean this term in a double sense. The disease and its prevalence can be understood and reacted upon only based on data, *and* it has provided the impetus for a tsunami—a pandemic—of data. While illness and death are experienced as individual tragedies, the particular virus cannot be seen by the affected patients and their relatives: it takes data to establish cause and effect. Furthermore, individual tragedies do not constitute a pandemic: it is their sum—the documentation of their global reach—that establishes the phenomenon as a pandemic. As the pandemic started a tsunami of data, it accelerated the existing dynamics of intensified data sourcing: even more people now wanted more data on more people—and yet other actors wanted to reuse the data for additional purposes (see also Felt, Öchsner, and Rae 2020). It generated a lot of conflict and tension.

These observations are in line with what I had already found, as well as what I have presented in the previous chapters. Indeed, I am not the only observer who saw a reason in the crisis for reiterating points they had made before, however different the particular points are. The philosopher Giorgio Agamben (2020), for example, quickly stated that the pandemic was an excuse for installing what he had theorized as a proclaimed state of exception: "It would seem that, terrorism having been exhausted as the cause of measures of exception, the invention of an epidemic could offer the ideal pretext for extending them beyond all limits" (1). The anthropologist Carlo Caduff, who had studied pandemic overpreparedness (2015), now wrote: "The response to the disease is driven by a fantasy of control that overestimates and overreacts. This fantasy has caused and is causing enormous harm" (Caduff 2020:10). The sociologist Slavoj Žižek (2020) commented that the pandemic was as much caused by the global political and economic systems as by any virus, adding that "the coronavirus epidemic has also triggered a vast epidemic of ideological viruses which were lying dormant in our societies: fake news, paranoiac conspiracy theories, explosions of racism" (39). In a sense, we might add, the pandemic also seemed to reinvigorate dormant analytical dispositions.

While confirming some of my own observations, the pandemic also challenged some of the analyses presented in the previous chapters. In chapters 1 and 2, I criticized the prophecies of disruption as being unrealistic, but now swift and drastic changes suddenly did look much more feasible. It was not disruption in the sense suggested by the dominant data promises, but an abrupt and sudden reorganization of healthcare still seemed at least partially achievable. Also, my description in chapter 2 of pervasive but invisible data infrastructures might have given the impression of a docile and trustful Danish population, but during the pandemic, there suddenly were people protesting and demonstrating in the streets about government interpretations and uses of health data. People were also protesting against reuse, in future research, of test tubes from coronavirus testing.

With people taking to the streets contesting government interpretations—and uses—of data, I realized that I had hitherto primarily described political uses of data as a way of preempting opposition and turning politics into technicalities (cf. Espeland and Stevens 2008; Merry 2016). This, as if data politics were what Ferguson (1994) once called an "anti-politics machine." Now I had to acknowledge that data also open up politics. Citizens such as Mathias were openly questioning governmental data analyses. In short, the pandemic made me aware of a new paradox of two competing but coexisting truths: *data close down debate and conceal political choices—and yet data also open up and unsettle political choices.*

I should not have been so surprised. Debates about various types of vaccination (Rose and Blume 2003; Halpern 2004; Decoteau and Underman 2015), as well as populationwide screening programs (Timmermans and Buchbinder 2013; Raz 2004; Sjönell and Brodersen 2009) have been important precursors to the forces released by the pandemic. The climate crisis can be seen as another example where conflicting interpretations of data generate divisive political struggles (Edwards 2010; Roeser 2012; O'Reilly, Isenhour, McElwee, and Orlove 2020). Still, the COVID-19 pandemic took contestations of data interpretations—and of the government's approach to data reuse—to new levels.

The Danish government took a strong and determined approach to slow the spread of the disease. The country was among the first in Europe to go into lockdown at a time when there appeared to be few carriers of the virus in the country. The lockdown was based on a data prediction. It was announced at a press conference one Wednesday evening, March 10, 2020, when Prime Minister Mette Frederiksen explained, "We have a very significant obligation to protect in particular the weakest in our society, the most vulnerable, people with chronic illnesses, cancer patients, older people. For their sake, the virus must not spread." She continued with what became a mantra, repeated again and again, politically as well as at dinner tables: "Now it is time to stand together, by keeping a distance" (Redaktionen 2020). At the press conference, the Minister of Health showed what was to become a famous graph, with a red curve and a green curve, which appeared in slightly different versions around the globe. The curves symbolized two possible scenarios: the red curve represented no intervention and many people in need of hospital admittance at the same time, while the green curve represented interventions that "flattened the curve" to spread out hospital admittances over time and ensure that the pressure on hospitals remained within capacity limits (see figure 6.1).

The lockdown literally emptied the usually busy streets of the city overnight. I live in central Copenhagen, and the morning after the press conference, a homeless young man who often hangs around my neighborhood stood confused in the empty street, shouting: "It's because of 4G. It's because of 5G. It's the immigrants!" The image of the man, vulnerable and distraught, trying to make sense of the silent city, came to serve as a premonition of the search for causes and meaning that was to erupt, as well as the blame games that would unfold next. Going back to my apartment, I also had to acknowledge that even though the prime minister emphasized solidarity, this crisis would also fuel existing inequalities and introduce new ones (Wahlberg, Burke, and Manderson 2021).

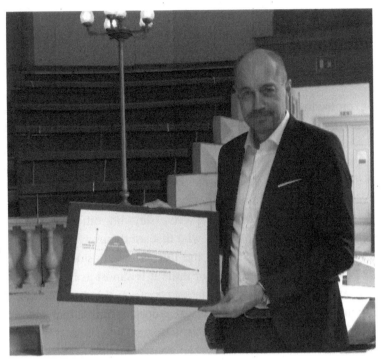

FIGURE 6.1

The red and green curves. Here, Minister of Health Magnus Heunicke is handing over the famous red and green curves used at the press conference to my colleagues at the Medical Museion, who have included it in their collections (credit: Julie Wouwenaar Tovgaard, Medical Museion).

Mickey Vallee (2020) comments on the pandemic that "strangeness and indeterminacy call for more data" (6). However, data cannot create certainty. They can be interpreted in many ways. In the mud of uncertainty, several types of doubt have found fertile soil. A way to cope with doubt is to turn to morality and politics. Data doubts, therefore, provide ample space for political tensions. In this chapter, I reflect on the ongoing pandemic as a data-political moment where data both conceal political choices and yet also open up new forms of political contestation. I return to the themes from the previous chapters and illustrate how promises, living, work, experience, and wisdom play out under COVID-19 and sustain, deepen, and sometimes challenge the points from the preceding chapters. First, however, I present a few reflections on why the pandemic gave rise to such an interest in data—and on the data that it made me and others generate with a rare sense of urgency.

PAN(DEM)IC: A TSUNAMI OF DATA

If the coronavirus pandemic has become a data pandemic, it is partly because of certain biological properties of the specific virus strain, SARS-CoV-2, which is causing the disease Corona Virus Disease 2019 (abbreviated as COVID-19). For example, it has an incubation period where carriers can infect others even if they themselves show no signs of the disease. Also, COVID-19 develops very differently in different individuals. Some hardly notice it, or they feel as if they have a light (or perhaps severe) flu, while others suffer a violent and painful death. Some patients, who first see themselves as only lightly affected, later experience strange and uncomfortable side effects such as loss of memory or sense of smell or taste. It is almost as if the same virus causes very different diseases in different people. As the virus mutates, these uncertainties multiply. Such biological properties mean that individuals cannot know their own risk, nor the risk they might pose to others. People cannot necessarily feel whether they are contagious or safe—so if they want to act, they need data. COVID-19 is not the only such disease, but it is rare for people around the entire globe to face this type of uncertainty at the same time. The pandemic created a sense of panic, partly as a result of this uncertainty operating at a new, much greater scale.

In response, a tsunami of new studies was hitting the shores of academia, news media, and governmental institutions. The burst of quickly produced data created the public spectacle of "watching the scientific sausage being made." In Denmark as well as many other countries, a public crash course in data analysis unfolded around figuring out ostensibly simple matters, such as how many citizens were carrying the virus. Newspaper articles, radio hosts, and blog posts explained how these statistics depended on, for example, test capacity and test strategy. Many of the people we interviewed would remind us that "one cannot compare test data from the spring of 2020 with those from the autumn, because many more people were being tested in autumn." They had learned not to compare figures produced under different circumstances. Similarly, many people realized that death tolls and delineations of risk groups were anything but straightforward. Mathias was right: it is difficult to determine how many die *with* or *of* COVID-19.[1] The most basic question about whether one's life was at risk could get no simple answer from the data, and yet there was no answer without data either. Everybody seemed to request more data.

I joined the data rush. I felt an urge to understand what was going on, and to do so, I turned to documentation. What did I do? In my general sense of bafflement, I first took pictures, recorded press meetings, collected policy papers, and took field notes on all types of experiences. However, my main commitment ended up being the collaboration mentioned in the introduction of this chapter, with two eminent epidemiologists in another section of my department, Naja Hulvej Rod and Katrine Strandberg-Larsen. They also introduced me to an ethnologist working with them, Amy Clotworthy, as well as other epidemiologists working in their respective groups. Within the first weeks of the lockdown, we constructed the Copenhagen Corona-Related Mental Health (CCMH) questionnaire to document some of the effects of the pandemic. It came to focus mainly on mental health because of Naja's and Katrine's expertise in this area, but it covered behavioral changes and people's sources of information about the pandemic as well. Later, we added attitudes to vaccinations to the studied topics.

It was when answering this questionnaire that respondents like Mathias were invited to volunteer for a phone interview as well. Amy and I were coordinating this qualitative element. Many researchers volunteered, and the project group grew. The CCMH questionnaire was translated into Dutch, English, and French by other groups. Many of the questionnaire elements were already being used in a large cohort study managed by Katrine, and we distributed the CCMH questionnaire to the cohort, as well as to the wider population through a time-series study administered by a survey company and through our project website. In this way, we hoped to be able to evaluate effects both diachronically in Denmark and synchronically among countries. The survey methodology and material have been described in separate papers (Clotworthy, Skovlund Dissing, Nguyen et al. 2020; Varga, Bu, Dissing et al. 2021). In the qualitative part, we ended up interviewing forty-eight individuals in Denmark, some of them several times.

In our interviews, most people expressed great support for the governmental approach, something also found in other studies.[2] Indeed, according to the Pew Institute, Denmark was at the top of the list of public satisfaction with the government's strategy compared to fourteen other countries (Devlin and Connaughton 2020). Even in the midst of a global crisis, there are people who have time for fabricating rankings. According to political scientist Michael Bang Petersen (2021), who did the most extensive studies of public attitudes in Denmark and served as an advisor to the government, the widespread popular support in Denmark was related to the way in which the governmental communication embraced uncertainty and stated up front that they would inevitably commit mistakes.

Petersen's studies, as well as our survey, furthermore suggested that people really did change their behavior radically (Clotworthy et al. 2020). According to our data, however, it came with a mental health price: increased loneliness, isolation, lower quality of life, and more anxiety and worry. Other studies around the world found a similar negative impact on mental health (Vindegaard and Benros 2020). We had distributed the survey in the general population and in Katrine's existing cohort study, but the numbers differed in the two "populations." In the general population, the young in particular seemed to be negatively affected, while data from the cohort study (where people had long been answering the same questions) did not fluctuate enough to suggest extraordinary pressure on the young. With different results in the two populations, Naja had to exert judgment. She decided to advise the authorities to do more to prevent mental health problems among the young. Eventually, restrictions on schooling were lifted before other restrictions in order to help the young cope with the pandemic.

My engagement in this project gave me hands-on experience with the challenges that civil servants like Torben and Flemming described in chapter 5. We had to acknowledge doubts and uncertainties and yet use data to help inform our decisions. We had to speak on behalf of the data we had, although we were aware that we were missing data on many other potentially important factors. For example, there might very well be more vulnerable people than those responding to our questionnaire (e.g., in eldercare, among unregistered migrants, and the homeless). Another resemblance to the challenges of civil servants was the ambition of isolating effects. Torben and Flemming were tasked with isolating healthcare performance, and we had wanted to isolate the effects of the lockdown strategies in different countries. However, data from the four countries did not suggest clear differences in mental health effects despite very different political strategies (Varga et al. 2021). If the questionnaire did measure the chosen mental health aspects in a valid way, it appeared that the type of lockdown was less significant than we had anticipated (and had we found a clear variation between the countries, it might have been caused by a parameter other than the lockdown strategy).

The questionnaire was made carefully, but under great time pressure. Some questions were not conceptualized and tested as we would normally do because getting started as soon as possible was a main priority. When we asked respondents which precautions they took to avoid infection, the reply options included, for example, "Increased handwashing and use of sanitizer." As the crisis continued, the term "increased" became dubious, but we could not change the wording because it would be difficult to publish in epidemiological journals if questions changed along the way. Although questions on loneliness were previously validated questionnaire items, they were not validated for this particular use. Maybe they were understood differently in the context of a shared societal lockdown, where loneliness might have become a more legitimate feeling to express? Still, if we were to create data in the midst of the crisis, we could not wait until the perfect solution materialized. In the end, we had to accept, as argued in chapter 5, that even though data can give rise to invalid conclusions, the situation can be worse without data.

COVID-19 also became a data pandemic by accelerating the datafication of my own research. We interviewed forty-eight people, but *I* did not interview them. It was a group endeavor. Three assistants were employed, Sofie Amalie Olsen, Sif Vange, and Nikoline Nygaard, to help with the "data collection" (a term I otherwise rarely use to refer to interviews). Sofie, for example, interviewed Mathias, whom I previously quoted, and Sif conducted a follow-up interview with him in September 2020. Later, Sofie á Rogvi joined to explore the growing opposition to the government strategy. Through the work of these talented assistants, interviews and ethnographic observations were turned into shareable *data*—decontextualized, digital, and transferable (Poirier, Fortun, Costelloe-Kuehn, and Fortun 2020). We obtained funding from the Velux Foundation, which also emphasized data sharing. Data sharing disentangles narratives from the intimate relation between interviewer and interviewee. It was new for me to, at least in this way, draw information from interviews I did not conduct myself. Amy and others were using the same interviews for other analyses. Even interview data in this way become multiple: serving many purposes at once.

"It feels strange that people who have confided in me, should see their thoughts used by others," Sofie á Rogvi said at one point when we spoke about placing interview transcripts in sharable folders. "It feels like *my* informants," she continued, holding her hands up like a hug or holding a baby. Sofie is not a "data hoarder" (Tupasela 2021a). She was expressing care. Although we all want to understand and represent our interviewees well, datafication can exert a sort of violence on the relations through which the data emerge. I do not wish to ignore or downplay the role that ethnographic encounters have had in extractive colonial practices (Clifford 1986), but I do wish to suggest that face-to-face encounters provoke ethical reflections in ways computer screens and data in columns do not. It is a relational care that we as a research community must consciously work to preserve if all our data are to be offered in machine-readable formats for secondary analyses as part of the open data movement. Data sharing facilitates some new and intriguing forms of analysis, but it comes with a price.

In short, COVID-19 is a phenomenon known through data, and it instigated a call for even more data, as well as deepened datafication. In the wake of this data tsunami, I began reflecting on my previous points about promises, living, experience and wisdom.

PROMISES: CHATBOTS, APPS, AND DIGITALIZATION

As the anthropologist Adriana Petryna (2002, 2005) has shown, any good crisis involves opportunities for those who seize them. The pandemic was no different. It was not just producers of masks, sanitizers, and vaccines who made a fortune, along with online shopping companies like Amazon and delivery services of various sorts. The pandemic also fueled the data promises that already had a strong grip on decision makers. Lockdowns instigated an immediate need for digital tools for communication, and the authorities instantly began working with 'data-driven' software to monitor and prevent COVID.

Some of these tools proved effective, such as the construction of data pathways that allowed the authorities to identify the long-term effects of the disease, side effects of vaccines, and pressures on healthcare resources. In other cases, however, investments seemed motivated by data promises that were able to overrule any call for evidence. Chatbots, for example, were almost instantly set up as online symptom checkers in many countries (Greenhalgh, Koh, and Ca 2020). In Denmark, one chatbot was supposed to serve as a digital replacement for GPs and thereby relieve the health services

(Danske Regioner 2021). One of the key data promises, that automated data processing could replace doctors, finally seemed to be materializing—and to be doing so overnight. Indeed, several hundred thousand Danes were now communicating with a computer rather than with a person. Christoffer Bjerre Haase, a PhD student of mine who is also a medical doctor, invited me and a couple of other colleagues to analyze the chatbot. It turned out to be a relatively simple algorithm. It focused only on capturing COVID-19 symptoms, which meant that if a patient had symptoms of another illness such as meningitis, the chatbot would not suggest any urgency. Still, the algorithm was disposed toward "better safe than sorry," and therefore almost every other symptom led to the same chatbot response: "You should see a doctor." How would this relieve the healthcare system? And how would its degree of success be evaluated? There was no way of capturing its potential mistakes, no way of figuring out whether it served its purpose. It was an evidence-free invention, and yet it was heralded as a great digital triumph (Haase, Bearman, Brodersen et al. 2020).

In the space of urgency, politics and science were mingling with ease, and in many ways that ease was not all that different from the general embrace of the new digital options described in chapter 1. Digital contact tracing apps were developed at great speed in many countries. The Danish authorities moved a little slower than most other countries on the implementation of these apps. There was no doubt that the government wanted a contact-tracing app, but numerous complaints from many sides about data security delayed the process (Mirzaei-Fard 2020). When a mobility tracker app aimed at identifying risk of exposure was introduced in Denmark in June 2020, it was basically the same as an earlier Norwegian version. Ironically, Norway had dropped this app for lack of proven effects just a week before it was implemented in Denmark (Datatilsynet 2020).

Yet the lack of evidence of effects did not disturb the Danish plan. The Danish delay was explained as a matter of ensuring a *safe* version (apparently more than an evidence-based one). It made it somewhat peculiar that while the population was told that this special Danish version did not constitute any digital risk, employees in the Ministry of Foreign Affairs were told not to download the app due to increased risks of hacking (Krogh 2020). Such double standards, along with more or less dubious attempts at using data collected for the combat of disease for security purposes, mushroomed in various versions in countries all around the globe (Harari 2020; Powers

2020), including China (Mozur, Zhong, and Krolik 2020), Singapore (Illmer 2021), and even Germany (Privacy International 2020), a country otherwise known for being cautious with data being repurposed for surveillance.

In June 2021, Lisbeth Nielsen, the director for the Danish Health Data Authority, was interviewed by a political magazine about the impact of the pandemic on the work with digital health data in Denmark. She emphasized the importance of the strong data infrastructures in place in Denmark already before the pandemic struck. She added that "nobody notices infrastructure when things work as they should" (in Lehmann 2021). Policymakers and the public have long been accustomed to think that "somebody" knows exactly how many patients have a particular diagnosis, for example, but the pandemic made the work going into producing such numbers more visible as the demand for real-time data became more urgent than ever before. The director explained:

> We are now on steroids in this data production. These days we make sizable reports daily [with] very detailed data on who is vaccinated, where, and which parishes have high infection rates. . . . Suddenly, it's the Prime Minister's office reading health data. I don't think they've done that before (in Lehmann 2021).

With the pandemic, the demand for health data exploded! Nielsen was also thrilled to see how the pandemic had pushed the agenda of digitalization and "data-driven decision making" (Ibid.). It took less than a week to introduce video consultations into general practice using the existing infrastructure (Danske Regioner 2020). Then, only two weeks after initiation of the first lockdown, it was also possible for psychologists to offer online therapy options on safe connections (Dansk Psykolog Forening 2020). In a book about the government's multi-level response to the pandemic, a group of retired top civil servants and academics observed, with a hint of envy, that "changes that would usually take years were implemented in weeks" (Østrup, Jørgensen, and Zwisler 2020: 261). Within a year, a whole range of new so-called self-service options were introduced to ensure physical distance between patients and staff, and citizens were invited to book their own tests and vaccinations, download their own proof of infection status, and so on.

Nielsen also saw in the pandemic response a confirmation of the legitimacy of previous political choices: "A couple of years ago, we were still discussing whether it was reasonable for people to see their own laboratory results—without a delay . . . We will never return to a situation where we have to discuss whether people can bear seeing their own data." Interestingly, she seemed to reach this conclusion because of a renewed digital conviction, not because of any new evidence (and more likely *despite* the emerging evidence—see chapter 5). Thereby, the pandemic response in Denmark has accelerated the transition toward wired medicine and self-care, which characterizes data living.

LIVING: RISK, TESTING, AND SOCIAL DISTANCING

With my mention of tracking apps that do not capture what they are supposed to, and yet which open up possibilities for surveillance in new ways, I have exemplified how the pandemic revived some of the common paradoxes of everyday data living: data both reveal *and* conceal; they both empower *and* disempower. These paradoxes have played out differently in different countries, depending on the preexisting (but largely invisible) infrastructures and healthcare options already in place. Infrastructures, and not just political leadership, have shaped the pandemic response—and determined who were left with which opportunities for obtaining help in a time of crisis (Bal, de Graaff, van de Bovenkamp, and Wallenburg 2020; Caduff 2020). In Denmark, a publicly funded healthcare system has ensured broad coverage, and existing data infrastructures have ensured an overview of developments. Test figures, hospital capacity numbers, daily numbers of hospital admissions, intensive care admissions, people on ventilators, and other forms of real-time monitoring not only were shared with the prime minister's office, but also were turned into direct updates and graphs shared online and with media outlets. Data were used for planning, but they also were publicly released so that news agencies could produce automated heat maps such as those in figure 6.2 (from the National Broadcasting Company), indicating the geographical distribution of positive tests and high-risk groups (based on age, comorbidity, and overweight). A real-time cohort was set up for research on safe servers to follow all those infected (and later, all the vaccinated) across all subsequent uses of healthcare (Pottegård, Bruun Kristensen, Reilev et al. 2020). It has been used to monitor the long-term effects of having had COVID-19 (Lund, Hallas, Nielsen et al. 2021), as well as the side effects of treatments and vaccinations. When reports appeared internationally about deadly side effects of the AstraZeneca vaccine, such as the so-called vaccine-induced thrombotic thrombocytopenia (VITT), it took a week to identify all healthcare contacts from everyone who

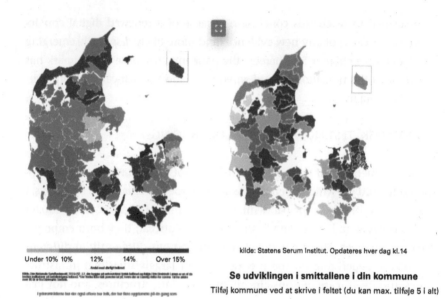

kilde: Statens Serum Institut. Opdateres hver dag kl.14

Under 10% 10%   12%   14%   Over 15%

Se udviklingen i smittallene i din kommune

Tilføj kommune ved at skrive i feltet (du kan max. tilføje 5 i alt)

FIGURE 6.2

Heat maps of viral risk. On the left, a map entitled "How many are at special risk of coronavirus infection," showing the concentration of high-risk groups (age, over-weight, comorbidity) published at the beginning of the pandemic. On the right, an interactive map entitled "Check infection rates of the past week in your municipality," showing the concentration of positive test figures per 100,000 inhabitants (from June 1, 2021). This map was updated throughout the pandemic. In contrast to the one on the left, it contains no legend linking the color coding with specific numbers: coloring continuously changed to show maximum difference between municipalities (credit: data analyst Nis Kielgast and graphics Simone Cecilie Møller, National Broadcasting Company).

had received the vaccine in Denmark and analyze their disease patterns.[3] Based on such calculations, first the AstraZeneca vaccine, and later the Johnson & Johnson vaccine, were left out of the Danish mass vaccination program.[4] The data infrastructures were operating "on steroids," as the director of the Danish Authority of Health Data put it.

These experiences with digital data infrastructures were mostly continuations of forms of data living that I already described in chapter 2, such as being connected to digital monitoring and communication devices. There was, however, a new way in which the pandemic inscribed itself in data living. It was the mass experience of living in the shadow of data predictions. With COVID-19, society as a whole had become an extended healthcare sector: work to fight disease was no longer confined to certain institutions or practices. "Morbid living" (Wahlberg 2018b) permeated the everyday behaviors of even those who had never been touched by disease.

In our interviews and in the survey, we learned about how people experienced the social changes brought about by the pandemic. We could observe some dramatic shifts in behavior. According to the survey, more than 95 percent of respondents reported increased use of handwashing and sanitizers and practicing physical distance with strangers. This was "thin data," ethnographically, but the information sent a clear signal. In our interviews, we learned more about what such a response meant to people and how they practiced these precautions. The interviews also indicated that sometimes we might not be measuring exactly what we thought we were with the CCMH questionnaire. For example, we could see that Pernille, in her response to the survey, stated that she did *not* practice increased handwashing and use of sanitizers. We assumed that that meant that she had decided not to follow the public guidelines, but when we interviewed her, she explained, "We already were doing that [before the pandemic], sanitizing our grocery shopping and all that. So we kind of had a head start on all of that." Such deviations in measurement are probably not a big deal when numbers are large enough, but it was amusing to see our own assumptions challenged.

What the numbers could not convey was what behavioral change *meant* to people. First and foremost, the sudden shift in behavior in the early months of the pandemic generated social conflict, both between strangers and in intimate relations: What was the adequate level of precaution? Most people felt that they were being too strict in the eyes of some and too lax in the eyes of others. They complained about others, but also about others complaining about them. In April 2020, Lise (age 81) remarked: "There are many young people who are out running . . . and some of them are ruthless; they only think of themselves while running." I read this and similar remarks about runners and began practicing a lot of distance when passing people on my own runs, only to have an older couple shouting aggressively after me: "We are not carrying the plague, you know!" Also, in April 2020, Chunhua (age 31), a woman of Chinese descent, said she had been wearing a mask long before it became official policy in Denmark. She reflected on feeling "weird": "We were a little concerned, . . . if we would make other people panic if they saw the mask." Others, indeed, commented on those using masks, and later, when that became mandatory, they would comment on those *not* wearing a mask. Even before the pandemic, masks were embedded in dense scientific symbolism. Writing on the history of masks, Lynteris (2018) says that they provide an "essentially atropaic promise of scientific control," where the mask assigns the wearer to particular communities (442; see also Lupton, Southerton, Clark, and Watson 2021, for a fine analysis of the social dynamics of mask wearing during the pandemic).

The sense of social anxiety wrote itself into intimate relations (Schiermer 2020). Interpretations of data predictions influenced who could spend time with whom, how, and where, and with every cycle of lockdown, reopening, and renewed lockdown, people had to renegotiate risk levels with family and friends. The interviews are permeated with examples of inconsistent personal choices aimed at balancing differing perceptions. Johan (age 64), for example, admitted that he saw his girlfriend's children in a very casual way, but he avoided his own children and grandchildren or saw them at a marked distance: "Last time I saw my daughter, son-in-law, and the grandchildren, the children stayed inside in the living room, and then we opened the door to the terrace and I could stand out there talking to them." Johan explained that his daughter and son-in-law were nurses and "knew much more about COVID" than his girlfriend's children, so he had to accept their rules when he was with them. He did not doubt their expertise, but when they were not around, he had decided to focus on other priorities.

People with chronic diseases would talk about the disempowering feeling of having to communicate about diseases that they usually tried hard to make sure did not determine how they lived their lives (see also Grabowski, Meldgaard, and Rod 2020; Clotworthy and Westendorp 2020; Lau, Kofod Svensson, Kingod, and Wahlberg 2021). Davis and Lohm (2020) noticed similar reactions in the wake of the swine flu outbreak in 2009 in the United Kingdom and Australia. On top of this, social distancing generated a common sense of *loss*. The people we interviewed spoke about not being able to attend funerals and of people who lost contact with their close relatives in their final year of life. Such tragic experiences have been recounted all over the world (Nagesh 2020; Videbæk 2020). When Sif Vange spoke to Mathias again in September 2020, he also commented on a sense of loss, but of a more mundane type:

> We can talk on the phone, we can talk on Skype, but it's just not the same as face-to-face cozy intermingling where you can read their bodily gestures and

their facial expressions. Body language is as important as what the mouth says, almost.

For most people, connections are not just informational. When society as a whole structures people's interactions on the premise of preventing disease, people will tend to experience their loss of social life in a much more direct manner than the preservation of biological life that the preventative measure serves.

WORK: LAY EPIDEMIOLOGISTS, CONTROL, AND OPPOSITION

Similar to the way that the pandemic affected how I thought about data living, it influenced my understanding of data work. Intensified data sourcing continues to create both more and less data work by moving it around among groups of people. I had already noticed the data work undertaken by patients (chapter 2), but my main focus had been on the work carried out by health professionals (chapter 3). Now all citizens faced much more data work, not least because the pandemic accelerated the ongoing transition toward digital self-service options, as observed by Lisbeth Nielsen. To avoid physical contact, patients increasingly had to (and to date still must) enter information from home (or through sanitized iPads or data entry stations in the clinic), rather than speaking to a nurse or secretary. It has had the consequence that citizens now do more of the data-work-of-production. Many citizens have also embraced data-work-of-analysis, mostly just in the form of comparing and interpreting numbers as Mathias did, but some citizens have kept Microsoft Excel spreadsheets of their own, with which they have been monitoring the veracity and consistency of official statistics. Citizens have also faced more data-work-of-instruction in the form of having to present health data to access social gatherings, cafés, and educational institutions. This is data-work-of-instruction because they might have been in line to get test results not to know their infection status, but to comply with rules. Some families have installed rules of their own that generate a form of data-work-of-instruction, such as to provide a digital certificate proving negative infection status when children move between divorced parents or as a ticket to enter a birthday party. Most important, however, the pandemic has generated much more data-work-of-use. Keeping up to date with the latest numbers became a daily occupation for practically every person I have encountered since March 2020. It is, therefore, data-work-of-use that I focus on in this chapter.

Mathias, for example, conveyed how he kept spending more time simply following data when he spoke to Sif in September 2020:

> I often check this homepage, I can't remember its name. There you can really see the curves, how it looks right now. . . . And "how many on respirators," "so many on intensive care, but not in need of respirator." Yes. And then there are the age groups, I care a lot about them . . . and the geography, of course. Obviously, we're somewhat egocentric: How is my part of Jutland doing compared to the other regions? . . . I didn't care that much in the beginning. It's something that was awoken in me during the past couple of months. 'Cause you're bombarded [with data] . . . and now I can't help checking them (*giggling*).

Mathias, like many others, has become a data consumer. The direct feeds from hospital systems to central databases were released every day at 2 p.m., and some people used them for informal betting. A morbid pastime, fit for morbid living, but also a new form of work: recreational data-work-of-use.

Just like the other types of data work, the work associated with data use is unevenly distributed. Those individuals, who do not agree with the tacit priorities of the government's strategy, spend countless hours looking for sources supporting their hunch. Apparently, they need data to justify their position. In Denmark, as in Canada and several other countries (Lupton et al. 2021), the opposition to restrictions came from both the right- and left-wing sides of the political spectrum. It has not been a bipartisan issue of party politics to the same extent as in the United States, though in Parliament, it has mostly been a particular right-wing party that gradually began formulating criticism of restrictions. At demonstrations, a common battle cry has been "Fuck the left wing, fuck the right wing, fuck the centrists. We are the people, and we have had enough!" The antielitist stance is often articulated on the homepages of the opponents (e.g., *danmarkforst.dk*, which informs readers that the so-called elite has planned the pandemic to carry out genocide on the populace using vaccination as the weapon). Regardless of their political position, however, the Danish opponents of restrictions have found themselves steeped in data use. It is as if the only legitimate opposition to policies building on data predictions was alternative uses of data.

I stumbled across this type of data work aimed at challenging governmental choices among opponents more or less by chance when I, in April 2020, came across a demonstration against the government strategy. It was so strange seeing some 50 to 100 people gathering at a time when the city was otherwise empty. I stood listening a while, at a distance. The speakers were presented as "experts," and the main theme was that the authorities were lying—a point made by citing statistics. In the months to come, and in particular from September onward, the opposition mounted. A group convened in front of Parliament every day with saucepan lids and spoons, banging and making noise. I decided to pass there on my running route and stop for brief chats with some of the demonstrators. I have sometimes seen as few as two or six people, and sometimes what I guessed amounted to several thousands. They appeared to be an unusual mix: left-wing herbalists and right-wing pro-Israel supporters, yoga trainers and thoroughly tattooed bodybuilders, young and old, but they were all talking to each other, and all were very interested in explaining themselves to a passerby like me. Often, when I have asked, "How did you get involved with this?" they have responded something like, "Oh, I've been involved for years!" Apparently, many of them see themselves as engaged in various forms of opposition, with long histories. Others described themselves as "awoken" by the pandemic—for the first time, aware of the politics shaping their daily lives.

I expected to see something about the continued demonstrations in the news, but the media remained remarkably silent. Several new political parties emerged in this period, again without getting much media attention. By mid-2021, no fewer than 121 new parties had begun collecting signatures to begin the process of featuring on the next parliamentary ballot (Krogh, Lehmann, and Lønstrup 2021)–in a country of just 5.8 million inhabitants. One opposition party which had been around for some years before the pandemic, but which now attracted much larger crowds, is called Earth, Freedom, Knowledge. It has for years been warning voters against an evil elite. In their party manifesto, they suggest "treating herbalism and conventional medicine equally" and "banning 5G from entering Denmark, because it is extremely dangerous to health" (JFK21 2021). However, now their main cause is "to bring an end to the illegal restrictions in conjunction with COVID-19, to work for herd immunity like in Sweden, and to remove the Act on Epidemics." In line with most of the other new parties, Earth, Freedom, Knowledge accused a proposed Act on Epidemics for installing mass surveillance. The final law was modified before being enacted, but it was not modified enough to satisfy many of those who have begun questioning the motives of the government. The pandemic has generated a burst of activism (Milan, Treré, and Masiero 2021; Callison and Slobodian 2021), but in the latest election (which was for municipality and regional representation), there was no increase in active voters. On the contrary, there was a slight decrease (Frost 2021). Mostly, this type of data activism challenges the basic legitimacy of existing political institutions.

When I first began hanging out at the margins of some of these demonstrations, I simply sought to understand their concerns. Gradually, it also become a micropolitical act. I wanted to maintain a dialogue with people whom I quickly realized feel silenced, ignored, and treated as outcasts (Tønder 2020). Dialogue came to feel like a necessity in an increasingly divided political atmosphere. One day in November 2020, I am speaking with two women, both retired, who offer me a leaflet. It is full of data derived from the Danish Health Authority, and it compares death statistics from smoking and COVID-19. I would have interpreted these data differently, but one of the women gives me a telling smile, saying: "Why don't they [pointing to the Parliament building] do anything about smoking? Perhaps because they smoke themselves?" I ask whether they doubt the published data on COVID-19, and like many other opponents, they are pretty confident that the disease exists and that the official Danish data are correct. However, they maintain that the data are "manipulated to scare you." I ask whether they think there is nothing to fear, and they respond as one voice: "No, we hug and shake hands and we're all right." Then much to my surprise, one of them adds: "It's just the old and weak ones who die," while her friend nods.

Statistically, these two women must belong to that very category. It then turns out they too have lost friends to COVID-19. They do not deny the deaths. One of them then takes a deep breath and explains that the real danger is "not to lose your life, but to stop having a life." She had seen friends isolated in their final year of life, and others dying of diseases other than COVID, but isolated and alone because of the lockdown measures. She accepts the statistics of COVID-19 but opposes valuing biological life over social life. She then adds that herbal tea is probably the best prevention. It later struck me as strange that she initiated the conversation by handing me a list of numbers from the Danish Health Authority if she believes that herbal tea delivers a cure. Would she have used data to argue her affinity for herbal tea before 2020? Is it the pandemic that has forced her to use official health data to argue her case? At the given point, however, a young man comes over and begins advising me on how to find the "real data" on www.bitchute.com, explaining that the site is also where I will see the truth about "the Muslim invasion." At that point, I decide to take off.

Attending these gatherings was like going down a rabbit hole and entering an alternative world, where everything takes on different colors and different meanings, gets filtered through different interpretations. If, in chapter 3, I observed how policymakers and clinicians could sometimes appear to live in separate worlds, now it was as if divergent segments of the population occupied different planets. Sofie á Rogvi and I decided to begin interviewing some of the opponents of the government's strategy, beginning with participants at these gatherings. Each mode of sampling creates its own public: data always reflect how they came into being. When we compared the interviews with our survey respondents (who, like the general population, were mostly supportive of the government strategy) to interviews with some of these opponents of the government, on the one hand, there was an interesting contrast in attitudes toward the government, while on the other hand, supporters and opponents were remarkably similar in other respects: both groups expressed doubt about official data analyses, they questioned the logic of specific restrictions, and both were looking for meaning and explanations using data. People on both sides had similar doubts, such as whether too much sanitizer could be harmful to health, granted that some bacteria are beneficial to human health (Hamblin 2020). As also found in a study from the United States, however, *opponents* often get to know much more about data analysis than supporters of the government's strategy (Lee et al. 2021). They needed to invest more in the data discourses to acquire a position from which to speak.

At a point when 95 percent of the respondents to our survey said "Yes" to wanting a vaccine (see figure 6.3), the majority of the people gathering at demonstrations seemed to be convinced that the vaccines were harmful tools of surveillance, or that the pandemic was manufactured to sell vaccines.[5] Personally, I am convinced that most opponents have misunderstood the science and the risks associated with the disease and the vaccinations, but in many ways, it is impossible to simply dismiss their analysis of the politics: most of them are convinced that big tech thrives on extractive practices, governments carry out mass surveillance, and a preposterously wealthy elite gladly uses any crisis as an opportunity to make money. Even if their concrete assumptions about COVID-19 cannot be backed empirically, these are relatively valid political assertions and legitimate viewpoints (see also Jackson 2002a; Wynne 1992). Vaccine hesitancy, Goldenberg (2021) argues, should not be understood as the result of

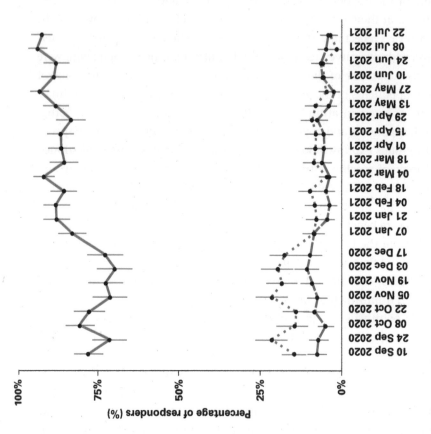

FIGURE 6.3

Graph of vaccination attitudes. Results from the survey after questions about interest in getting vaccinated were added: solid line means "yes," dashed line "no," and dotted line "not sure." Willingness rose after the authorities decided to withdraw two vaccinations from the program due to risk of blood clots—that is, the VITT syndrome. (Credit: Tibor Varga.)

a knowledge deficit. Rather, it "is the result of unsuccessful science-public relations. The success of those relationships, like all relationships, hinges on trust" (17). Unlike me, many opponents have had experiences that dispose them toward mistrust of the government and the authorities. Now, to make space for themselves, people in this marginal position have to use data to justify their opposition.

Gradually, the saucepan demonstrations were replaced by more aggressive demonstrations led by an organization called Men in Black (Olsen 2021). An element of violence erupted from these events, which was moderate by international standards but it finally caused mainstream media to begin reporting on the opposition. While there were some at these events who claimed that the virus does not exist, others simply opposed the implicit values written into the data politics ruling their lives. Speakers at these events also opposed how mouth swab samples are stored and offered to researchers. They talk about how Denmark is on a route to becoming a surveillance state and a dictatorship. In this period, my husband, who is a schoolteacher, also observed how ordinary parents began opposing the testing of their children at schools because of its implied data sourcing.

When Sofie á Rogvi and I decided to interview some of the people producing the most popular data representations for the media, Piet from the National Broadcasting Company explained how the pandemic had given rise to reactions from readers like no previous topic ever had. He had had to respond to more than a thousand complaints and was surprised by the detail with which people argued their points. Line and Noah from TV2, the media corporation in Denmark that has had the most traffic on news about the pandemic, similarly told us about an unprecedented response from the public. Line and Noah were also the ones telling about people who monitor and comment on any deviance in official numbers based on their own Microsoft Excel spreadsheets (as I mentioned previously). Members of the public were also telling Line and Noah how important the daily figures had become for them. Piet compared these massive public reactions to the absence of response to news about a controversial impeachment trial of a former minister. The impeachment trial was big news politically and revolved around the illegal separation of refugee families. This is a very controversial topic indeed, but according to Piet there was virtually no public reaction to their news reporting:

> It's difficult to get upset about [our reporting on] that [trial] because we say "some say this" and "others say that." But if we write "There were 1700 new cases of infection yesterday," then it opens up a discussion, because somebody can say, "Well, this American professor says that you can't measure it in this way" . . . It is quite simply easier to disagree with [data]. And everything has been on speed during coronavirus, also people's . . . misinformation. And there is some really, really thorough misinformation out there. . . . They provide so many numbers and they cross-reference each other.

It is indeed an interesting observation: controversial political topics are less controversial from a news perspective than a simple test figure based on the latest available health data.

The pandemic certainly gave rise to an explosion of "alternative facts" (Gruzd and Mai 2020; Islam, Sarkar, Hossain Khan et al. 2020), where those eager to find alternative analyses did so on international platforms. These platforms are designed to track people's interests and feed them what they want (Pariser 2011; van Dijck 2013). During the pandemic (as well as during the US presidential election in 2020), most platforms claimed to combat misinformation, but their very business model was to keep people connected to harvest their data (Crawford 2021; Zuboff 2019; Sadowski 2019b). It also implies that every time citizens *look* for information, they have to *provide* information about themselves and their interests. In this way, the data work goes full circle: when wanting to *use* data analyses, citizens *produce* data for big tech. Big tech then uses these data to feed people similar stories (Pariser 2011). As people, confused and distraught, are trying to make sense of the crisis, they are fueling the platform data economy.

The pandemic turned every citizen into a lay epidemiologist, but rather than establishing scientific authority, it opened up this authority for scrutiny. While the official data governance has sought to tighten societal control, it has simultaneously facilitated societal disintegration; and when official data interpretations are deemed meaningless, people have construed alternative stories using data. In this way, the paradoxes of data work have proliferated anew, no longer just in hospital wards, but in everyday life and among ordinary citizens.

EXPERIENCE: CURVES, HEAT MAPS, AND THE PURSUIT OF MEANING

With all the new data-work-of-use, data experiences became a daily pastime. How did people experience the data? In his pre-COVID analysis of pandemic preparedness, Caduff (2015) analyzes the many times a pandemic has been announced without materializing, noting that it takes a lot of work to create "the perception of an event as already in the process of happening even though it is yet to come" (62). Predictions convey probabilities. They can be wrong. For people to build their actions on scientific predictions of risk in a way that makes the suggested precautions meaningful, they have to trust the data used to make the argument—or, at least, the people presenting the data. As I just showed, not everybody did that. People are not like computers, which can be wired to use particular sources. Human beings make embodied, emotional decisions.

Homepages with virological visualizations have mushroomed,[6] and as citizens were bombarded with data, many began adding their own (Bowe, Simmons, and Mattern 2020). Data solidified their position as aesthetic objects expressing both danger and beauty (Carusi 2020). Throughout the pandemic, the paradox of dematerialization and rematerialization has played out, as the pandemic as an abstract phenomenon with no immediate presence or frame of experience has rematerialized through visualizations pored over on tablets, computers, and phones in people's living rooms. Later, with a variant called omicron, many people experienced a light version of the disease that for some made the scare of the numbers appear alien and detached from their own experience. In 2020, when official numbers were still released each day at 2 p.m., Noah explained how they could see people began logging in from around 1:30 p.m., to get ready. TV2's data on daily "views," Noah said, reveal that "we have created a habit in people's lives." Line elaborated: "It's without precedent . . . [Our COVID figures] have been viewed 190 million times. And we're five million Danes. It is insane how many people there are who log on again and again and again and again . . . This number, it's outrageous! You'll find no parallels anywhere [in news history]." Noah adds: "Before coronavirus, the single story getting the most clicks had 1.3 million." And those numbers were just website clicks (news can also be accessed through the app and other outlets).

In terms of shaping political choices, however, the most prominent data visualization was probably the graph with the red and green curves shown in figure 6.1. The two curves build on interpretations of different interventions in two states in the United States during the Spanish flu pandemic in 1918 (Wilson 2020; Strochlic and Champine 2020). The evidence behind the two curves has been questioned (Markel, Lipman, Navarro et al. 2007);

it *is* difficult to isolate intervention and effect, as discussed in chapter 5 and earlier in this chapter. However, the point is that rather than analyzing the evidential status of the curves, most people used them to *make sense* of the restrictions. How people experience data informs their path of action. When we interviewed Pernille the second time in October 2020, she reflected on the red-and-green curves, saying: "I found it really overwhelming. I thought 'My God! Will so many people be infected?' And I thought, we'd better act a little more carefully." Pernille, who sanitized her groceries even before the pandemic, already was very careful. For her, the curves spoke to a sense of danger already present in her life. In January 2021, Jeppe (age 24) similarly mentioned the curves as being powerful, but in a less emotional register: "I thought it made really good sense. Really, I'm a math teacher, so I guess it was the math in it that made me think, 'it is logical.' There are these two options: it can look all wrong or all good. From a mathematical perspective." In this quote, Jeppe does not analyze the underlying data, and he does not question the normative assumptions. For him, the curves seem to make the lockdown meaningful by conveying a sense of mathematical precision.

Sebastian (age 34) who was interviewed in October 2020, said: "I thought some really bright people must have made these graphs somewhere. And therefore I think that you have to trust them." He did not find comfort in the mathematical simplicity of the curves as Jeppe did. Instead, he saw them as symbols of sophisticated work by clever people. For Sebastian, the curves were "signs" of science as much as science communication. He added that it was images from Italy of overburdened hospitals and rows of military vans with coffins that made the danger feel real: "When you see these scenes from Italy, then you think, okay, it probably makes sense to do something to stop this virus." The same data representation, including the red-and-green curves, comes to make sense to people through different pathways of sense-making.

As I was reading the interview transcripts, I began realizing how I also read the daily COVID numbers in an emotional register. I could get worried looking at curves that take a bend regardless of the levels of infection, sometimes even ignoring my own analytical precautions about numbers that should not be compared. Apparently, I am no different than Torben and Flemming from chapter 5. Similar disregard for careful data analysis has unfolded when I have been communicating with friends in other countries. In June 2021, for example, Sydney went into lockdown at the same time as Denmark was lifting restrictions—although the infection rates were higher per capita in Denmark than in Sydney. I could simultaneously sympathize with my friends in Sydney who worried about rising numbers and feel relieved about the much-higher Danish numbers that had at least stabilized. Even when we train ourselves to use data with analytical care, they work on many of us through an emotional register.

Data do not contain any clear message about what is the "right level" of risk. They gain power through human interpretation. Similarly, data cannot create trust on their own. As one data analyst remarked with a hint of humor, alluding to the data that he worked hard to communicate as truthfully as possible: "I only trust the numbers I myself have manipulated!" During the pandemic, I have noticed how people rarely lean on data alone when explaining their choices. They describe themselves as part of a community, using expressions such as "being in this together" and "we are all in the same boat" and speaking about their local communities or Denmark as a whole as "managing this pretty well." Anders (age 54) said in November 2020 that he was proud of his local community, and he then confirmed his trust in the authorities and in particular the director of the Danish Health Authority, Søren Brostrøm, in this way:

> If the health services and Søren Brostrøm says, "Just do it, God damn it," then I do it. No doubt. He doesn't tell me to do anything for his own sake. He's telling me for my own sake. That's how naïve I am (laughing) . . . When anybody says "Jump!" I just ask, "How high?" It has worked before for me.

Anders is not naive, but he is convinced that he is better off following advice than trying to figure out for himself what to do. Beate (age 24), conversely, did not find any reason to trust the authorities. Sofie á Rogvi interviewed Beate because of her stated opposition to the government approach. Beate is one of the few who are convinced that it is all a conspiracy: "I believe 100 percent that coronavirus is planned. It is to, well, in a way, to decimate the weak, because they are too expensive for the rest of society. They are doing that." Who "they" are is not clear in this quote, but that is partly her point: the people pulling the strings are hiding from view. Beate was also convinced that vaccines are introduced to "control people." Just as Anders seemed to trust the authorities based on past experience, Beate did *not* trust them, also based on past experience. They both depended on communities of interpretation to make sense of the data. Both the opponents and the supporters of governmental policies glean information from their communities of belonging—it is just different communities—and they do so based on their experiences of whom they trust to be on their side. People learn from people, not just data.

Governments are no different. A study of government responses to the pandemic showed that shifting policies did not build on data or new evidence, but rather on mimicking the responses of other governments: "In times of severe crisis, governments follow the lead of others and base their decisions on what other countries do" (Sebhatu, Wennberg, Arora-Jonsson, and Lindberg et al. 2020: 21201). When the Danish government decided to adopt a mask policy, it came just weeks after the authorities had released an analysis stating that there was no evidence of effect. As the government decided to follow the World Health Organization (WHO) and surrounding countries and impose masks, the authorities then released a new report based on practically the same studies as their previous report, but now saying that public masking might have a positive effect. Just like citizens, governments listen to people they respect, not to data alone.

I remarked previously that supporters and opponents were questioning the logic of government interpretations and restrictions in similar ways, though they differed in their willingness to obey the rules. Both sides articulated similar reflections when trying to make sense of the pandemic. Citizens use numbers to produce meaning, and they seek to make numbers meaningful. They do not only analyze death tolls and infections rates—they try to make sense of them in a normative way. This was obvious, for example, when we asked people in the interviews to reflect on "Why do you think we are in this situation?" Among the responses, several supporters of the government approach said things that were not that different from Beate, who saw coronavirus as a tool for decimating the weak. While Beate was just twenty-four and thought with horror about the decimation of the weak, the seventy-six-year-old Hanne, who supported the government's approach, said:

> There are . . . these people saying that we all need to be vaccinated, we should do this and that, because "people are not allowed to die." But we're all going to die at some point, God damn it, if the old ones—yes, I know I sound a bit cynical, but that's my way of expressing myself—if the old ones are not allowed to die, where will you make space for the newborns? . . . We have had yellow fever, and the plague, and we have had—well, it's not like I'm religious, but the Earth might need to clean out and make space once in a while.

For Beate, the pandemic was somebody's plan; for Hanne, it was nature's response. Similar to Hanne, Edith, at seventy-nine-years-old, said that the pandemic might be a way of ending meaningless life:

> You can't help getting a little philosophical and ask, "Is it worth it?" It is this cynical assessment that pops up once in a while . . . I mean, I can't in good conscience say that anybody should purposefully be killed, but I could sometimes say that we should hold back on the preservation of life.

For Edith, the pandemic made sense as a way of making lives end in a society that kept old people alive at any price but offered them only biological life, not a life worth living. Other supporters of the government's approach saw in the pandemic a reason to question overpopulation, globalization, hygiene standards, and a wide range of political priorities. They do not understand the pandemic as just a matter of data analysis: they are trying to make sense of the changes around them in morally and politically embedded ways, and through the communities in which they see themselves as belonging. In line with the esteemed scholars with whom I began this chapter, they saw in the pandemic crisis a reason for rearticulating their opinions and used these opinions to make sense of the crisis. Žižek (2020) suggests that such longing for meaning is a mistake:

> We should resist the temptation to treat the ongoing epidemic as something that has a deeper meaning: the cruel but just punishment of humanity for the ruthless exploitation of other forms of life on earth. If we search for such a hidden message, we remain premodern: we treat our universe as a partner in communication (14).

Still, human beings tend to search for meaning, and how they orient themselves in the world shapes the kind of spaces they come to inhabit. Just as we have never been modern, to paraphrase Latour (1993), we have never stopped being premodern, if premodern means longing for meaning. People are not computers; they are embodied and emotional beings trying to make sense of the world around them.

WISDOM: PRIORITIES, PROTECTION, AND CAUTION

The pandemic also reinvigorated the key paradox of data as sources of knowledge: data clearly were used for drawing invalid conclusions, while the whole pandemic situation simultaneously appeared worse in countries with limited available data and no respect for data predictions. It takes competence and care to use data well. What, then, was the wise way to respond to the viral threat? What was a wise use of data? Which countries took the right approach? Which losses, tragedies, and lives—or ways of life—count in such a calculation?

Answers to normative questions about who took the right approach cannot be data driven (Weible, Nohrstedt, Cairney et al. 2020). Data can, and in many cases should, inform assessments of relative merits, but they cannot settle questions about which goals that are worth pursuing. Furthermore, data are extremely difficult to interpret when making comparisons among different contexts. From the outset, the Danish governmental strategy focused on protecting the weak and vulnerable, at least rhetorically, but what type of weakness? Prime Minister Frederiksen focused on virological vulnerability when announcing the lockdown, but just weeks later, when commenting on how to open the country back up, she said that it was time to prioritize those harmed by the lockdown: people with mental illness, children in families with abuse, the homeless, and other vulnerable people (Outzen 2020). It was a different type of vulnerability—a different aspect of the pandemic. Even while talking about those negatively affected by the lockdown, she nevertheless insisted on prioritizing biological life more highly than social and economic life; in her words: "What is more important than anything else is to save as many lives as possible!" In a sense, it looks as if Agamben (1995, 2020) was right when seeing his thoughts about a reduction to "bare life" played out in relation to the pandemic. Still, I cannot see it as just an excuse for installing a state of exception. The prime minister had to choose priorities, and at least she was clear about them. Frederiksen furthermore complicated the notion of a reduction to "bare life" when she added that the real danger was actually not just the loss of lives, but the loss of faith in the institutions that we depend on to live our lives with a sense of basic security: "As a society, we simply cannot afford to let the institutions we otherwise trust break down" (quoted in Outzen 2020). Biological life here gives way to a form of collective life: trust in societal institutions as a common good. Whether she succeeded on that parameter remains difficult to ascertain (Petersen 2021).

As the pandemic has unfolded, however, it has become clear that collectives, in order to prioritize and care for some, exclude and ignore others. All around the world, governments have valued some lives more than others, as many refugees, sex workers, drug users, and others in marginal positions have come to realize (Outsideren 2020; Heissel 2020; WHO 2020; Faber and

Hansen 2020; Sørensen 2020). In the Global North, people in low-income jobs have been working throughout the pandemic in warehouses, delivery services, and as "self-employed" assistants in the platform economy, where they have had to face viral risks so that others could work safely from home. Meanwhile the platform owners have profited enormously from the boom in online trade (BBC News 2020). Measures to protect older people in privileged countries also involved the redistribution of risk globally. One report even suggested that as a consequence of changed economic conditions aimed at protecting older people in the Global North, the global child mortality rates would go up, in particular in the Global South (Roberton, Carter, Chou et al. 2020). In 2022, Oxfam released a report stating that, in the course of the pandemic,

> the world's 10 richest men have doubled their fortunes, while over 160 million people are projected to have been pushed into poverty. . . . The cost of the profound inequality we face is in human lives. As this paper shows, based on conservative estimates, inequality contributes to the deaths of at least 21,300 people each day (Ahmed 2022: 9)

It seems that at least some of the activists expressing mistrust of government restrictions got something right when sensing that the pandemic would benefit the elite at the expense of people like themselves. In Frank Snowden's book about the history of epidemics, he succinctly observes that "every society produces its own specific vulnerabilities" (Snowden 2019b: 7), which any epidemic then exposes.

Measures to protect human life also implied a massive loss of animal life. Just in Denmark, a mass slaughter of mink took place in November 2020, when a mutation of SARS-CoV-2 became associated with mink farming (Hagemann-Nielsen 2020). Almost three times as many Danish minks as there are Danish citizens were culled and mostly buried in mass graves (admittedly, they were to be killed anyway, but not in this way). It brought an end to mink farming in Denmark, as the particular Danish Saga mink breed is now extinct, and it was carried out in such haste that no legal mandate was in place. In a world of viral entanglement, protection of human life also has implications for animals, and as Svendsen (2022) vividly argues: prioritization cuts across species and sacrifices some for the benefit of others. Data cannot tell you which dimensions to prioritize, nor can they delineate the collective that needs to choose priorities. It takes "Data Wisdom" to make such choices.

PARADOXES OF PANDEMIC POLITICS

To sum up the lessons of COVID-19 for the politics of intensified data sourcing, it has stimulated a *data pandemic,* where data, just like the virus, have experienced exponential growth on a global scale. The pandemic fueled already-dominant data promises and put data integration, surveillance technologies, digitization, self-service, and home monitoring "on speed." Again, data promises could claim benefits based on the hope of *future* evidence. In many cases, the pandemic implied abandoning even established norms of evidence without reflecting on what to put in its place (Hoffman 2020), as when several countries, including the United States, quickly decided to lower the evidence threshold for new treatments to speed up any mitigating options (Meyer 2020). Many researchers began to base conclusions on preprints rather than wait for peer-reviewed papers. Nevertheless, in Denmark the pandemic also illustrated the benefits of highly integrated data infrastructures (Pottegård, Bruun Kristensen, Reilev et al. 2020). The existing digital options for communication, furthermore, made the transition to healthcare at a distance much more seamless than in many other wealthy and technologically advanced countries. I think it is also evident, even though the global pandemic is not over as I am writing this, that data—and data predictions—have helped save lives.

The pandemic widened the scope of data living and instigated a boom in data work. Looking at data representations became a daily occupation for most citizens. Looking at data is an embodied act, not just an analytical achievement. Although examining more or less the same graphs, people had remarkably different data experiences. The pandemic also made many more citizens realize that their samples and health data *are* being reused, and it is now obvious that not everybody agrees with this reuse—not even in Denmark. Many citizens gained a new data literacy and suddenly understood terms such as "false positive tests" and "R-number," but for many, this increased data literacy also provided more awareness of how difficult it is to interpret data. Data do not speak for themselves after all. It might have changed the future conditions for data politics: a more general awareness seems to be emerging around data as carriers of values and priorities.

In the previous chapters, building mostly on fieldwork conducted prior to the pandemic, I have emphasized how data can be used to close political conflicts or depoliticize decisions. Now, I have realized how the public data spectacle also opened up political conflicts. Many supporters of the government would question the same issues as opponents and still see opposition as "irrational." For those disagreeing with the moral and political values shaping the government approach, however, data became the hook on which to hang their complaints. In paradoxical ways, *data simultaneously close down and open up political contestation*. The undetermined space of data probability can end up being filled with moral certainty. The window of epistemic doubt is closed with political and moral stances as people decide who to trust, which community to join.

It is dangerous when societies fall into antagonistic camps of people unable to communicate because they subscribe to different "facts" or different communities of fact-making. If the authorities wish to establish a conversation with an increasingly hostile opposition, it is probably not useful to maintain that opponents *simply* misunderstand the data, even when they do. Policymakers and researchers must be willing to discuss the valuations shaping their own data analyses, as also suggested by Oreskes (2019) in relation to other data conflicts. Without honesty about values and political priorities, data can unleash violent and divisive forces. Here might rest a more general lesson for data politics. Bickerton and Accetti (2021) talk about *technopopulism* as a type of governance that presents itself as a simple technical solution to the management of state affairs. It is "populist" because it claims to govern for *the* people as a singular entity with one set of interests. In technopopulist regimes, those in office present themselves as the clever interpreters of data. Data, however, never serve all citizens equally well. Any data analysis involves priorities. To use data wisely, therefore, is also to dare to reflect on—and articulate—the priorities shaping the analyses and to open up these priorities for political debate. The political scientist Anna Durnová (2019) similarly suggests that for science to retain legitimacy in politics, scientists must refrain from claiming neutrality. We must all acknowledge the normative—and even emotional—aspects of various data analyses, exactly because "public debates on science mediate values and beliefs through emotional appeals" (Durnová 2019: 46). Human beings do not simply compute data messages; they engage them with a meaning-seeking and emotional intent. Their embrace of data also depends on their relationship to those who produce the data representations. Among those who reject certain data, we find many people with the experiences of not being heard, not being cared for, and not sharing a vision of the Good Life with those in power. They do not feel respected. When, conversely, people experience institutions as embodying care and respect, they are more likely to accept the data that these institutions use to do their job (Taylor 2020).

My own work is also informed by norms, of course, and I should be honest about them. They revolve around solidarity, justice, and mutual recognition, as I will explain when I turn to the ethics of intensified data sourcing in the conclusion. Humans (and nonhuman forms of life) are so fully and utterly entangled that it is necessary to build communities in which we can live together, even when wanting to live different lives. A virus knows no borders. It does not acknowledge race, gender, or class. Some forms of virus even move between species. It is the ways in which we erect borders and differentiate—based on parameters such as race, gender, and class—that shape the forms of suffering that a virus eventually instigates. We need social institutions that are able to care for all if we are to respond to viral threats in ways in which everybody is willing to join the fight. This is a normative point, and as I sum up my overall argument next, I elucidate how I think that a more explicitly normative approach to data politics can help conserve the benefits of intensified data sourcing and reduce the risks.

CONCLUSION: DATA PARADOXES

What are the drivers for, and the implications of, intensified data sourcing? I have been pondering this question for years now, and rather than clear-cut answers, my pursuit of answers has led me to a set of paradoxes. Every time I have identified one driver and one implication, I have realized that intensified data sourcing also involves very diverse—sometimes almost completely opposite—drivers, as well as very different implications for other people elsewhere, or the same people at a later stage or connected to a different agenda. I therefore believe that instead of hoping for simple answers—for example, taking the form of predictions about what intensified data sourcing can be expected to do everywhere and anytime—practitioners and scholars need to remain curious about what is at stake in any local situation. For many anthropologists and science and technology studies (STS) scholars, this attention to locality is already on the menu. The key question is how an improved understanding of the complex challenges of intensified data sourcing also can inform practical solutions and facilitate better future uses of data. I believe that awareness of paradoxes can destabilize premature conclusions and nudge both scholars and practitioners to contemplate additional dimensions of a problem. Paradoxes are complicated, though, because they suggest complexity. Complexity does not easily guide actions. How can we train not just social scientists, but also data scientists, technology developers, administrators, and policymakers to care about local specificities? How can insights from anthropology, STS, and critical data studies help practitioners and scholars from other fields to think about solutions in new ways?

To avoid a deadlock of complexity, I will make two moves. After summarizing my argument about the paradoxical drivers for and implications of intensified data sourcing, I first suggest a new metaphor with which to think about data. Some might say that it is an analogy rather than a metaphor, but I leave such issues to philosophers. Instead of the common value-oriented metaphors of oil and gold, I propose to think of data as drugs. My intention is to stimulate curiosity and encourage better questions with which to explore local implications. My second move is to suggest some alternatives to the dominant framing of the ethics of intensified data sourcing. With a different normative framework, I hope to inspire reflections on how to regulate intensified data sourcing in a balanced manner aimed at the common good. Before I outline any alternatives, however, I summarize my analysis.

WHEN DATA PROMISES HIT THE GROUND: THE STORY IN BRIEF

Contemporary healthcare in high-income countries is becoming increasingly data intensive. A wide range of different stakeholders want more data, of better quality, on more people, and they want to use them for more purposes. Consultants, information technology specialists, administrators, and policymakers happily articulate what I have called "data promises." In reports, strategy papers, and policy documents, at conferences and during high-profile meetings and workshops, these proponents of data intensification suggest an imminent future where doctors are replaced by statisticians and robots and healthcare governance becomes data-driven through processes that simultaneously ensure economic growth. The result is said to be disruption of healthcare as we know it. As an echo of Facebook's early motto, "Move fast and break things" (Halting Problem 2017), a new healthcare system is proclaimed to be about to rise like a phoenix from the ashes of the desired blaze.

Despite the high hopes, the bold data promises have a hard time materializing on the ground. An important motivation for me in writing this book has been the plain observation of a series of significant gaps. These are gaps between the promises of disruption and hard-to-change everyday practices; between a sort of data gospel about automation and concrete and often manual data work; and between prophecies of future seamlessness and present-day experiences with hitches and hassles. Of course, data *do* perform important—and expected—tasks in healthcare organizations, all in line with declared purposes. Data *do* boost research outputs. Data tools *do* deliver more precise diagnostics, treatment, and adequate monitoring of patients. They *do* facilitate increased political and administrative control. Data *do* help to ensure consistent growth rates in the medical industry.

However, investments in data do not always deliver, and sometimes what they do deliver is curiously different from what the promises suggested. Furthermore, most of the new data practices are much more mundane, low-tech, and time-consuming than data promises suggest. Patients and citizens respond to questionnaires. They are asked to rate their ability to self-care on a scale from one to ten. They use monitoring devices and upload results to central databases. Doctors and nurses spend increasing amounts of time looking at data, or trying to find data in the expanding databases. Administrators depend on increasing amounts of data to produce reports on organizational performance, but they sometimes do so while being well aware that these data do not convey an adequate impression of the performance they want to measure. Academic and industrial researchers are obtaining easier access to data, but some new users of data do not know what the data mean. It is all pretty far from the promised magical high-tech dust that was supposed to fall as glitter on the old cumbersome clinical routines.

In place of the total disruption of everyday healthcare practices, we see investments in something slightly duller and more conventional: *digitization* and *information infrastructures*. In place of disruption, there is infrastructural integration. At first glance, infrastructural integration speaks to old dreams of a "world brain" of all available information (see chapter 5). However, after years of data integration, the predominant experience in Denmark seems to be that no system can capture "all data on everything" (see chapter 3). Nor is it possible to reach agreement on what data mean, who should use them, and for what purposes. With the integration of multiple sources of data come not only more information, but also a haze of data, or what Andrejevic (2013) calls "infoglut." Data integration is never complete, and data are never transparent. The vision of completeness as a step toward a transparent "world brain" of all available information is what Jasanoff and colleagues call a "sociotechnical imaginary" (Jasanoff and Kim 2013; Hurlbut, Jasanoff, and Saha 2020). It works through the ambitions it installs more than the results it delivers.

Though infrastructural changes sound duller than total disruption they are very important. Intensified data sourcing means that data are now serving research, clinical, governmental, and industrial purposes. This multiplication of purposes is an important transformation. The four purposes overlap (one purpose can become a means for another), and the same actors can be dedicated to several purposes, or even all four of them. I have grouped them in this way to illustrate how various stakeholders want to use data to pursue at least four goods: knowledge, health, governance, and wealth. Each type of good has a less benevolent counterpart. Instead of knowledge, data can be used to create a haze that generates unnecessary doubt or help researchers achieve bibliometric targets without delivering insights. Instead of health, data practices can make clinicians pursue patient satisfaction or other performance measurements. Instead of good governance, data can be used for surveillance and control. Instead of wealth, data may serve plain greed and the unrestrained accumulation of capital. My main point, however, is that even when we accept just the benevolent intentions, we have to acknowledge that the four purposes do not always align.

How are we to understand the friction between these purposes? Cutting across all chapters, I have pointed to the *ontological multiplicity* of data as a key feature of intensified data sourcing. I am well aware that ontological multiplicity is a somewhat convoluted expression, and yet I have found it necessary to use it to reorient the otherwise epistemological problematization of data. My point is that data do not just *mean* several things; they *are* several things, or rather they *do* several things simultaneously. Health data might be data on a patient's disease at the same time that they are data on the treating physician, the hospital, and the laboratory that delivered a test. Data can affect each of these arenas differently, depending on who uses them for what. To accept ontological multiplicity involves investigating data, not just for what they signify, but for the diverse effects they may have in several arenas at the same time, or how effects can shift for the same actors over time. Because intensified data sourcing implies that data serve an increasing number of purposes, they become like cogs operating in several machines at once (to repeat the image from chapter 5). The machines are producing different things, but they depend on the same parts. Such friction can make machines collapse.

I have described a shift from curated transfers of information to automated pooling. This shift accelerates the speed of all the motors in which data operate. In the period of curated transfers, where selected pieces of clinical information went into central registries, there was limited feedback when data were reused for a new purpose. Researchers accessing data through Statistics Denmark did not report when they found an error in clinical reporting because they were not allowed to disturb a different system. As the various systems become increasingly interconnected, disturbances begin to proliferate. Some of these disturbances are beneficial for patient treatments. Patients can notify clinicians when they discover inaccurate reporting of symptoms; people working with quality controls can ensure higher degrees of consistency in treatment; and doctors can correct their own prescription patterns through automated feedback comparing them to others—to mention just a few of the examples from the preceding chapters.

Other disturbances, however, risk undermining the clinical function of patient data. When clinicians complain about drowning in meaningless data work, that is an important red flag indicating possibly perilous disturbances. When researching physicians seek to boost their research by using their position in reference groups for quality databases to increase everyday clinical demands of documentation and have these demands integrated into electronic medical record systems, then research aims are taking precedence over clinical aims. When politicians and administrators govern through forms of data-work-of-instruction that make clinicians overrule their own best judgment to comply with standardized demands, that is no longer *good* governance. It puts clinical goals at risk. Similarly, the increased emphasis on using data as vehicles of economic growth also risks jeopardizing the public legitimacy and stability of the integrated data infrastructures (Skovgaard, Wadmann, and Hoeyer 2019; Skovgaard and Hoeyer 2022; Sterckx, Rakic, Cockbain, and Borry 2015; Vezyridis and Timmons 2017, 2021).

Data promises draw on powerful ideas about informatization, but bodies and healthcare organizations are always more than information. The care for suffering bodies is difficult to disrupt. The complexity and multidimensionality of bodies cannot be turned into data. Suffering bodies need care. Furthermore, even data infrastructures are material. The bit economy is full of atoms, to turn Nicholas Negroponte's famous distinction against his own vision (Negroponte 1995). Digital data are not just ephemeral, cloudlike creatures. Danish news media even report cases where health data occasionally need to be transported as atoms, literally driven on trucks to supercomputers, because it would take too long via broadband (Møllerhøj and Engelhardt 2013). The constant appetite for data also has important ecological ramifications: digital data tools depend on mining of rare minerals, constant replacements of hardware, and an excessive consumption of electricity (Benko 2015; Crawford 2021). The internet is already consuming approximately 9 percent of the world's energy usage (Jensen 2020a). Within a few years, data centers are expected to increase the Danish energy consumption with 22 percent (Maguire and Winthereik 2021). Just as datafication does not eliminate bodily suffering, it does not deliver an escape from the climate catastrophe. It is not an option to live a life as just bits, but no atoms.

In the introduction, I suggested that if people want to see what intensified data sourcing looks like in real life, they should go to Denmark. Indeed, hundreds of delegations from all over the world already do just that. Denmark is a showcase for data infrastructures of the sort that the global data promises now inspire elsewhere: digitized healthcare and highly integrated information infrastructures. It is a country readily embracing what I called "wired medicine" in chapter 2—a term coined to capture the changing nature of healthcare in the Global North. However, in light of what I just wrote about the inability to reach the promised land of the data gospel, it should be clear that foreign policymakers will not get what they hope for by copying the Danish setup. Furthermore, even if they manage to establish similar database opportunities in their own countries, other nations will get something very different. With this book, I have argued that data always affect people's lives through local instantiation of infrastructures. This means that even similar software packages conjoined on comparable digital networks will do different things in different contexts. An information infrastructure is never just software and hardware; it is also a social texture shaped by political, economic, and legal histories. It is, therefore, not possible to do a controlled experiment in Denmark and then scale it up and expect it to have the same results in the United States or Japan.

Nevertheless, there is a lot to learn from studying Danish levels of data integration. The Danish experiences suggest a range of potential implications. For example, despite promises of seamless automation, intensified data sourcing generates new forms of work. I have suggested grouping data work into four types: *production, analysis, instruction,* and *use.* Data are not free. Besides the expenses related to work, intensified data sourcing depends on infrastructures that are expensive to establish and maintain. The more complex an infrastructure gets, the more repair work it demands. Nevertheless, policy papers often present data as a form of commons out there—available and free. I therefore believe that my argument about the ongoing transformations being different from the disruption evoked by data promises carries a more general insight that reaches beyond Danish borders.

Infrastructural changes may have profound effects. Academic observers, media, and policymakers have a well-known tendency to simultaneously overestimate technological transformations in the short run (as when expecting a total disruption) and underestimate their long-term implications. Technologies of data are no different. With the early registries and their curated one-way transfers of information to central databases, narratives remained local and in the custody of the clinicians. With the gradual shift toward automated pooling of data, even the narrative part of patient documentation is now "potentialized" for infinite future reuse (Taussig, Hoeyer, and Helmreich 2013; Bowker 2005).

As clinicians no longer control who gets access to what, notions of professional confidentiality may transmute in ways that we cannot imagine yet. Also, data are used in organizational decision making in ways that are destabilizing ideas about knowledge. Much to the regret of clever and experienced data analysts, the increased focus on becoming data-driven has meant that the political and administrative top management have become increasingly content with quick and dirty uses of data. The time and resources needed to make sense of data are lacking. By centralizing data infrastructures and opening them up for multiple and simultaneous forms of (superficial) data reuse, the conditions for politics are thereby changing. Power balances shift. When data serve as handmaidens of decision-makers, intensified data sourcing also affects something even more basic for the human perception of the world: what counts as true. Intensified data sourcing thereby undermines the epistemic authority of data that gave them their appeal and authority in the first place. In *The Postmodern Condition*, Lyotard noted how the computerized database gained authority through a notion of data serving as references to particular aspects of the outside world. Databases were dissolving this reference, Lyotard (1984) argued. According to Poster (1990), the point was that "increasingly meaning is sustained through mechanisms of self-referentiality and the non-linguistic thing, the referent, fades into obscurity" (13). Intensified data sourcing seems to involve an organizational willingness to accept dissolving referentiality.

It may sound abstract, but I am pointing to something very concrete. In systems ruled through data, health professionals and bureaucrats have to manipulate data. It took more than a century to build the social robustness of claims based on data and to make people trust a data analysis (Oreskes 2019; Daston and Galison 2010; Zuboff 1989). Anthropology and STS have taken issue with this robustness and its implied objectivity. However, now is also the time to express concern about what will happen if trust in data disappears (Poirier 2021). If it becomes an everyday organizational reality that data cannot be trusted, then what steps into the place of trust? What fills the void? These changes might be more profound than what is suggested by terms such as "smart healthcare."

I do not suggest the resuscitation of blind trust in data. It is not useful to claim objectivity and cover up opinion as facts. I think that greater acknowledgment of the *limits* of data can help preserve all the benefits of intensified data sourcing. The first step is to acknowledge that healthcare must build on several types of knowledge. It is important to talk about tactile skills, action skills, and—perhaps—about *associative thinking* as elements of both clinical and organizational judgment. Similarly, it is important to acknowledge *data experiences*. Data work on people. They work on embodied beings. Humans are poorly understood when viewed simply as faulty computers. They form judgments in other ways. These ways need training (Kahneman, Sibony, and Sunstein 2021). Training depends on strong institutional cultures. To get out of the promissory cloud and back onto the ground, therefore, is also to get back into the body. It is to get back to a serious engagement with how human beings think, work, and thrive. In contemporary healthcare, clinicians and administrators must be able to read and analyze data, but they must also be able to identify the proper space for data among other sources of knowledge. In an even more general sense, the notion of evidence must be broadened. Both clinicians and regulators need to expand the range of knowledge forms that inform their understanding of evidence—and include new big data methodologies, as well as understanding of the social dynamics of data reuse.

As the COVID-19 pandemic struck, bodily engagement with data became a daily experience for most citizens. The pandemic created a data-political moment of unprecedented strength. Politics based on data predictions made the need for careful data analysis more obvious than it might ever have been before. In some ways, the pandemic also became a reason to rethink several of my points, not least the one about the inertia of healthcare. With the sudden lockdowns, rapid reorganization of healthcare suddenly looked possible. In addition, the pandemic challenged the image of a population comfortable with extreme data integration. Suddenly, some people took to the streets—they challenged test regimes and complained about reuse of data for research. Not only did citizens now question data infrastructures, they also questioned the values informing the data predictions that ruled their lives. Data predictions are analytical products that come in the form of probabilities. Both the proponents and opponents of government politics filled the void of epistemological certainty with a form of moral certitude. This moral certitude precluded a dialogue between what was becoming two sides of a conflict. Data politics thereby seems to involve a particular risk of social bifurcation. Dealing with this risk is likely to prove to be one of the major challenges of our times.

As I have recounted my argument, I have drawn out the most important points from the preceding chapters, but none of these points is without contradictory examples. Throughout the book, therefore, I have told the story through paradoxes. I now recapitulate these paradoxes and my reason for insisting on paradoxical narratives.

PARADOXES: LEARNING TO APPRECIATE OPPOSING STORIES

I believe that paradoxes are useful vehicles for thinking because they inspire us to acknowledge that several transformations can take place simultaneously. Paradoxical narratives stand in contrast to how data discourses usually frame knowledge products. The lure of data promises partly stems from the hope of being able to close a case with a statistical argument. It flattens the dimensions of a problem. It reduces complexity. As Luhmann (1999) has insightfully suggested, most of us have an urge to reduce complexity. Many clinicians have a deep desire for certainty. This is understandable. Clinicians carry the lives of patients in their hands. They want to be sure that they establish the right diagnoses and administer the right treatments. Administrators and politicians also want certainty. They are frustrated about not knowing whether they are prioritizing the right initiatives. When they want to become data-driven, they seek affirmation of their decisions. Paradoxes, in contrast, inspire analysts to be prepared for the unexpected. That can be scary. My hope is that anticipation of paradoxes can make complexity more fun, and in a sense more manageable. If conflicting trends are what to expect, there is a comfort in finding them. The comfort of certitude, however, is not within reach.

I have found paradoxes attractive because for me, they have offered a way of overcoming the division between two positions that have shaped debates about data in the scholarly literature, as well as among the people I have studied: the pro and con positions, the semireligious data gospel, and the unforgiving criticism among data critics. The "Data Wisdom" that I would like to see in healthcare organizations cannot grow in soil fertilized only with hopeful gospel or fearful dread. Paradoxes serve as an invitation to contemplate "both and" rather than "either or."

In table 7.1, I list the paradoxes I have discussed in the preceding chapters. These paradoxes represent what I believe are the most important implications of intensified data sourcing in healthcare. I have added an extra paradox to the list: *data move too freely, and data never move freely enough.* This final paradox is an addition that represents a fundamental conundrum of all data integration. I described it in chapter 2 as being embedded in the paradox of empowerment/disempowerment when referencing Brown and Duguid's classic work on "sticky" and "leaky" data (Brown and Duguid 2000). Still, it deserves its own mention in the list because it cuts across all chapters and is endemic to intensified data sourcing: with an increasing

Table 7.1
The paradoxes of intensified data sourcing

Data promises thrive on a claimed need for evidence	. . . and . . .	data needs and initiatives are rarely backed by such evidence.
Data empower citizens	. . . and . . .	data disempower citizens.
Data uncover patient concerns	. . . and . . .	data cover up patient concerns.
Data mean less work	. . . and . . .	data create more work.
Data create meaningless tasks	. . . and . . .	data are used as meaning-making tools.
Data intensification tightens organizational control	. . . and . . .	data intensification facilitates organizational disintegration.
Data become successful through standardization	. . . and . . .	data are never able to standardize human experience.
Data dematerialize interactions	. . . and . . .	data rematerialize interactions.
Data are used to draw invalid conclusions	. . . and . . .	lack of data can be worse.
Data close down and conceal political choices	. . . and . . .	data open up and unsettle political choices.
Data move too freely	. . . and . . .	data never move freely enough.

number of stakeholders, people will not agree on who should use data for what. What appears to some as too-restricted access will be too lax from the perspective of others. This is not a particularly Danish point: it is a consequence of the ontological multiplicity of data used for an increasing range of purposes.

I do not suggest paradoxical thinking as some form of analytical panacea. For me, the figure of the paradox arose as a response to specific challenges associated with data doing different things in different work practices (production, analysis, instruction, and use) aimed at producing different values (knowledge, health, governance and wealth). As I have argued toward the end of each chapter, opposing stories tend to be politically expedient: in the tension between opposing narratives, stakeholders can select the truths that fit their agenda in that moment. The politics of data unfolds in the tension between opposing narratives. Should this paradoxical approach be useful for other social phenomena or practices, it will have to prove it through concrete analysis. It cannot serve as a theoretical dogma replacing empirical engagement.

The various data uses and registers of value have each been carefully theorized by leading scholars in STS, anthropology, sociology, and critical data studies. Paradoxical thinking was for me a way of bringing together the insightful work on how data intensification operates in and affects *research* (Biruk 2018; Prainsack 2017; Leonelli 2016), the *clinic* (Hunt, Bell, Baker, and Howard 2017; Wiener 2000; Wachter 2017), the *administration* of healthcare (Jerak-Zuiderent and Bal 2011; Pollitt, Harrison, Dowswell et al. 2010; Pedersen 2019a; Bonde, Bossen, and Danholt 2018; Hogle 2019), health *politics* (Adams 2016a; Ashmore, Mulkay, and Pinch 1989; Bigo, Isin, and Ruppert 2019; Merry 2016; Murphy 2017) and the commercial actors associated with *industry* (Mcfall 2019; Daemmrich 2004; Sadowski 2019b; Sharon 2016). It is necessary to conjure these strains of work because the predominant effect of intensified data sourcing is the way in which infrastructural integration makes such otherwise different practices interact.

I am, of course, not the first to write about data paradoxes. Xiao-Li Meng, a statistician, has used the term "data paradox" to describe the counterintuitive fact that exponential growth in data can lower, rather than increase, statistical strength because of increased data velocity and variety and inadequate statistical theorizing (Meng 2018). Media researchers have used the term "big-data paradox" to describe how even with "seeming big data, the data at the individual level is often extremely limited for most users" (Liu, Morstatter, Tang, and Zafarani 2016: 141). Others refer to "data paradoxes" in a different sense, more akin to "irony" or "sad observation" (Davis 2017; Kaźmierska 2020). This also seems to be the case when the legal scholar Frank Pasquale (2015) talks about how blackboxing of information sources embodies the "paradox of the so-called information age: data is becoming staggering in its breadth and depth, yet often information most important to us is out of our reach, available only to insiders" (191, see also Tanner 2017). I agree with these observations, but this is not how I use the term "paradox" in this book. I think of data paradoxes as instances where *opposing narratives about what data do are both partly true*. With this take on data paradoxes, I wish to prepare the mind for discovering the unexpected, unwarranted, and contradictory effects of new data initiatives.

The embrace of multiplicity and complexity should not make analysts shy away from articulating clear trends. For example, I do think that it is worth noting how healthcare systems marked by intensified data sourcing—*in general*—come to prioritize research, administration, and commercial interests at the expense of the clinic and patient care. I agree with Kieran Healy (2017), who says that social scientists who only wish to bring nuance to the table risk missing the most important message. Conversely, I am also aware that there are ethnographers who would have wanted to see more detail, more ethnographic presence—more nuance, as it were—in the preceding pages. My analytical ambition has constantly been a synthesis of the drivers for, and the implications of, intensified data sourcing rather than a detailed study of any individual data uses. I wanted to understand what happens when more people want more data and use them for more purposes. I wanted to describe the interplay of policy, practice, and experience. The book was therefore never to be a nuanced ethnography of a particular patient group, clinic, research laboratory, governance office, or country. Paradoxes make it possible to bring together and understand even conflicting local narratives from diverse sites as elements of the same social forces of intensified data sourcing. Rather than dissolving into endless variance (nuance), I think of paradoxical thinking as a way of exploring intensified data sourcing and the shift toward wired medicine in a more comprehensive manner.

Despite the many good reasons for embracing paradoxes, I am aware that they may appear as overly byzantine figures of thought. They do not easily translate into practice. I have therefore thought about how to make it easier to pose questions that are relevant in local contexts where people work. As stated already, my suggestion is a new metaphor: *data as drugs*.

METAPHORS: OIL, GOLD, OR DRUGS?

Metaphors work as implicit frames of thought (Lakoff and Johnson 1980). I have several times alluded to my discontent with the dominant metaphors for data: "gold" and "oil." They make the attention revolve around wealth and profit, and thereby tacitly distort how policymakers and administrators prioritize the four types of goods that data are supposed to generate. Sally Wyatt (2022) has criticized the oil and mining metaphors. She points out how they not only lead people to ignore important questions related to how data are made rather than found, but also how people who refer to data as oil do not use the metaphor very well. They ignore, for example, how the oil industry is a source of pollution and a main factor in the climate crisis. They forget the externalities of wealth creation. Kate Crawford (2021) forcefully fleshes out how the data industry mirrors the exploitive mining industry delivering the raw materials for its digital infrastructure, saying that "those who profit from mining do so only because the costs must be sustained by others" (26). It is, as she points out, also how some forms of commercial data extraction tend to work. If used well, the metaphors might do a better job of stimulating reflections. However, as Wyatt argues, unexamined metaphors do not generate genuine thinking; they foreclose it.

I therefore suggest a different metaphor: *drugs*. It can inspire a wider range of questions. In many ways, data already form a part of treatments on par with drugs. Data *are* drugs, as it were. In chapter 2, on data living, I discussed how people like Lone undertake daily data monitoring and sometimes even think that they need a data holiday, just as Kane Race (2009) describes HIV patients taking breaks from their medication. For many chronic patients, a treatment regime without data is no more an option than a life without drugs. By pointing to drugs as a *metaphor* for data, however, I aim at something different. By thinking of data *as* drugs, I suggest using experiences with drugs to pose better questions when examining local data practices.

What does a drug metaphor offer the study of data? Most importantly, we are already accustomed to thinking about drugs as being steeped in paradox. They can be life-saving *and* they cost lives. They are expensive *and* they sometimes help save money. Drugs can do good *and* have bad side effects. They can heal *and* create addiction. They can be used *and* abused. Each of these paradoxes translates well to how we could think about data practices. Furthermore, a drug metaphor acknowledges that data are not some form of preexisting resource to be drilled out of the ground. Like drugs, data must be produced. Data result from activity, work, investments. A drug metaphor can help us remember that data are never obtained for nothing. The drug metaphor also acknowledges that there are potential benefits: drugs are extremely useful when used correctly. We thereby avoid debates about being for or against data.

When tuning in on the specific implications of a data initiative, the study of drugs has produced insights into mechanisms that can inspire questions that are also relevant when investigating data practices. For instance, it is well known that for drugs, there is a *dose-response curve* in the pharmaceutical effect (where you can get too much or too little of a given drug). Here, the metaphor might make policymakers consider the risks and benefits associated with both too many and too few data—whether in administration or clinical practice—and serve as an antidote to the attitude of "the more the merrier" that shapes many contemporary data initiatives. Drugs are also known to have side effects, and similarly, certain uses of data have unintended and detrimental effects, such as when people gain unauthorized access to patient data or use them for purposes that harm the individual. In an article on confidentiality, Grossman (1977) once made an analogy between data and drugs, noting that "personal data can be poisonous to the patient, depending on who uses it and how it is used" (43).

In relation to drugs, *polypharmacy* is known to involve serious risks of negative drug interactions. Similarly, multiple uses of data also involve risks of negative interactions, and a drug metaphor could inspire reflection on the risk of negative synergy in data initiatives. With drugs, commercial interests sometimes benefit from lacking *diagnostic accuracy* for prescriptions and from inflated off-label prescriptions. Similarly, the companies selling standard data tools sometimes seem to profit from lacking "diagnostic accuracy" with respect to data needs in healthcare organizations. It is a well-known problem with drugs that commercial research focuses on *initiation* rather than *discontinuation* of pharmaceutical treatment (Sismondo 2008; Wadmann 2014b). We can use this insight proactively in relation to data by directing attention and funding toward identifying when data collections cease to work. It ought to be on the agenda for administrators to establish practices for data discontinuation. Finally, drugs are known for having a placebo effect (Andersen 2011): they make people feel better even when the drug delivers no cure (or, as some would say it, the belief that a drug will bring a cure shapes its effects). Similarly, data proponents often seem unable to question the benefits of their own initiatives. They sometimes even feel an improvement that is so substantial that they ignore critiques from clinicians, as described in chapter 3.

Data tools are not only comparable to pharmaceutical drugs in the sense that they should be prescribed with care (not too many, not too few), studied for what they do in practice (make them subject to careful evaluation), and discontinued when no longer needed. Data practices are also comparable to drugs in a different sense of the word, namely *narcotics*: data can intoxicate and disturb the sense of reality. They can deliver kaleidoscopic visions of organizational reality. They can dissolve the sense of referentiality. Like drugs, data practices can get people addicted. Substance abuse can be dangerous. Data tools are often designed to ensure a form of technological lock-in, where it is difficult, even almost impossible, to shift to a different system. Addiction also comes across as a fear of losing control or overview if a data practice stops.

The drug metaphor and its narcotic associations can also help to shift attention to the more affective dimensions of data that I focused on in chapter 4. A drug metaphor might help stimulate reflections on how data work *feels*. Drugs—pharmaceuticals *and* narcotics—affect your moods. Data are no different. Drugs affect how people view themselves and others (Lane 2007) and can be associated with feelings of pride and shame. Again, data are no different. I found that in hospitals, health professionals sometimes strive to reach arbitrary goals because doing so *feels* better than working with no goal. Data can incite and arouse people—and create excitement and transitory moments of social cohesion. Unfortunately, as is the case with drugs, this can be followed by serious hangovers and withdrawal symptoms. Furthermore, drug experiences are not stable; they develop over time. Why should data experiences be any different? It is worth noting that Wyatt (2018) has warned against the use of the addiction metaphor in relation to digital technology because that construes social problems as individual deviance. She is right. We need an approach to data that performs better than the governance of illicit drugs. Data addictions should not be blamed on individuals. I will return to this point in my discussion of ethics later in this chapter.

A *drug* metaphor—covering both standard pharmaceutical and narcotic connotations— also should inspire consideration of *externalities*, including exploitive global relations of exchange, the risk of pollution, and environmental impact, and it should inspire more work on how to *regulate* intensified data sourcing. For drugs, there are regulatory regimes in place—however faulty they might be—and widespread agreement that there is a need to know something about whether and how drugs work before introducing them in the clinic (Petersen and Tanner 2015; Daemmrich 2004; Faulkner and Kent 2001). Data tools, conversely, are promoted without a similar interest in whether they work and what they do, and they are governed by much more lenient regulatory frameworks than drugs. In 2019, the US Food and Drug Administration (FDA) published an action plan stating that rather than assessing the safety and effect of health apps, they would authorize selected big tech companies to develop them (US Food & Drug Administration 2019; Lievevrouw, Marelli, and Van Hoyweghen 2021). Imagine if the pharmaceutical industry were granted the same authority to control its own products. Data tools can rarely be tested in randomized clinical trials (RCTs) as drugs can, but still, it is dangerous to go full speed on a digital transformation aimed at using data tools for treatments without establishing proper regulatory oversight. It is also well known that drugs have more than biological effects and need to be studied from multiple disciplinary perspectives (Van der Geest, Whyte, and Hardon 1996; Whyte, Van der Geest, and Hardon 2003; Greene 2007; Dumit 2012). Similarly, data reach into areas of life that computer scientists rarely have the tools to explore. Different disciplines must collaborate if we are to use data wisely in healthcare.

In short, data are no less important for health services than drugs are. They deserve the same attention. I also hope that the drug metaphor can prompt new types of curiosity aimed at exploring their likely paradoxical implications. Although we are typically told that we should use data to look for *answers*, the most important form of knowledge that any practitioner needs is the ability to pose relevant *questions*. I propose that the drug metaphor will help policymakers and administrators articulate questions that are relevant for their own practices and data initiatives. I have suggested some of them as easy prompts in table 7.2—not to foreclose curiosity, but to sustain it. As Strathern (2007) observes: "We are in great peril if we do not cultivate curiosity in what is around us" (21).

Table 7.2

How a drug metaphor might prompt questions with which to explore local data practices

Metaphorical Observation	Questions with Which to Explore Data
Drugs are expensive to produce.	What are the costs of data, and how are they distributed?
There is a dose-response curve in the drug effects and a need for policies of discontinuation.	When do you collect too many and when too few data—whether in administration or clinical practice—and when it is time for data discontinuation?
Drugs have side-effects.	What are the unintended consequences of data initiatives?
Drugs have placebo effects.	How will we know the effects of data initiatives? Can data prove their own worth?
In drug development, industrial partners have weighty economic interests influencing their advice.	What should count as conflict of interest when companies provide advice on data initiatives?
Drugs have emotional effects and work through embodied experiences.	How do people's data experiences vary, and how do they shape what data do?
Drug use can lead to addiction and abuse and have delusional effects on some people.	When do data tools give rise to lock-in? When do they disturb perception? What counts as abuse?
Drugs need regulation.	How are data tools to be regulated?

ETHICS: THE INTOLERABLE INDIVIDUALIZATION OF RESPONSIBILITY

While this book has focused on the drivers for and implications of intensified data sourcing, my interests have—of course—also been informed by more normative questions. They have simmered beneath each of the chapters: Who is held accountable for data promises? How can the standardization involved in data living make room for human diversity? What is a fair distribution of data work? How can data experiences become recognized as more than a failure of people to behave like computers? What is "Data Wisdom"? I have been pondering these questions because I think that it is important to build and maintain healthcare systems that respond to patient hopes, needs, and concerns, regardless of their backgrounds and resources. However, questions of this type differ in significant ways from the usual framing of ethical issues in data-intensive healthcare.

I needed to first flesh out in detail my argument here before I can go on to explain my dissatisfaction with the dominant framing of ethics and, in particular, the regulatory "solutions" that it has given citizens. To the extent that "ethical concern" serves as the typical counterweight to data promises, there is a need to rethink data ethics. It is therefore with ethics and its relatively meager solutions that I end this conclusion. For some readers, it may seem like a long detour right before the end, but in many ways, it has been the goal all the way through: to recalibrate the way that we think about how to regulate data in healthcare in ways that better balance the forceful data promises.

The ethics of health data have been dominated by discourses about consent, privacy, and data literacy (Sterckx et al. 2015; Dickenson 2013; Dickenson, van Beers, and Sterckx 2018; van Dijk 2020; Piasecki, Walkiewicz-Żarek, Figas-Skrzypulec et al. 2021). The urge to make citizens understand and take control of their own data lives can be found even among scholars who point to the escalating complexity of information infrastructures (Gray, Gerlitz, and Bounegru 2018; Kitchin 2021; Brunton and Nissenbaum 2015). When policymakers address institutional and political concerns, they similarly talk about individual competence and choice. Alternatively, they circumvent ethics and focus on data security.[1] These are all important and relevant issues, but in order to address the concerns associated with intensified data sourcing, the scope of ethics must be broadened.

During the past five years, I have served as "ethics advisor," as informal discussant on "ethics," as speaker on "the ethics of data sourcing" at conferences, and as member of all sorts of "ethics committees." In these forums, I have become dissipated by the intolerable insistence on limiting ethics to questions of individual autonomy and, in consequence, individual responsibility. Again and again, I have heard people who specialize in information technology and work full time with data suggesting that to protect themselves, ordinary citizens should "just" do this or that—typically while pointing to a counterintuitive use of a system designed to make users do exactly the opposite. These extremely well-paid experts, who *build* these evermore complex systems, have the audacity to suggest that *all* citizens should be able to learn to maneuver complex systems as cleverly as they themselves do. It is not going to happen (Obar 2017).

Furthermore, there is no unambiguously prudent way to live with data. Thanks to intensified data sourcing, data are many things at the same time, part of many different projects, and they serve many purposes, most of them beyond the control of any particular individual. People continue to use expressions such as "my data," but the very expression "my data" is an oxymoron. Data are always data on somebody or something else too. Nevertheless, data ethics continues to emphasize individual control and responsibility.[2]

It is important not to forget about individuals. There are good reasons for caring about individual control (Dickenson, van Beers, and Sterckx, et al. 2018). People thrive when they feel recognized and respected as individuals. Patients often have to confide sensitive information to healthcare staff to get help. They care about where this information might end up. As intensified data sourcing affects the conditions of confidentiality and secrecy (Wadmann, Hartlev, and Hoeyer 2022), institutions need to find new ways to respect patient norms and expectations (Nissenbaum 2011). Such norms differ between places and communities (Johansson, Bentzen, Shah et al. 2021). There is a need to rethink how to make individual patients feel recognized and respected. Simmel (1950) noted that "writing is opposed to all secrecy . . . it involves an unlimited, even if only potential, 'publicity'" (352). As patient information has become digitized, this potentiality is magnified (Manderson, Davis, Colwell, and Ahlin 2015). Data can be repurposed and shared, but they also can be leaked and hacked. Still, patients wish to exert some form of influence over who knows what about them. They continue to expect some form of confidentiality and control.

What have the authorities in Denmark done to ensure such control? What does the common ethical framing offer patients? In Denmark, as in most other countries, patients must provide an informed consent for the treatment of their information as a condition of care.[3] They constantly sign informed consent sheets (or, more commonly, click on consent buttons electronically) to verify that healthcare information can be stored. When patients need healthcare, this does not come across as a genuine choice. Rather, they are obliged to do an extra piece of data-work-of-production to legitimize exactly the type of data transfers that most patients want: communication with and between their doctors. Then, once the data enter the databases, they are available for other purposes related to research, governance, and industry. In most cases, data can be used for these purposes without additional consent. Informed consent thereby becomes a pseudo-choice that does not provide patients with any real control.

As a reaction to various citizen complaints about lacking individual control, the authorities have offered citizens various technical solutions over the years, such as the "privacy marking" option of medical records mentioned in chapter 5 and some opt-out registries. I mentioned in chapter 1 how the Danish parliament in 2014 deleted the largest opt-out registry to date because 'too many' had opted out. What type of control do the remaining opt-out registries offer patients? Opting out does not imply deleting any information; it involves being featured in an *extra* registry. In some cases, the opt-out registry can expose patients in new ways. In terms of privacy, patients can be better protected when hidden in large population datasets than when singled out as autonomous decision-makers.

There are opt-out registries for tissue-based research and for withholding genetic information from research, and even some for local record systems. An opt-out registry turns difficult decisions about legitimate reuse of tissue and data into an individualized responsibility, where patients need to know that they can opt out in the first place and then realize that they can opt out of only some uses. The main opt-out registries focus on research. Opting out of *all* research, while remaining in the archives for other purposes, is not necessarily a meaningful choice (Holm and Madsen 2009). Patients might wish to support academic research into cancer, but not commercial research into psychiatric diseases. Or they might wish to support research, but not administrative control regimes aimed at monitoring their physicians. If the point is to let patients influence how their data are used, much more fine-grained and dynamic options are needed (Holm and Ploug 2017; Kaye, Whitley, Lund et al. 2015). The most common experience when interviewing patients, however, is that they want to focus on their own treatment, not on administering data reuse. Options aimed at data control are likely to serve only the most resourceful citizens. Responsibilization of the individual nevertheless remains the standard response in data politics.

Informed consent in general does more to protect the institutions and companies thriving on data sharing than the individuals providing their consent (Hoeyer and Hogle 2014; Hoeyer 2005; Hoeyer and Tutton 2005; see also Rothman 1991). This point remains relevant for the ethics of data-intensive medicine as well. With the open data movement and the FAIR principles, the use of informed consent as a means of protection becomes even more ineffective. FAIR means that research participants first provide informed consent to specified research projects, and then when the project ends, the data are to be made available to other researchers with other research questions in anonymized form. A pharmaceutical company or a competing academic research group might use data from an academic study for purposes that run directly against the ones listed on the original consent form. In such cases, FAIR is not *fair*. Danish policymakers claim that anonymization constitutes a technical fix to the problem with informed consent, but to reuse data generated for a different purpose where there was an explicit consent is not respectful. It is not recognizing people as contributors to research.

Furthermore, if enough data are available, nobody is anonymous. Moreover, people have interests other than controlling their own data. Predictive data tools target people regardless of whether they were part of the group providing consent in the first place (Taylor, Floridi, and van der Sloot 2017; Taylor 2017). Many research projects facilitate data predictions that can target individuals based on particular traits, such as their weight, blood pressure, sexuality, ethnicity, income, or place of residence (Holmberg, Bischof, and Bauer 2013; Amelang and Bauer 2019). In some cases, such tools can deprive groups of people access to benefits, treatments, or insurance. Data tools that are not designed well may even hit the wrong target (Altman 2019; Lipworth, Mason, Kerridge, and Ioannidis 2017). When data profiles are traded in automated systems, individuals can have their identities mixed up with strangers without knowing, and with no opportunity to object (Pasquale 2015). In some cases, it might not be privacy breaches, but invalid conclusions based on the wrong data, which constitute the primary risk to patients.

There is no safe way to administer your data in data-intensive healthcare, not even for the data-literate individual. Absence of data about a person is also a data profile, as Lone discovered when she had her driver's license cancelled because she tried to "protect" herself by not sharing her data (see chapter 2). I once called a data broker to find out why I received a certain invitation via surface mail, only to learn that they were selling my profile as a person who is "*not* on Facebook, Twitter, or LinkedIn." It may all sound relatively innocent, but in automated systems of law enforcement, a data absence can also translate into the profile of "likely to be criminal"' or a "terrorist," and in credit scoring and in the insurance industry, data absences can be very expensive (Sætnan 2018; O'Neil 2016). How should informed consent ever protect people against these harms?

When data operate as cogs in multiple machines, including machines aimed at monitoring and controlling people, the very ambition with data reuse can be to overrule individual choice, and then informed consent is little more than a shimmer of false control, generating massive amounts of data work. I described in chapter 4 the impossibility of reading terms of agreement before consenting, and how it left me with no real choices. Instead, click-to-consent involves an intolerable responsibilization of citizens. When insisting on consent, the healthcare system has come to mirror the absurdity of the wider space of the Internet, where agreeing to cookies is a precondition for access to platforms with a voracious appetite for people's data (Fourcade and Kluttz 2020). There is a dire need for tools other than data literacy and individual "choice" if governments wish to protect—and respect—citizens in data-intensive societies.

The ethics of data-intensive healthcare, therefore, is in need of an alternative to the trope of individual responsibility. I stated in chapter 6 that I believe that research must be honest about the values shaping its findings. My own research—and my quest for a *response-able* healthcare system—is informed by ideas about justice (Reardon 2017), solidarity (Prainsack and Buyx 2017), and recognition (Taylor 1994). These are values that focus on ensuring equal opportunity, conserving common goods, and showing respect for individual differences. The point of combining these ideas is to acknowledge that people have individual stakes in data sourcing, but not to hold them individually responsible for living in systems that they cannot control. I believe that policymakers who wish to preserve legitimacy could benefit from focusing on the values of justice, solidarity, and recognition. It could inspire them to build more socially robust systems. Data *can* serve solidarity, justice, and recognition. Data *can* be considered what Widdows and Cordell (2011) call a "community good," increasing in value (and value dimensions) through aggregation. It takes concerted effort, however, as well as a willingness to monitor and explore the unintended consequences of data integration.

To ensure continued legitimacy, I believe that there is a need to begin thinking in much more radical ways about potential solutions. Such solutions should preserve aggregated data as a common good, ensure fairness, and make people with diverse values feel recognized. I present a list with a few suggestions in table 7.3. They are intended as prompts or, you might say, as provocations. I do not present them as a new coherent governance model because no government would adopt such a model anyway. I outline them only as ideas so they may circulate and perhaps translate in locally meaningful ways. I do not wish to replace local innovation with standard proposals. The point with this list is merely to suggest that guided by justice, solidarity,

Table 7.3

A nonexhaustive list of alternative ethics framings building on solidarity, justice, and recognition

---

Prioritize clinical uses of data over reuse of data for secondary purposes and make sure that reuse of data does not endanger patient interests. Make priorities between different types of reuse. Even legitimate interests in detecting various forms of fraud might backfire if people lose faith in the healthcare system and the doctors and nurses treating them.

Give access to health data for research purposes only on condition of a proven ability to understand the data. If researchers do not understand data well, they produce useless (or even potentially harmful) results. Make sure to fund documentation of metadata where needed.

Invest in user interfaces ensuring that patients are granted proper options of choice, and build those options on careful research into the hopes and concerns of the affected people rather than the hunches and gut feelings of civil servants and IT developers. People should feel recognized and respected when seeking to influence their own data representations, and the available options must be as easy to use as the interfaces through which data are sourced in the first place.

Retain options for the use of population data for research purposes aimed at promoting the common good on the condition that the research can be carried out in ways that ensure the anonymity of each individual.

Ban data profile markets with very few, well-regulated, and transparent exemptions.[4] In what sense can selling people's data profiles ever be seen as representing a common good? Selling data profiles has undermined a number of other common goods, such as independent media, trust in healthcare providers, and collective sharing of risk in the insurance industry.

When making data investments, consider what economists call "externalities" and make carefully balanced investments with an eye to the need for repairs and renewal of equipment. Do data technologies carry the risk of technology lock-in and monopolies? Do they depend on technologies that carry high environmental risk? How much energy will data storage consume, and what is the climate impact? Can they be used for surveillance? Do the technologies emerge through exploitive global relations?

---

and recognition, new regulatory solutions may transpire—solutions that acknowledge the need to protect individuals, prioritize among data reuses, help build more robust data analyses, make citizens feel respected and accommodated, and harness the benefits of data while acknowledging the costs.

With these alternative framings of ethical issues, I suggest focusing on making data reuses *fair* so that data provided in good faith are not later used against individuals, and already disadvantaged groups do not face greater risk than others. I suggest administering data resources with care as collective goods to be consumed in *solidarity*. And I suggest working to ensure that people feel *recognized* and their expectations of confidentiality are respected. The list of suggestions in table 7.3 might look far from feasible in the current political atmosphere, but I maintain that they are more realistic than the imaginary "total disruption through datafication," which is featured in many policy papers, strategy papers, and consultancy reports.

THE POLITICS OF INTENSIFIED DATA SOURCING IN HEALTHCARE AND BEYOND

The data-political dynamics that I have identified in this book relate to a particular sector and build on work in a particular context of highly integrated data infrastructures. Still, I believe that some of these dynamics have a broader relevance for datafication in other contexts and other social arenas in Denmark and beyond (Amoore & Piotukh, 2015; Madsen, Flyverbom, Hilbert, & Ruppert 2016; Petersen, 2019). Data promises sweep across not only health, but also *education* (Kwet 2019; Hartong and Förschler 2019; Fernandez and Lutz 2019; Gorur 2011), *social work* (Høybye-Mortensen 2015; Lyneborg 2019; Parton 2008), *media* and *entertainment* (Fuchs 2016; van Dijck 2013), *law enforcement* and *defense* (Adelman 2017; Möllers 2021; Slayton 2021; Shklovski, Troshynski, and Dourish 2015; Haggerty and Ericson 2000; Grünenberg 2020; van Eijk 2021), *migration* and *biometric border control* (Grünenberg 2020; Trauttmansdorff and Felt 2021; Grünenberg, Møhl, Fog Olwig, and Simonsen 2020), *credit* and *finance markets* (Pasquale 2015; O'Neil 2016; Riles 2013; Mackenzie 2021), and *city planning* and *traffic control* (Halpern 2014; Poirier 2021). Data intensification characterizes both public and private sectors. Still, even a country as data-intensive as Denmark is not data-driven. Rather, it is a data-pursuing society. The governance of human lives should not be data-driven—it should *use* data. With care. It involves learning to look *at* data and what they do, not just to *use* data as tools of observation. I am confident that this is relevant not only in Denmark, and not only in healthcare.

Data promises gain political strength partly due to a strong tradition for searching for technological solutions to societal challenges. Technological solutions are supposed to be simple fixes. STS scholar Andrew Barry (2001) notes: "We live in a technological society . . . to the extent that specific technologies dominate our sense of the kinds of problems that government and politics must address, and the solutions that we must adopt" (2). It is better to look for *socially* robust solutions than for technological fixes. To investigate social dynamics carefully implies also listening to dissenting voices. In the messianic space of semireligious dataism, people who divert from the standards designed by a tiny minority of tech experts are treated as renegades. Societies that wish to embrace new technological opportunities must be able to build more accommodating solutions; otherwise, they risk stimulating dichotomous spaces of truth-telling where opposing parties are unable to agree on anything. The major threats to data intensification might be the pompous and self-contained data gospel, more so than technological failure; and claims of neutrality in data forecasts, more so than acknowledgment of doubts and values.

Most people expect technologies to fail occasionally, and they know that experts have opinions. To have faith in technology, citizens must trust the good intentions of the companies and governments. When politicians and industry representatives abuse data to legitimize decisions that serve their self-interest, when complaints from citizens and clinicians are ignored or sidestepped as coming from dimwitted laggards, when quick and dirty analyses proliferate, and when policymakers ignore local knowledge because it does not feature in their data set, then everything that citizens and patients stand to gain from data intensity is at risk. When instead policymakers, administrators, and clinicians ask the right questions, when they care for those who are in need, when they face mistakes with openness and courage, then data can come to serve the interests of future patients, in all their diversity. With "Data Wisdom,", I contend, it is possible to build healthcare systems that meet this challenge.

NOTES

1. Many will recognize the voices of people like Eric Topol (a cardiologist and scientists known for his bestselling books about the future of healthcare) or Leroy Hood (a biologist and scientists known for his ambitions for a type of medicine, which is predictive, preventive, personalized and participatory) filtering through these promises (Hood and Flores 2012; Hood et al 2015; Topol 2010, 2015). I nevertheless leave them without references here because this is how they typically appear: as facts in no need of a reference.

2. Interestingly, the Danish word for "computer science" is *datalogi* (the study of data). The word *datalogi* was invented in 1966 by Peter Nauer and is today used in the Nordic languages, whereas Anglophone speakers say "computer science." The term "computer science" puts semantic emphasis on the hardware, whereas the French *informatique* and the German *Informatik* slither toward software, though they do not focus on data in the same way, as a basic unit of computation.

3. The image of the Internet as a global arena for free speech is becoming increasingly difficult to uphold as online communication is increasingly subjected to censorship and an increasing number of Internet lockdowns (Freedom House 2021). There is no longer *one* Internet (if there ever even was such a thing), but multiple Internets subject to different types of control and censorship. Furthermore, concomitantly with the rise of promises of a "data-driven" future, venture capitalists very far from Barlow's old counterculture have become deeply entangled in the economic structures of Silicon Valley. Some of them are affiliated with the most conservative political forces in the United States. They also subscribe to a future beyond the grip of the state, but for them, it means beyond taxation and beyond democratic control (Chafkin 2021).

4. Since Mol's important work has been subject to diverse receptions, it is probably better to clarify the nature of my argument. I suggest that multiple uses of the

same data turn these data into particular types of semantico-material actors: they do different things in different organizational practices (simultaneously or over time). Unlike the reception of Mol that emphasizes multiplicity as a basic ontological condition relevant for basically all phenomena, I thus point to a shift in the work that data come to do in healthcare organizations. My intention is not to criticize the more general reflections on ontological multiplicity. Indeed, you could say data have always been multiple, just as any other phenomenon can be claimed to be so. However, as a consequence of current political and organizational processes in healthcare, we see a shift in the agential properties of data whereby the ontological multiplicity acquires a different political salience in need of our attention.

5. I draw on a range of very different materials, including personal experiences as citizen and patient, informal professional encounters, interviews, and participant observation, as well as media and policy representations. These materials call for different ethical and methodological reflections. When I refer to named persons in media stories, I use the name occurring in the story or report for the sake of transparency (full names for people in official roles and first names only for citizens and patients). I provide pseudonyms for people whom I interviewed. For some, anonymity has been paramount, and they have asked to appear under a different gender, have no name given, or both, so that it is harder to combine different quotes and potentially reidentify them. I have translated Danish into English from both written and oral sources, discussing difficult passages with colleagues and the language editor Julie Dyson.

CHAPTER 1

1. Promises also shape the business opportunities for health tech companies outside the governmental sector (Fiore-Gartland and Neff 2016). In a particularly conspicuous scandal, a woman named Elizabeth Holmes managed to raise nine billion US dollars for a company called Theranos by promising to deliver omnipotent diagnostics with new data-intensive technology—but it turned out that there was no such technology (Hartmans and Leskin 2020). It was just a promise. Other companies have raised venture capital by claiming to develop sophisticated artificial intelligence (AI) but actually employing poorly paid people in India to do the work more or less manually (Statt 2019). This type of politics operates in a realm of potentiality (Taussig, Hoeyer, and Helmreich 2013). Companies and policymakers imbue data with potential; a potential for future certainty. They do not, however, impose the criteria of evidence on the quest of data per se.

2. This means that the international ICD-10 manual specifies a taxonomy of disease that is adopted into a national classification system, making it possible to use a code to describe a hospital visit. In ICD-10, for example, there is a broad range of codes (M00–M99) for diseases of the musculoskeletal system and connective tissue, and under them, M15–M19 is used for "arthrosis," M13 for "other arthritis," and M15–M19 for "osteoarthritis." In Danish coding, there will be a "D" in front of the code

to signal that the code refers to "diagnostics." There are other overarching coding letters referring to different types of codes, signaling either administrative information (A), type of treatment (B, E, K, N, U, W), or pharmaceutical information (M). A code can have a maximum of ten digits. It nevertheless creates a complex coding language with many thousands of codes. The code DM138A, for example, means that it is a disease (D) and arthritis (M13) and a subcategory of "other arthritis" related to allergy (8A). Other codes describe which services has been delivered and where. It has become a specialist competence to read such codes, not least since they change over time.

3. The fact that digitalization enhances traceability, and thereby interacts with litigation practices, has been part of the history of digital communication practices from very early on. A US white paper from 1997 says about e-mail: "In contrast with telephone conversations, e-mail is self-documenting: Copies of e-mail can be printed or attached to the patient's electronic record. Finally, since many malpractice claims can be traced to faulty communication, good communication is part of good insurance" (Kane and Sands 1997: 105).

4. The only person I have encountered who has considered whether data are worth the investment was Jens, a strategy developer. He had wanted to measure whether his data governance tools had any effect, but his boss responded that measurements were for documenting the achievement of political goals, not to evaluate administrative tools. The Deloitte report mentioned in this chapter is another exception. It states, however, that it cannot determine the cost of data production because there is no written agreement on data standards (a so-called service-level agreement) on which to base the calculation.

5. Danish GPs were using a piece of software that was generally seen as very helpful for generating an overview of patients, but it relied on pooling, and after a conflict about how the data began being reused for purposes that many GPs disagreed with, it was discovered that the pooling was unlawful. The database—which was, in an uncanny premonitory way, entitled DAMD—turned out to be damned. It had to be deleted. This case illustrates the need for engaging the political, legal, and social dynamics of data integration, not just the technical facilitation of data (Langhoff, Amstrup, Mørck, and Bjørn 2018; Wadmann and Hoeyer 2018).

CHAPTER 2

1. Henriette Langstrup has kindly agreed to let me reuse elements of this conversation and our shared work, which has previously appeared in a coauthored chapter in a book on patient activism edited by Susi Geiger (Hoeyer and Langstrup 2021).

2. The investigative journalist Adam Tanner refers to something he terms the "data paradox" in American medicine: "Our health-care system gives us little of what we want and need—easy access to our comprehensive medical records to help professionals with our treatment. But it has also given us much of what we fear—others

trafficking our records" (Tanner 2017: 37). It may sound similar, but as will become clear, I do not claim that the same is taking place in Denmark. Instead, data are pooled primarily to facilitate governance, and this takes place within the remits of the public healthcare system, not through commercial data sales. The ambition of turning health data into assets that can fuel the economy remains a policy "promise" more than an actual motor explaining who or what accesses Lone's data.

3. Besides high-tech practices such as genomic medicine, P4 medicine translates into more mundane invitations to self-care. One example is a 2014 government health policy program called "The Sooner the Better" (*Da; Jo før, jo bedre*) (Regeringen 2014) with an "investment" of 5 billion DKK in the period 2015–2018. This suggested that GPs should be given data tools so they can profile their patients and discuss lifestyle issues with high-risk individuals. Most researchers working with prevention consider preventive consultations to have only limited effect (Jørgensen and Brunak 2014; Hollands et al., 2016). The majority of citizens targeted in this manner suffer from complex combinations of social inequalities rather than a lack of medical advice on what to eat or how to exercise (Marmot et al., 2010). Still, data-intensive care can make some patients visible in new ways while covering up the problems that these patients are actually dealing with. Data uncover and cover up.

4. I leave aside the usual arena for debates about data trouble—the commercial platforms. Again, my interests revolve around intensified data sourcing in healthcare systems and welfare services. On commercial platforms, the price for a seamless user experience is your data (van Dijck, Poell, and De Wall 2018). Those data are occasionally used against your interests, and sometimes you are cornered by harmful and misguided profiling (Pasquale 2015; Ebeling 2016; Goriunova 2019; O'Neil 2016). In that sense, they represent a parallel paradox: seamlessness empowers the user experience and disempowers citizen rights.

5. The Danish healthcare sector is not simply "tax-financed." Officially, approximately 80 percent of the health expenses are paid by taxes, although it can be debated what counts as "total expenses." Intricate systems of partial out-of-pocket payment operate for dentists, pharmacy bills, psychologists, and other items and services. The welfare state ambition implies that systems are put in place to adjust for social inequality in relation to out-of-pocket payments (e.g., subsidies to low-income households), and these systems add to data demands to ensure that the right citizens get the right subsidies. Around 35 percent of citizens also have employer-paid health insurance giving access to various forms of private health promotion and/or private hospitals ahead of the public waiting list. Another 40 percent have a form of private insurance to cover part of the out-of-pocket payment simply called *danmark* (the country name, but noncapitalized), which is a membership association aimed at equaling out peaks in expenditure for the individual (Clausen 2020). Many have both types of insurance. Of course, each of these numbers could be questioned. Still, the type of health promotion allowed by insurance companies, where activity trackers become mandatory—a system that is becoming more prominent in countries

like the United States and Switzerland—remains rare in Denmark (Martani, Shaw, and Elger 2019).

6. GPs, as well as many specialists (such as neurologists or ophtalmologists), are typically run as private businesses, although citizens seldom realize this because their bills are paid by the regions and municipalities they live in. Their prices and terms of services are negotiated between the Regions and the unions of the specialists in collective agreements. It is also through these agreements that GPs and specialists become obliged to use electronic patient records and convey information for national registries and other data infrastructures.

7. Statistics Denmark (similar to Statistics Sweden, Statistics Norway, and Statistics Finland) provides platforms for researchers and administrators to combine data sets across sectors and explore correlations in a logged and controlled environment.

8. As of October 30, 2020, 6,680 people were registered not to have their blood and tissue samples used for research purposes, and 3,062 registered that they did not want their genome information used. Following debates about the storage of COVID-19 samples, the number of those opting out increased so that by June 2022, 12,022 had registered to avoid having their blood and tissue reused, and 7,773 to avoid having genomic data used for research (see chapter 6).

9. The private sector is thoroughly digitized too, building on the public data infrastructure. In the 1960s, the Nordic banks were already collaborating with public authorities on the digitization of the financial sector. A computerized billing method was introduced in 1968 in Denmark, and in updated formats today, it ensures an almost fully digitized billing system. In 1983, a national credit card (Dankort) introduced digital payments, and Denmark quickly had the highest number of digital payments in the world. It operates with no fee, in contrast to VISA and Mastercard. In 2000, a national digital postal service system called E-Boks was invented. It operates as a company, but on a public legal mandate: in 2005, state authorities decided to use E-Boks to correspond with all public employees, and in 2012, a law made it the default means of communication between the state and all citizens. As a consequence, surface mail is such a rarity that hospitals and GPs can no longer rely on it for sending tissue samples as they once did. In a further move toward pervasive digitalization, in 2010, a national secure access and multifactor identity system called EasyID (*Da; NemID*) was developed by a consortium of companies in response to a public tender request. It is currently replaced by an updated version called MyId (*MitID*). Today, it is used by both authorities and commercial service providers. It is yet another setup that the European Union is considering implementing across the whole union in modified forms (European Commission 2020b).

10. I asked my gym why, and though the man at the counter was at first a little annoyed by the folly of such a stupid question, he kindly asked around. He found out that it was because "their systems were set up in that way." As I probed further, I was told that it was easier for them to always update people's addresses from the Civil

Registration System (known simply as CPR) than maintaining their own registrations manually. In consequence, those without a CPR number cannot go to the gym.

11. When a nongovernmental organization (NGO) started a clinic for people without a CPR number on the island of Funen, they were approached by approximately seventy unregistered migrants a year (DR Nyheder 2019b). This will seem to most people like a small number, and that is part of what causes the misery: it is indeed small, small enough for organizational interfaces to assume that *everybody* has a number. There are procedures for tourists and others passing through the country who can have an artificial number if visiting a hospital, but those rules do not apply to people who are not supposed to be in the country.

CHAPTER 3

1. As explained in the introduction, people from published sources are identified with their real names, interviewed persons with pseudonyms, and some, at their request, anonymously.

2. A similar name is used in Norway, Helseplattformen, and in Finland, Epic has sold an integrated social care and healthcare system and given it the name Apotti. The company also has customers in the Netherlands, but otherwise it mainly operates in the United States at the time of writing.

3. Part of this analysis has been published in an article coauthored by Sarah Wadmann (Hoeyer and Wadmann 2020). I am grateful for our discussions and her permission to allow me to reuse elements here. Besides analyzing policy documents, Sarah and I interviewed sixty-nine persons: five working on developing the frameworks for data collection at the state level; at the regional level, thirteen data analysts, along with five other people, working with data integration tasks; three hospital managers; four clinical department managers; four staff nurses at hospitals; one hospital-based quality manager; three nurses subspecializing as quality coordinators working in hospital departments; twenty-two physicians working in hospitals and general practice; eight hospital-employed nurses; three hospital secretaries; and three audit workers. Wadmann also undertook four days of observation on two different wards and one day of observation of a management seminar. See also (Wadmann et al. 2018; Holm-Petersen, Wadmann, and Andersen 2015).

4. For example, Google's DeepMind algorithms are touted to be able to warn physicians of acute kidney injury (Tomašev, Glorot, Rae et al. 2019). Danish emergency calls are monitored with artificial intelligence (AI) designed to alert doctors of the risk of cardiac arrest based on patterns in previous calls, including speech pace and judder (Blomberg, Folke, Ersbøll et al. 2019, see also chapter 5). Such tools use data from other patients to make predictions that operate in in real time and react to data produced with new patients.

5. The management, at least, has remained positive and optimistic. Promises persevere. Despite problems with patient safety, staff burnout, lost efficiency, and

data that remain stuck in the system, the Capital Region announced in 2017 that the introduction had been "satisfactory" (Højer and Flach 2017). A national audit concluded that the administration had failed in its implementation, it had omitted necessary tests, and the system had caused a serious reduction in efficiency and productivity (Statsrevisorerne og Rigsrevisionen 2018). Still, the administration decided to grant a bonus of 100,000 DKK to the director for the implementation (Larsen and Nielsen 2018). The administration points to consultancy reports and surveys that they interpret as proof that the system is better than its rumor (Hildebrandt 2017c).

6. Some science and technology studies (STS) scholars have discussed this type of dialogue as a productive type of "data friction" where new hybrid insights are produced (Bonde, Bossen, and Danholt 2019; Edwards, Mayernik, Batcheller et al. 2011). My point here is primarily that the friction generates extra (but invisible) work for the clinicians (Boyce 2016).

7. A particular case has fueled these concerns. A doctor was taken to court for a prescription that was, according to the doctor, given verbally due to high work pressure. The medicine was never given to the patient, with fatal consequences. The doctor could not prove the verbal prescription, and it escalated the debate about the need to prioritize "covering one's ass" over organizational solidarity when under pressure (Folkmann 2017; L. Lange 2017; Nathan 2017; Redaktionen 2018).

8. An edict often referred to as "Campbell's Law" states: "The more any quantitative social indicator is used for social decision-making, the more subject it will be to corruption pressures and the more apt it will be to distort and corrupt the social processes it is intended to monitor" (Campbell, 1979: 85). In Donald Campbell's framing, the power dynamics relate to people trying to optimize their own position and income. This is probably true, but it is only one element of the story, as my focus on the pursuit of meaning suggests.

CHAPTER 4

1. I looked up the legal framework at home and found a regulation of the business area from 1994 stating an obligation to keep records. It does not mention using the CPR number for record keeping (Sundheds-og Ældreministeriet 1994).

2. I have, of course, done many other things. The data infrastructures I set out to study are funded, regulated, and sustained by organizations that document their decisions and actions. Taking an ethnographic response to documents (as in Riles 2006), I therefore traced policy papers, budget agreements, legal documents, and guidelines. Hundreds of policy papers, copies of internal memos, distributed slides, and even video presentations on YouTube and elsewhere have made it into my archive. Along with analyzing documents, I have participated in conferences, meetings, workshops, and public hearings. Based on all of these sources, I have identified actors for interviews, and through these interviews, I found other papers and

additional actors with whom I needed to engage in order to understand the workings of Danish health data infrastructures.

3. A significant amount of work has been done on the topic of "numeracy" by scholars with a behavioral approach coming from, among other disciplines, psychology (Nelson, Reyna, Fagerlin et al. 2008). This is a strand of work with a lot of merit in explaining how difficult it is for some people to use numerical data when making decisions. Still, I have deliberately not drawn upon numeracy here because I do not share the ambition in this literature of finding an instrument with which to measure the size of the "deficit in understanding." I wish to focus on what people *do* understand, and how they do it.

4. I have been inspired by the Chatham House Rules for meetings (www.chathamhouse .org), where participants in meetings can use the information provided, but they cannot reveal the identity of speakers and other participants. It has rarely been relevant—or possible—to go back and ask for informed consent to use concrete examples, but the point has not been to cite a particular colleague for anything, but rather to let everyday encounters inform my understanding of the link between what Mills (2000 [1959]) called personal trouble and societal issues (8). It would be against my sense of research integrity to ignore what I know as a person when writing up my analyses as a researcher. It does not matter how I came to know something. I therefore draw on every experience, including at meetings, but avoid conveying anything that could expose people who have not agreed to participate in my research.

CHAPTER 5

1. The eight goals are (1) integrated patient pathways, (2) better care for chronic patients and older people, (3) improved survival and safety, (4) high quality of treatment, (5) quick access to diagnosis and treatment, (6) improved patient empowerment, (7) more health-adjusted years of life, and (8) a more efficient healthcare system (Sundheds- og Ældreministeriet, KL, and Danske Regioner 2018).

2. Several times, I have heard researchers complain about receiving different data on the same phenomenon when requesting them from different sources. Data are no better than the infrastructures through which they are collected. If some systems do not report to certain databases, the data will have gaps, but people will not always know that because they see only the data that make it all the way through to the interface in which they work. See also Hjertholm, Flarup, Mahncke Guldbrandt, and Vedsted (2017).

3. Case-mix is developed in health economics and helps with adjusting for variance in the population compositions between various areas. It is time consuming to apply case-mix, and it makes the numbers less straightforward to understand because they are presented as weighted figures. When doctors once complained in a letter to the editor in a medical journal about naive data uses that ignore the importance of case-mix (Krasnik 2021), the regional quality agency replied that they did in fact produce

annual reports with case-mix figures (Jensen, Settnes, Lund Jensen et al. 2021). These annual reports, however, do not feed into everyday performance management. Speed and accuracy are not always compatible, and when data need to serve many competing purposes, and in "real time," no standard will fit them all (Winthereik 2004).

4. The conditions for access to psychological therapy have been changed several times, and in 2020, depression and anxiety gave direct access to psychologists on the public purse. However, this again necessitated a commitment to a diagnosis. Apparently, there is no such thing as a free chat. Experiments with digital access to therapy is hoped by some to help solve this problem, as patients can approach the psychiatrist directly without referral.

5. Muller (2018) suggests the following types of error: measuring the most easily measurable; measuring the simple when the desired outcome is complex; measuring inputs rather than outcomes; degrading information quality through standardization; gaming through creaming; improving numbers by lowering standards; improving numbers through omission or distortion of data; and cheating (23–25).

6. Data quality in registries, for example, is assessed in terms of "validity and completeness" (Schmidt, Schmidt, Sandegaard et al. 2019), "completeness, inaccuracy, ambiguity" (Laudon 1986: 137–138); "completeness, accuracy and comparability" (Chan, Fowles, and Weiner 2010); or "completeness, correctness, concordance, plausibility, and currency" (Weiskopf and Weng 2012). Quality is typically assessed by comparing data sources (White 1999)—data against data.

CHAPTER 6

1. Even when going into the individual death certificates, doubts only proliferate. In many cases, the "real" source of death cannot be known. Counting the dead is not as easy as it sounds (Kielgast, Hecklen, and Møller 2021).

2. See, for example, a project run by psychologists (https://ku-corona-diary.netlify .app/2020/04/07/what-are-all-the-people-doing/) and one run by political scientists (https://hope-project.au.dk/).

3. In Denmark, 600 people had received two doses of the vaccine and 150.000 the first dose at the time when the vaccinations were halted. The European Medicines Agency (EMA) acknowledged vaccine-induced thrombotic thrombocytopenia (VITT) syndrome, but it continued recommending vaccine use because it asserted that the overall death rates in society could be reduced with continued vaccinations. In Denmark, the authorities decided that people at risk for VITT would not face similar dangers to their own health from COVID-19, so they withdrew vaccines associated with VITT from the official program.

4. The Johnson & Johnson vaccine was later offered in a parallel program for voluntary use for people wishing to get a vaccination before it was their turn in the mass program.

5. As with the doubts articulated by Mathias, many people turned out to be less clear-cut in their stance on vaccines. The vaccination rate in December 2021, before children below twelve years could get the vaccine, was 77 percent, and in January 2022, when children above five years were included in the program, the rate was 82 percent. At the same time, however, only 60 percent of the population had opted for the third booster shot.

6. See, for example, COVID-19 Dashboard by the Center for Systems Science and Engineering at Johns Hopkins University, https://gisanddata.maps.arcgis.com/apps /opsdashboard/index.html#/bda7594740fd40299423467b48e9ecf6; https://www.world ometers.info/coronavirus/; https://ncov2019.live/; https://nextstrain.org/; and "Tracking Coronavirus COVID-19," https://app.developer.here.com/coronavirus/ (accessed July 10, 2021).

CONCLUSION

1. Data security is immensely important, and presumably something is still lacking in the case of Denmark. In 2022, a governmental report found that the Danish Health Data Authority met only fourteen of twenty defined security standards for public authorities (Statsrevisorerne 2022). While clearly more care is needed here, my point is that such standards do little to solve the social and ethical challenges with intensified data sourcing.

2. I do not mean to suggest that individuals hold *no* responsibility for their actions, or that responsibility is not important. New technologies typically interact with responsibility in important ways (Schicktanz and Raz 2012). The question is what responsibility implies. Schicktanz and Schweda (2012) point out that when carefully analyzed, relations of responsibility are much more defined and restricted. Responsibility typically has seven dimensions (or *relata*, as they put it): "Someone (*subject*) is in a particular time frame (*time*) retrospectively/prospectively (*temporal direction*) responsible for something/someone (*object*) against someone (normproofing *instance*) on the basis of certain normative standards (*standard*) with certain sanctions or rewards (*consequences*)" (133, italics in the original). This is altogether different from expecting individual citizens to behave wisely.

3. In this section I use the term informed consent to cover various concepts figuring in laws regulating research, healthcare and data protection, though GDPR for example only uses the term "consent". There are important legal differences between the various regulations and remaining elements of confusion (Dove and Chen 2020; Gefenas, Lekstutiene, Lukaseviciene et al 2021). My argument is not a legal one, however, but aimed at the thinking around individual responsibility embedded in the concept.

4. When this book was submitted to the publisher the European Union had not yet adopted the Digital Service Market Act which takes timid steps in this direction.

REFERENCES

Aanestad, Margunn, and Tina Blegind Jensen. 2011. "Building nation-wide information infrastructures in healthcare through modular implementation strategies." *Journal of Strategic Information Systems*, 20: 161–176.

Abrahamson, Eric. 1996. "Management fashion." *Academy of Management Review*, 21: 254–285.

Achiumi, Tendaya. 2020. *Report of the Special Rapporteur on contemporary forms of racism, racial discrimination, xenophobia and related intolerance Note by the Secretary-General*. OHCHR and United Nations.

Ackerman, Sara L., Katherine Weatherford Darling, Sandra Soo-Jin Lee, Robert A. Hiatt, and Janet K. Shim. 2016. "Accounting for complexity: Gene-environment interaction research and the moral economy of quantification." *Science, Technology, & Human Values*, 41: 194–218.

Adams, Vincanne. 2016a. "Introduction." In Vincanne Adams (ed.), *Metrics: What counts in global health*. Duke University Press: 1–17

Adams, Vincanne. 2016b. "Metrics of the global sovereign: Numbers and stories in global health." In Vincanne Adams (ed.), *Metrics: What counts in global health*. Duke University Press: 19–54

Adelman, Rebecca A. 2017. "Security glitches: The failure of the universal camouflage pattern and the fantasy of "identity intelligence." *Science, Technology & Human Values*, 43: 431–463.

Agamben, Giorgio. 1995. *Homo sacer: Sovereign power and bare life*. Stanford University Press.

Agamben, Giorgio. 2020. "Giorgio Agamben: The coronaviris and the state of exception," *Autonomies*, March 3, 2020.

Ahmed, Nabil. 2022. *Inequality kills: The unparalleled action needed to combat unprecedented inequality in the wake of COVID-19*. Oxfam.

Aiello, Allison E., Audrey Renson, and Paul N. Zivich. 2020. "Social Media- and Internet-Based Disease Surveillance for Public Health', *Annual Review of Public Health*, 41: 101–18.

Akrich, Madeleine. 1992. "The de-scription of technical objects." In Wiebe E. Bijker and John Law (eds.), *Shaping technology/building society*. MIT Press: 205–224.

Albinus, Niels-Bjørn. 2021. "Brug af kunstig intelligens skal aflaste mammaradiologer," *Dagens Medicin*, October 29, 2021, Kræft section: 9.

Allen, Arthur. 2019. "Lost in translation: Epic goes to Denmark," *Politico*, June 6, 2019. https://www.politico.com/story/2019/06/06/epic-denmark-health-1510223.

Alm, Emanuelle, Niclas Colliander, Gustav Gotteberg, Frederik Lind, Ville Stohne, and Olof Sundström. 2016a. *Digitizing Denmark: How Denmark can drive and benefit from an accelerated digitized economy in Europe*. Boston Consulting Group.

Alm, Emanuelle, Niclas Colliander, Frederik Lind, Ville Stohne, Olof Sundström, Maikel Wilms, and Marty Smits. 2016b. *Digitizing the Nethlerlands: How the Netherlands can drive and benefit from an accelerated digitized economy in Europe*. Boston Consulting Group.

Almarsdóttir, Anna Birna, Janine Morgall Traulsen, and Ingunn Björnsdóttir. 2004. "'We don't have that many secrets'—the lay perspective on privacy and genetic data." In Gardar Árnason, Salvör Nordal and Viljálmur Árnason (eds.), *Blood and data—ethical, legal and social aspects of human genetic databases*. University of Iceland: 195–202.

Altman, Douglas G. 2019. "The scandal of poor medical research," *British Medical Journal*, 308: 283.

Alvesson, Mats, and André Spicer. 2012. "A stupidity-based theory of organizations," *Journal of Management Studies*, 49: 1194–1220.

Amelang, Katrin, and Susanne Bauer. 2019. "Following the algorithm: How epidemiological risk-scores do accountability," *Social Studies of Science*, 49: 476–502.

Ames, Morgan G. 2019. *The charisma machine: The life, death, and legacy of one laptop per child*. MIT Press.

Amoore, Louise, and Vohla Piotukh. 2015. "Life beyond big data: Governing with little analytics," *Economy and Society*, 44: 341–366.

Andersen, Lars Ole. 2011. *Før Placeboeffekten. Indbildningskraftens virkning i 1800-tallets medicin*. Museum Tusculanums Forlag.

Anderson, Benedict. 1983. *Imagined communities*. Verso.

Anderson, Chris. 2008. "The end of theory: The data deluge makes the scientific method obsolete," *Wired*, June 23: 1–3.

Andrejevic, Mark. 2005. "The work of watching one another: Lateral surveillance, risk, and governance." *Surveillance & Society*, 2: 479–497.

Andrejevic, Mark. 2013. *Infoglut: How too much information is changing the way we think and know*. Routledge.

Andrejevic, Mark, Alison Hearn, and Helen Kennedy. 2015. "Cultural studies of data mining: Introduction," *European Journal of Cultural Studies*, 18: 379–394.

Angell, Marcia, and Arnold S. Relman. 2002. "Patents, profits & American medicine: Conflicts of interest in the testing & marketing of new drugs," *Daedalus*: 102–111.

Angwin, Julia, and Steve Stecklow. 2010. "'Scrapers' dig deep for data on Web," *Wall Street Journal*, October 12, 2010.

Annas, George J. 2014. "The songs of spring: Quest myths, metaphors, and medical progress." In P. Macneill (ed.), *Ethics and the arts*. Springer Netherlands: 225–233.

Anthony, Callen. 2021. "When knowledge work and analytical technologies collide: The practices and consequences of black boxing algorithmic technologies," *Administrative Science Quarterly*, 66: 1173–1212.

Appel, Hannah, Nikhil Anand, and Akhil Gupta. 2018. "Temporality, politics, and the promise of infrastructure." In Nikhil Anand, Akhil Gupta, and Hannah Appel (eds.), *The promise of infrastructure*. Duke University Press: 1–38.

Armstrong, David. 2007. "Professionalism, indeterminacy and the EBM Project," *BioSocieties*, 2: 73–84.

Árnason, Arnar, and Bob Simpson. 2003. "Refractions through culture: The new genomics in Iceland," *Ethnos*, 68: 533–553.

Asad, Talal. 1994. "Representation, Statistics and Modern Power," *Social Research*, 61: 55–88.

Asdal, Kristin, and Christoph Gradmann. 2014. "Introduction: Science, technology, medicine—and the state: The science-state nexus in Scandinavia, 1850–1980," *Science in Context*, 27: 177–186.

Asdal, Kristin, and Ingunn Moser. 2012. "Experiments in context and contexting," *Science, Technology, & Human Values*, 37: 291–306.

Ashmore, Malcolm, Michael Mulkay, and Trevor Pinch. 1989. *Health and efficiency: A sociology of health economics*. Open University Press.

Babbage, Charles. 1830 [2018]. *Reflections of the decline of science in England*. Alpha Editions.

Bal, Roland, Bert de Graaff, Hester M. van de Bovenkamp, and Iris Wallenburg. 2020. "Practicing Corona—towards a research agenda of health policies," *Health Policy*, 124: 671–673.

Ballestero, Andrea, and Brit Ross Winthereik. 2021. "Analysis as Experimental Practice." In Andrea Ballestero and Brit Ross Winthereik (eds.), *Experimenting with ethnography: A companion to analysis*. Duke University Press: 1–12.

Bansler, Jørgen. 2021. "IT-projektet der kørte af sporet." In Niels Bentzon and Jacob Rosenberg (eds.), *Destruktiv Digitalisering. En debatbog om Sundhedsplatformen 2016–2021*. FADL's Forlag: 27–53.

Barassi, Veronica. 2020. "Datafied times: Surveillance capitalism, data technologies and the social construction of time in family life," *New Media & Society*, 22: 1545–1560.

Barlow, John Perry. 1996. "A declaration of the independence of cyberspace." Electronic Frontier Foundation.

Barnes, Deborah E., and Lisa A. Bero. 1998. "Why review articles on the health effects of passive smoking reach different conclusions." *JAMA*, 279: 1566–1570.

Barry, Andrew. 2001. *Political machine:. Governing a technological society*. Athlone Press.

Barth, Fredrik. 2002. "An anthropology of knowledge," *Current Anthropology*, 43: 1–18.

Baudrillard, Jean. 2021 [1994]. *Simulcra and simulation*. University of Michigan Press.

Bauer, Susanne. 2013. "Modeling population health," *Medical Anthropology Quarterly*, 27: 510–530.

Bauer, Susanne. 2014. "From administrative infrastructure to biomedical resource: Danish population registries, the 'Scandinavian laboratory,' and the 'epidemiologist's dream,'" *Science in Context*, 27: 187–213.

Baugh, Peter. 2017. "'Techplomacy': Denmark's ambassador to Silicon Valley," *Politico*, https://www.politico.eu/article/denmark-silicon-valley-tech-ambassador-casper-klynge/ accessed April 7, 2020.

Baun, Line G. 2017. "Garvet kirurg på Riget siger op på grund af Sundhedsplatformen," *DR. dk*, February 17.

BBC News. 2020. "Coronavirus: Amazon workers strike over virus protection," BBC News, March 31, 2020, Business section. https://www.bbc.com/news/business -52096273.

Beaulieu, Anne, and Sabina Leonelli. 2022. *Data and society: A critical introduction*, SAGE.

Bech-Bruun. 2019. *Muligheder for at lempe juridiske barrierer for anvendelse af sundheds-data*. Bech-Bruun.

Beck, Ulrich. 1999. *Risikosamfundet*. Hans Reitzels Forlag.

Beck-Nielsen, Claus. 2003. *Claus Beck-Nielsen (1963–2001): En biografi*. Gyldendal.

Bekelman, Justin E., Yan Li, and Gary P. Gross. 2003. "Scope and impact of financial conflicts of interest in biomedical research: A systematic review." *JAMA*, 289: 454–465.

Benders, Jos, and Kees van Veen. 2001. "What's in a fashion? Interpretive viability and management fashions." *Organization*, 8: 33–53.

Benko, Jessica. 2015. "Making and unmaking the digital world." *New York Times Magazine*: 55.

Bentzon, Niels, and Jacob Rosenberg. 2021. *Destruktiv Digitalisering: En debatbog om Sundhedsplatformen 2016–2021*. FADL's Forlag.

Berg, Marc, and Els Goorman. 1999. "The contextual nature of medical informa-tion," *International Journal of Medical Informatics*, 56: 51–60.

Bernsen, Markus. 2019. *Danmark Disruptet. Tro, Håb og Tech-giganter*. Gyldendal.

Bessette, J, M. 2001. "Acountability: Political." In Smelser, Neil J. and Paul B. Baltes (eds.) *International Encyclopedia of the Social & Behavioral Sciences*. Elsevier Ltd: 38–41.

Biagioli, Mario, and Alexandra Lippman. 2020. "Introduction: Metrics and the new ecologies of academic misconduct." In Mario Biagioli and Alexandra Lippman (eds.), *Gaming the metrics: Misconduct and manipulation in academic research*. MIT Press: 1–23.

Bickerton, Christopher J., and Carlo Invernizzi Accetti. 2021. *Technopopulism. The new logic of democratic politics.* Oxford University Press.

Bigo, Didier, Engin Isin, and Evelyn Ruppert. 2019. "Data Politics." In Didier Bigo, Engin Isin and Evelyn Ruppert (eds.), *Data politics: Worlds, subjects, rights.* Routledge: 1–17.

Birch, Kean. 2017. "Rethinking value in the bio-economy: Finance, assetization, and the management of value." *Science, Technology & Human Values*, 42: 460–490.

Birch, Kean, DT Cochrane, and Callum Ward. 2021. "Data as asset? The measurement, governance, and valuation of digital personal data Big Tech." *Big Data & Society*, January–June: 1–15.

Biruk, Crystal. 2018. *Cooking data: Culture and politics in an African research world.* Duke University Press.

Björnberg, Arne, and Ann Yung Phang. 2019. *Euro Health Consumer Index 2018.* Health Consumer Powerhouse.

Blair, Ann M. 2010. *Too much to know: Managing scholarly information before the modern age.* Yale University Press.

Blocker, Gene. 1974. *The meaning of meaningslessness.* Martinus Nijhoff Publishers.

Blomberg, Stig Nikolaj, Fredrik Folke, Annette Kjær Ersbøll, Helle Collatz Christensen, Christian Torp-Pedersen, Michael R Sayre, Catherine R Counts, and Freddy K Lippert. 2019. "Machine learning as a supportive tool to recognize cardiac arrest in emergency calls." *Resuscitation*, 138: 322–329.

Bodenhorn, Barbara, and Gabriele vom Bruck. 2006. ""Entangled in histories": An introduction to the anthropology of names and naming." In Gabriele vom Bruck and Barbara Bodenhorn (eds.), *The anthropology of names and naming.* Cambridge University Press: 1–30.

Bohlin, Ingemar. 2011. "Evidensbaserat beslutsfattande i ett vetenskapsbaserat samhälle: Om evidensrörelsens ursprung, utbredning och gränser." In Ingemar Bohlin and Morten Sager (eds.), *Evidensens många ansikten.* Arkiv Förlag: 31–68.

Bonde, Morten, Claus Bossen, and Peter Danholt. 2018. "Translating value-based health care: An experiment into healthcare governance and dialogical accountability." *Sociology of Health & Illness*, 40: 1113–1126.

Bonde, Morten, Claus Bossen, and Peter Danholt. 2019. "Data-work and friction: Investigating the practices of repurposing healthcare data." *Health Informatics Journal*, 25: 558–566.

Borgman, Christine L. 2015. *Big data, little data, no data—scholarship in the networked world.* MIT Press.

Bossen, Claus. 2014. "Journaliseringsteknologi." In Lotte Huniche and Finn Olesen (eds.), *Teknologi i sundhedspraksis.* Munksgaard: 155–178.

Bossen, Claus, Yunan Chen, and Kathleen H. Pine. 2019. "The emergence of new data work occupations in healthcare: The case of medical scribes." *International Journal of Medical Informatics*, 123: 76–83.

Bossen, Claus, Kathleen H. Pine, Federico Cabitza, Gunnar Ellingsen, and Enrico Maria Piras. 2019. "Data work in healthcare: An Introduction." *Health Informatics Journal*, 25: 465–474.

Bovens, Mark, and Stavros Zouridis. 2002. "From street-level to system-level bureaucracies: How information and communication technology is transforming administrative discretion and constitutional control." *Public Administration Review*, 62: 174–184.

Bowe, Emily, Erin Simmons, and Shannon Mattern. 2020. "Learning from lines: Critical COVID data visualizations and the quarantine quotidian." *Big Data & Society*, July–December: 1–13.

Bowker, Geoffrey C. 2005. *Memory practices in the sciences*. MIT Press.

Bowker, Geoffrey C, and Susan Leigh Star. 1999. *Sorting things out—classification and its consequences*. MIT Press.

Boyce, Angie M. 2016. "Outbreaks and the management of "second-order friction": Repurposing materials and data from the health care and food systems for public health surveillance." *Science & Technology Studies*, 29: 52–69.

boyd, danah, and Kate Crawford. 2012. "Critical questions for big data: Provocations for a cultural, technological, and scholarly phenomenon." *Information, Communication & Society*, 15: 662–679.

Boysen, Mette. 2016. "Morten Hedegaard efter opsigelse: Jeg har aldrig prøvet noget lignende." *Dagens Medicin*, December 1, 2016, Karriere section.

Breit, Eric, Cathrine Egeland, and Ida Bring Løberg. 2019. "Cyborg bureaucracy: Frontline work in digitalized labor and welfare services." In John Storm Pedersen and Adrian Wilkinson (eds.), *Big data: Promise, application and pitfalls*. Edward Elgar Publishing: 149–169.

Brinkmann, Svend. 2014. "Doing without data." *Qualitative Inquiry*, 20: 720–725.

Brodersen, John, Lisa M. Schwartz, Carl Heneghan, Jack William O'Sullivan, Jeffrey K. Aronson, and Steven Woloshin. 2018. "Overdiagnosis: what it is and what it isn't." *BMJ Evidence-Based Medicine*, 32: 1–3.

Brown, Hannah, Adam Reed, and Thomas Yarrow. 2017. "Introduction: Towards an ethnography of meeting." *Journal of the Royal Anthropological Insitute*: 10–26.

Brown, John Seely, and Paul Duguid. 2000. *The Social Life of Information*. Harvard Business School Press.

Brown, Nik, Alison Kraft, and Paul Martin. 2006. "The Promissory Pasts of Blood Stem Cells." *BioSocieties*, 1: 329–348.

Brown, Nik, and Mike Michael. 2003. "A sociology of expectations: Retrospecting prospects and prospecting retrospects." *Technology Analysis and Strategic Management*, 15: 3–18.

Brunsson, Nils. 1989. *The organization of hypocrisy—talk, decisions and actions in organizations*. John Wiley & Sons.

Brunsson, Nils. 1999. "Standardization as organization." In Morten Egeberg and Per Lægreid (eds.), *Organizing Political Institutions*. Scandinavian University Press: 109–128.

Brunton, Finn, and Helen Nissenbaum. 2015. *Obfuscation: A user's guide for privacy and protest*. MIT Press.

Bruun, Maja Hojer, and Ayo Wahlberg. 2022. "The anthropology of technology: The formation of a field." In Maja Hojer Bruun, Ayo Wahlberg, Rachel Douglas-Jones, Cathrine Hasse, Klaus Hoeyer, Dorthe Brogård Kristensen and Brit Ross Winthereik (eds.), *Palgrave handbook of the anthropology of technology*. Springer: 1–33.

Büchner, Stefanie. 2018. "Digitale Infrastrukturen—Spezifik, Relationalität und die Paradoxien von Wandel und Kontrolle." *AIS-Studien*, 11: 279–293.

Buckingham, Marcus, and Ashley Goodall. 2015. "Reinventing performance management." *Harvard Business Review*, 93: 40–50.

Busch, Lawrence. 2011. *Standards: Recipes for reality*. MIT Press.

Busch, Lawrence. 2017. "Looking in the wrong La(place)? The promise and perils of becoming big data." *Science, Technology & Human Values*, 42: 657–678.

Caduff, Carlo. 2015. *The pandemic perhaps: Dramatic events in a public culture of danger*. University of California Press.

Caduff, Carlo. 2020. "What went wrong: Corona and the world after the full stop." *Medical Anthropology Quarterly*, 34(4): 467–487.

Callahan, Daniel. 2009. *Taming the beloved beast: How medical technology costs are destroying our health care system*. Princeton University Press.

Callison, William, and Quinn Slobodian. 2021. "Coronapolitics from the Reichtag to the Capitol." *Boston Review*, January 12, 2021, Politics section.

Callon, Michel, and John Law. 2005. "On qualculation, agency, and otherness." *Environment and Planning D: Society and Spaces*, 23: 717–733.

Callon, Michel, and Fabian Muniesa. 2005. "Economic markets as calculative collective devices." *Organization Studies*, 26: 1229–1250.

Campbell, Donald T. 1979. "Assessing the Impact of Planned Social Change," *Evaluation and Program Planning*, 2: 67–90.

Carsten, Janet. 2011. "Substance and relationality: Blood in contexts." *Annual Review of Anthropology*, 40: 19–35.

Carusi, Annamaria. 2014. "Personalised medicine: Visions and visualisations." *Tecnoscienza*, 5: 172–179.

Carusi, Annamaria. 2016. "In silico medicine: Social, technological and symbolic mediation." *Journal of Philosophical Studies*, 30: 67–86.

Carusi, Annamaria. 2020. "Things and trends: Images of COVID-19." *BMJ Blog*, Medical Humanities, https://blogs.bmj.com/medical-humanities/2020/04/22/things-and-trends-images-of-covid-19/.

Carusi, Annamaria, and Giovanni De Grandis. 2012. "The ethical work that regulations will not do." *Information, Communication & Society*, 15: 124–141.

Castells, Manuel. 2010. *The rise of the network society*. Wiley-Blackwell.

Chafkin, Max. 2021. *The contrarian: Peter Thiel and Silicon Valley's pursuit of power*. Max Bloomsbury Publishing.

Chan, Kitty S., Jinnet B. Fowles, and Jonathan P. Weiner. 2010. "Electronic health records and the reliability and validity of quality measures: A review of the literature." *Medical Care Research and Review*, 67: 503–527.

Cheney-Lippold, John. 2017. *We are data: Algorithms and the making of our digital selves*. New York University Press.

Christofides, Emily, and Kieran O"Doherty. 2016. "Company disclosure and consumer perceptions of the privacy implications of direct-to-consumer genetic testing." *New Genetics and Society*, 35: 101–123.

Clante, Caroline, and Marie Allerslev Eriksen. 2021. "Michala var kollega til dræbt læge: Nu kæmper hun for mere beskyttelse." *DR Nyheder*, April 28, 2021.

Clark, A. J. 1937. "Individual variation in response to drugs." *British Medical Journal*: 307–310.

Clausen, Line Egede. 2020. *Datainfrastrukturer i forandring* (Data infrastructures in transition) Københavns Universitet.

Clifford, James. 1986. "On ethnographic allegory." In James Clifford and George E. Marcus (eds.), *Writing culture: The poetics and politics of ethnography*. University of California Press: 205–228.

Clotworthy, Amy, Agnete Skovlund Dissing, Tri-Long Nguyen, et al. 2020. "'Standing together—at a distance': Documenting changes in mental-health indicators in Denmark during the COVID-19 pandemic." *Scandinavian Journal of Public Health*, 49: 79–87.

Clotworthy, Amy; Rudi Westendorp. 2020. "Risky business: How older 'at risk' people in Denmark evaluated their situated risk during the COVID-19 pandemic." *Anthropology & Aging*, 41: 167–176.

Collen, Morris F. 1986. "Origins of medical informatics." *Western Journal of Medicine*, 145: 778–785.

Collen, Morris F. 1991. "A brief historical overview of Hospital Information System (HIS) evolution in the United States." *International Journal of Bio-Medical Computing* 29: 169–189.

Comte, Auguste. 1988 [1830–1842]. *Introduction to positive philosophy*. Hackett Publishing Company.

Connerton, Paul. 1989. *How societies remember*. Cambridge University Press.

Cool, Alison. 2016. "Detaching data from the state: Biobanking and building big data in Sweden." *BioSocieties*, 11: 277–295.

Cool, Alison. 2019. "Impossible, unknowable, acocuntable: Dramas and dilemmas of data law." *Social Studies of Science*, 49: 503–530.

Crawford, Kate. 2014. "The anxieties of big data." *The New Inquiry*: 1–11.

Crawford, Kate. 2021. *Atlas of AI*. Yale University Press.

Creager, Angela N. H. 2021. "To test or not to test: Tools, rules, and corporate data in US chemicals regulations." *Science, Technology & Human Values*, 46: 975–997.

Cruz, Taylor M. 2017. "The making of a population: Challenges, implications, and consequences of the quantification of social difference." *Social Science & Medicine*, 174: 79–85.

Czarniawska, Barbara. 2005. "Fashion in organizing." In Barbara Czarniawska and Guje Sevón (eds.), *Global ideas: How ideas, objects and practices travel in the global economy*. Liber & Copenhagen Business School Press: 129–146.

Daemmrich, Arthur A. 2004. *Pharmacopolitics: Drug regulation in the United States and Germany*. University of North Carolina Press.

Dagiral, Eric, and Khetrimayum Monish Singh. 2021. "Governance and accountable citizenship through identification infrastructures: Database politics of Copernicus (France) and National Register of Citizens (India)." *Science, Technology & Society*, 25: 368–385.

Dahdah, Marine Al, and Rajiv K. Mishra. 2020. "Smart cards for all: Digitalisation of universal health coverage in India." *Science, Technology & Society*, 25: 426–443.

Dahler-Larsen, Peter. 2012. *The evaluation society*. Stanford University Press.

Dalsgaard. 2019. "Mistænkt for lægedrab i Tisvilde havde flere lægers navne på en liste." *DR Nyheder*, September 2, 2019, Indland section.

Dansk Psykolog Forening. 2020. "DR og DP indgår aftale om teknisk løsning for videokonsultationer via sundhed.dk." Dansk Psykolog Forening, https://www.dp.dk /danske-regioner-og-dansk-psykolog-forening-indgaar-aftale-om-teknisk-loesning -for-videokonsultationer-via-sundhed-dk/.

Danske Regioner. 2015. *Handlingsplan for personlig medicin*. Danske Regioner.

Danske Regioner. 2020. "Videokonsultationer skal mindske smitterisikoen hos de praktiserende læger." *Danske Regioner*, March 17, 2020, Corona/COVID-19 section.

Danske Regioner. 2021. "En ny digital løsning fra regionerne skal aflaste læger i hele landet." Danske Regioner, March 24, 2021. https://www.regioner.dk/services /nyheder/2020/marts/ny-digital-loesning-fra-regionerne-skal-aflaste-laeger-i-hele -landet.

Danske Regioner, and Dansk Industri. 2019. *HealthTech:DK. Danmark som førende HealthTech-nation*. Danske Regioner and Dansk Industri.

Das, Veena. 2000. "The practice of organ transplants: Networks, documents, translations." In Margaret Lock, A. Young, and Alberto Cambrosio (eds.), *Living and working with the new medical technologies: Intersections of inquiry*. Cambridge University Press: 263–287.

Daston, Lorraine. 2020. "Ground-zero empiricism." *Critical Inquiry*, 47: S55–S57.

Daston, Lorraine, and Peter Galison. 2010. "Epistemologies of the eye." In *Objectivity*. Zone Books: 17–53.

Datatilsynet. 2020. "Midlertidig stans av appen Smittestopp," https://www.datatilsynet .no/aktuelt/aktuelle-nyheter-2020/midlertidig-stans-av-appen-smittestopp /?utm_source=ActiveCampaign&utm_medium=email&utm_content=Smittestop-ap p+er+landet%3A+S%C3%A5dan+fungerer+den&utm_campaign=Technorama+%28 uge+25%29.

Davies, Gail, Emma Frow, and Sabina Leonelli. 2013. "Bigger, faster, better? Rhetorics and practices of large-scale research in contemporary bioscience." *BioSocieties*, 8: 386–396.

Davis, Mark, and Davina Lohm. 2020. *Pandemics, publics, and narrative*. Oxford University Press.

Davis, Sara L. M. 2017. "The uncounted: politics of data and visibility in global health." *International Journal of Human Rights*, 21: 1144–1163.

Dean, Mitchell. 2010. *Governmentality: Power and rule in modern society*. SAGE.

de Boer, Bas. 2020. "Experiencing objectified health: Turning the body into an object of attention." *Medicine, Health Care and Philosophy*, 23: 401–411.

Decoteau, Clarie Laurier, and Kelly Underman. 2015. "Adjudicating non-knowledge in the Omnibus Autism Proceedings." *Social Studies of Science*, 45: 471–500.

Deming, William Edwards. 1986. *Out of the crisis*. Center for Advanced Engineering Studies.

Denis, Jérôme, and Samuel Goëta. 2017. "Rawification and the careful generation of open government data." *Social Studies of Science*, 47: 604–629.

Derrida, Jacques. 1995. "Archive fever: A Freudian impression." *Diacritics*, 25: 9–63.

Desrosiéres, Alain. 1998. *The politics of large numbers: A history of statistical reasoning*. Harvard University Press.

Deville, Joe, Michael Guggenheim, and Zuzana Hrdlicková. 2016. "Introduction: The practices and infrastructures of comparison." In Joe Deville, Michael Guggenheim, and Zuzana Hrdlicková (eds.), *Practising comparison logics, relations, collaborations*. Mattering Press:17–39.

Devlin, Kat, and Aidan Connaughton. 2020. "Most approve of national response to COVID-19 in 14 advanced economies. But many also say their country is more divided due to the outbreak." Washington, D.C., Pew Research Center: 1-22.

Dewey, John. 1929. *The quest for certainty. A study of the relation of knowledge and action*. G. P. Putnam's Sons.

Dewey, John. 1998. "The problem of truth." In Larry A Hickman and Thomas M Alexander (eds.), *The essential Dewey, volume 2: Ethics, logic, phsycology*. Indiana University Press: 101–130.

Dickenson, Donna. 2013. *Me medicine vs. we medicine: Reclaiming biotechnology for the common good*. Columbia University Press.

Dickenson, Donna, Britta van Beers, and Sigrid Sterckx. 2018. "Introduction." In Britta van Beers, Sigrid Sterckx, and Donna Dickenson (eds.), *Personalised medicine, individual choice and the common good*. Cambridge University Press: 1–16.

Didier, Emmanuel. 2009. *America by the numbers: Quantification, democracy, and the birth of national statistics*. MIT Press.

Digitaliseringspartnerskabet. 2021. "Visioner og anbefalinger til Danmark som digitalt foregangsland." Regeringen: 1–99.

Digital Vækstpanel. 2017. *Danmark som digital frontløber*. Erhvervsministeriet.

Di Nucci, Ezio. 2021. *The control paradox: From AI to populism*. Rowman & Littlefield.

Domingos, Pedro. 2015. *The master algorithm*. Penguin Books.

Donaldson, M. S., J. M. Corrigan, and L. T. Kohn. 2000. *To err is human: Building a safer health system*. National Academies Press.

Douglas-Jones, Rachel, Antonia Walford, and Nick Seaver. 2021. "Introduction: Towards an anthropology of data." *Journal of the Royal Anthropological Insitute*, 27: 9–25.

Dourish, Paul. 2004. "What we talk about when we talk about context." *Personal and Ubiquitous Computing*, 8: 19–30.

Dove, Edward S., Jiahong Chen. 2020. "Should consent for data processing be privileged in health research? A comparative legal analysis" *International Data Privacy Law*, 10: 117–131.

DR Nyheder. 2018. "FN kårer Danmark som verdensmester i offentlig digitalisering." July 19, 2018, Indland section.

DR Nyheder. 2019a. "Amazon erobrer pladsen som verdens mest værdifulde selskab." *DR Nyheder*, January 8.

DR Nyheder. 2019b. "De er illegalt i Danmark og nu åbner Røde Kors for endnu mere lægehjælp til dem." *DR Nyheder*, March 12, 2019, Fyn section.

DR Nyheder. 2020. "Danmark er det dyreste land i EU." *DR Nyheder*, June 21, 2020, Indland section.

Dumit, Joseph. 2012. *Drugs for life: How pharmaceutical companies define our health*. Duke University Press.

Durnová, Anna. 2019. *Understanding emotions in post-factual politics: Negotiating truth*. Edward Elgar Publishing.

Dørge, Henrik. 2017. "Mere arbejde, færre børn." *Weekendavisen*, January 20: 5.

Easton, David. 1953. *The political system: An inquiry into the state of political science* Alfred A. Knopf.

Easton, David. 1965. *A framework for political analysis*. Prentice-Hall.

Ebeling, Mary F. E. 2016. *Healthcare and big data. Digital specters and phantom objects*. Palgrave Macmillan.

Ecks, Stefan. 2008. "Three propositions for an evidence-based medical anthropology." *Journal of the Royal Anthropological Insitute*, 14: 77–92.

Edwards, Paul N. 2010. *A vast machine: Computer models, climate data, and the politics of global warming*. MIT Press.

Edwards, Paul N., Matthew S. Mayernik, Archer L. Batcheller, Geoffrey C. Bowker, and Christine L. Borgman. 2011. "Science friction: Data, metadata, and collaboration." *Social Studies of Science*, 41: 667–690.

Egilman, David S. 2005. "Suppression bias at the Journal of Occupation and Environmental Medicine." *International Journal of Occupational and Environmental Health*, 11: 202–204.

Eichler, Hans-Georg, Brigitte Bloechl-Daum, Karl Broich, et al. 2018. "Data rich, information poor: Can we use electronic health records to create a learning healthcare system for pharmaceuticals?" *Clinical Pharmacoloty & Therapeutics*, 105: 912–922.

Ejbye-Ernst, Anders. 2019a. "I 10 år har de løber hurtigere, mens opgaven er vokset—nu skal de øge tempoet med 8 pct." *Dagens Medicin*, December 13: 6–8.

Ejbye-Ernst, Anders. 2019b. "Myten om de 8 procent." *Dagens Medicin*, October 25, 2019, 4–7.

Epstein, Steven. 2007. *Inclusion: The politics of difference in medical research*. University of Chicago Press.

Erikson, Susan L. 2012. "Global health business: The production and performativity of statistics in Sierra Leone and Germany." *Medical Anthropology*, 31: 367–384.

Erikson, Susan L. 2016. "Metrics and market logics of global health." In Vincanne Adams (ed.), *Metrics: What counts in global health*. Duke University Press: 147–162.

Espeland, Wendy Nelson, and Mitchell L Stevens. 2008. "A sociology of quantification." *European Journal of Sociology*, 49: 401–436.

European Commission. 2020a. "A European health data space." European Commission.

European Commission. 2020b. *A European strategy for data: Communication from the Commission to the European Parliament, the Council, the European Economic and Social Committee and the Committee of the Regions*. European Commission.

European Commission. 2020c. *Europe's moment: Repair and prepare for the next generation* European Commission.

Evans, S. R. 2016. "Electronic health records: Then, now, and in the future." *IMIA Yearbook of Medical Informatics*: S48–S61.

Faber, Stine Thidemann, and Claus D. Hansen. 2020. "Betydningen af køn og kønsnormer i det epidemiske samfund: COVID-19 i et kønsperspektiv." In Ole B. Jensen and Nikolaj Schultz (eds.), *Det epidemiske samfund*. Hans Reitzels Forlag: 117–132.

Fainzang, Sylvie. 2002. "Lying, secrecy and power within the doctor-patient relationship." *Anthropology and Medicine*, 9: 118–133.

Farrington, Conor, and Rebecca Lynch. 2018. "Personal medical devices: People and technology in the context of health." in Rebecca Lynch and Conor Farrington (eds.), *Quantified lives and vital data: Exploring health and technology through personal medical devices*. Palgrave Macmillan: 3–16

Fassin, Didier. 2018. *The will to punish*. Oxford University Press.

Faulkner, Alex. 2009. *Medical technology into healthcare and society: A sociology of devices, innovation and governance*. Palgrave Macmillan.

Faulkner, Alex, and Julie Kent. 2001. "Innovation and regulation in human implant technologies: Developing comparative approaches." *Social Science & Medicine*, 53: 895–913.

Fedak, Kristen M., Autumn Bernal, Zachary A. Capshaw, and Sherilyn Gross. 2015. "Applying the Bradford Hill criteria in the 21st century: How data integration has changed causal inference in molecular epidemiology." *Emerging Themes in Epidemiology*, 12: 1–9.

Feldman, Martha S., and James G. March. 1981. "Information in organizations as signal and symbol." *Administrative Science Quarterly*, 26: 171–186.

Felt, Ulrike, Susanne Öchsner, and Robin Rae. 2020. "The making of digital health: Between visions and realizations." *University, Society, Industry*, 9: 89–101.

Ferguson, James. 1994. *The anti-politics machine: "Development," depoliticization, and bureaucratic power in Lesotho*. University of Minnesota Press.

Fernandez, Anne Lutz, and Catherine Lutz. 2019. "Roboeducation." in Catherine Besteman and Hugh Gusterson (eds.), *Life by algorithms. How roboprocesses are remaking our world*. University of Chicago Press: 44–58.

Finkelstein, Eric A, Benjamin A. Haaland, Marcel Bilger, Aarti Sahasranaman, Robert A. Sloan, Ei Ei Khaing Nang, and Kelly R. Evenson. 2016. "Effectiveness of activity trackers with and without incentives to increase physical activity (TRIPPA): A randomised controlled trial." *Lancet Diabetes & Endocrinology*, 4: 983–995.

Fiore-Gartland, Brittany, and Gina Neff. 2016. "Disruption and the political economy of biosensor data." In Dawn Nafus (ed.), *Quantified: Biosensing technologies in everyday life*. MIT Press: 101–122.

Fiske, Amelia, Alena Buyx, and Barbara Prainsack. 2020. "The double-edged sword of digital self-care: Physician perspectives from northern Germany." *Social Science & Medicine*, 260: 113174.

Fiske, Amelia, Barbara Prainsack, and Alena Buyx. 2019. "Data work: Meaning-making in the era of data-rich medicine." *Journal of Medical Internet Research*, 21: e11672.

Fleck, Ludwik. 1979. *Genesis and development of a scientific fact*. University of Chicago Press.

Folketinget. 2014. "Forslag til lov om ændring af lov om Det Centrale Personregister." Folketinget.

Folkmann, Anne Sophie Hyldedal. 2017. "Læger efter dødsfald: Utroligt der ikke blev lavet større fejl i det kaos." *Jyllands-Posten*, September 28.

Forsvaret. 2018. *Statistiske oplysninger: Udfaldet, gennemsnitshøjden og BMI Body Mass Index) på forsvarets dag/session*. Forsvaret.

Fortun, Michael. 2008. *Promising genomics: Iceland and deCODE Genetics in a world of speculation*. University of California Press.

Foucault, Michel. 1973. *The birth of the clinic—an archaeology of medical perception*. Vintage Books.

Foucault, Michel. 1991. "Governmentality," In Graham Burchell, Colin Gordon, and Peter Miller (eds.), *The Foucault effect: Studies in governmentality*. University of Chicago Press: 87–104.

Foucault, Michel. 1997. "On the genealogy of ethics: An overview of work in progress," In Paul Rabinow (ed.), *Ethics: Essential works of Foucault, 1954–1984, volume 1*. Penguin: 253–280.

Foucault, Michel. 2002. *Overvågning og Straf. Fængslets Fødsel* (Discipline and punish: The birth of the prison). Det Lille Forlag.

Fourcade, Marion, and Daniel N Kluttz. 2020. "A Maussian bargain: Accumulation by gift in the digital economy." *Big Data & Society*, January–June: 1–16.

Frandsen, Morten. 2019. "Tusindvis af danskere får receptpligtig medicin fra engelske net-apoteker." *DR Nyheder*, December 26, 2019, Indland section.

Frank, Arthur W. 2012. *Letting stories breathe: A socio-narratology.* University of Chicago Press.

Frank, Lone. 2000. "When an entire country is a cohort." *Science*, 287: 2398–2399.

Frank, Lone. 2003. "The epidemiologist's dream: Denmark." *Science*, 301: 163–163.

Franklin, Sarah. 2006. "The IVF-stem cell interface." *International Journal of Surgery*, 4: 86–90.

Franklin, Sarah. 2007. *Dolly mixtures: The remaking of genealogy.* Duke University Press.

Frykman, Jonas, and Orvar Löfgren. 1987. *Culture Builders - A Historical Anthropology of Middle-Class Life.* Rutgers University press: New Brunswick and London.

Freedom House. 2021. "Freedom in the net 2021. The global drive to control big tech." Washington, Freedom House: 1–42.

French, Martin. 2014. "Gaps in the gaze: Informatic practice and the work of public health surveillance." *Surveillance and Society*, 12: 226–243.

Frenkel, Michal. 2005. "The politics of translation: How state-level political relations affect the cross-national travel of management ideas." *Organization*, 12: 275–301.

Friis, Jan Kyrre Berg Olsen. 2020. "Enactive hermeneutics and smart medical technologies." *AI & Society*: 1–9.

Friis, Jan Kyrre Berg Olsen. 2021. "Radiology as skillful coping and enactive hermeneutics." In Samantha J. Fried and Robert Rosenberger (eds.), *Postphenomenology and imaging: How to read technology.* Rowman & Littlefield/ Lexington Books: 127–148.

Frost, Karl Emil. 2021. "Valgdeltagelsen faldt i næsten alle kommuner: Forsker frygter øget demokratisk ulighed." *Altinget.dk*, November 28, 2021.

Frost & Sullivan. 2017. *Digitalization in healthcare: Emergence of digital health portals.* Frost & Sullivan.

Fuchs, Christian. 2016. "Introduction." In *Reading Marx in the information age: A media and communication studies perspective on Capital, volume 1.* Routledge: 1–12.

Fuchs, Christian. 2018. *Digital demagogue: Authoritarian capitalism in the age of Trump and Twitter.* Pluto Press.

Gabrielsen, Ane Møller. 2020. "Openness and trust in data-intensive care: The case of biocuration." *Medicine, Health Care and Philosophy*, 23: 497–504.

Gadsbøll, Niels. 2017. "10 gode råd til at overleve Sundhedsplatformen." *Dagens Medicin*, August 25:19.

Gardner, John, and Clare Williams. 2015. "Corporal diagnostic work and diagnostic spaces: Clinicians' use of space and bodies during diagnosis." *Sociology of Health & Illness*, 37: 765–781.

Garfinkel, Harold. 1984. *Studies in ethnomethodology*. Polity Press.

Gefenas, Eugenijus, J. Lekstutiene, V. Lukaseviciene, M. Hartlev, M. Mourby, and K. Ó. Cathaoir. 2021. 'Controversies between regulations of research ethics and protection of personal data: informed consent at a cross-road', *Medicine, Health Care and Philosophy, 25*: 25-30.

Gehl, Robert W. 2019. "Emotional roboprocesses." In Catherine Besteman and Hugh Gusterson (eds.), *Life by algorithms: How roboprocesses are remaking our world*. University of Chicago Press: 107–121.

Geiger, Susi. 2020. "Silicon Valley, disruption, and the end of uncertainty." *Journal of Cultural Economy*, 13: 169–184.

Geiger, Susi, and Nicole Gross. 2019. "A tidal wave of inevitable data? Assetization in the consumer genomics testing industry." *Business & Society*, 60: 614–649.

Geissler, P. W. 2013. "Public secrets in public health: Knowing not to know while making scientific knowledge." *American Ethnologist*, 40: 13–34.

General Secretariat of the Council: Working Party on Public Health. 2015. *Council conclusions on personalised medicine for patients*. General Secretariat of the Council.

Gitelman, Lisa, and Virginia Jackson. 2013. "Introduction." In Lisa Gitelman (ed.), *"Raw data" is an oxymoron* MIT Press: 1–14.

Gjødsbøl, Iben Mundbjerg, Bo Gregers Winkel, and Henning Bundgaard. 2019. "Personalized medicine and preventive health care: juxtaposing health policy and clinical practice." *Critical Public Health*, 31: 327–337.

Gjørup, Jes, and Henrik Hjortdal. 2007. "Tilgiv os—vi vidste ikke, hvad vi gjorde." *Politiken*, March 29: 7–8.

Goldenberg, Maya J. 2021. *Vaccine hesitancy: Public trust, expertise, and the war on science* University of Pittsburgh Press.

Goodwin, Dawn. 2010. "Sensing the way: Embodied dimensions of diagnostic work." In Monika Büscher, Dawn Goodwin, and Jessica Mesman (eds.), *Ethnographies of diagnostic work. Dimensions of transformative practice*. Palgrave Macmillan: 73–92.

Goriunova, Olga. 2019. "The digital subject: People as data as persons." *Theory, Culture & Society*, 36: 125–145.

Gorur, Radhika. 2011. "ANT on the PISA trail: Following the statistical pursuit of certainty." *Educational Philosophy and Theory*, 43: 76–93.

Gottlieb, Samatha D. 2013. "The patient-consumer-advocate nexus." *Medical Anthropology Quarterly*, 27: 330–347.

Grabowski, Dan, Julie Meldgaard, and Morten Hulvej Rod. 2020. "Altered self-observations, unclear risk perceptions and changes in relational everyday life: A qualitative study of psychosocial life with diabetes during the COVID-19 lockdown." *Societies*, 10: 1–13.

Graeber, David. 2018. *Bullshit jobs: A theory*. Simon & Schuster Paperbacks.

Gray, Jonathan, Carolin Gerlitz, and Liliana Bounegru. 2018. "Data infrastructure literacy." *Big Data & Society*, July–December: 1–13.

Green, Sara, Annamaria Carusi, and Klaus Hoeyer. 2022. "Plastic diagnostics: The remaking of disease and evidence in personalised medicine." *Social Science and Medicine 304*: 1–9.

Green, Sara, and Henrik Vogt. 2016. "Personalizing medicine: Disease prevention *in silico* and *in socio*." *Journal of Philosophical Studies*, 30: 105–145.

Greene, Jeremy A. 2007. *Prescribing by numbers: Drugs and the definition of disease.* Johns Hopkins University Press.

Greene, Jeremy A., and Andrew S. Lea. 2019. "Digital futures past the long arc of big data in medicine." *New England Journal of Medicine* 381: 480–485.

Greenhalgh, Trisha, Gerald Choon Huat Koh, and Josip Ca. 2020. "Covid-19: A remote assessment in primary care." *BMJ*, 368: 1–5.

Gregory, Kathleen Marie. 2020. *Findable and reuseable? Data discovery practices in research.* Maastrict University.

Gregory, Kathleen Marie, Paul Groth, Andrea Scharnhorst, and Sally Wyatt. 2020. "Lost or found? Discovering data needed for research." *Harvard Data Science Review*, 2: 1–51.

Grimes, David A. 2010. "Epidemiologic research using administrative databases: Garbage in, garbage out." *Obstetrics & Gynecology*, 116: 1018–1019.

Grommé, Francisca, and Evelyn Ruppert. 2020. "Population geometries of Europe: The topologies of data cubes and grids." *Science, Technology & Human Values*, 45: 235–261.

Gross, Matthias. 2010. *Ignorance and surprise.* MIT Press,

Grossman, Maurice. 1977. "Confidentiality in medical practice." *Annual Review of Medicine*, 28: 43–55.

Gruzd, Anatoliy, and Philip Mai. 2020. "Going viral: How a single tweet spawned a COVID-19 conspiracy theory on Twitter." *Big Data & Society*, July–December: 1–9.

Grünenberg, Kristina. 2020. "Wearing someone else's face: Biometric technologies, anti-spoofing and the fear of the unknown." *Ethnos*, 87: 223–240.

Grünenberg, Kristina, Perle Møhl, Karen Fog Olwig, and Anja Simonsen. 2020. "Issue introduction: IDentities and identity: biometric technologies, borders and migration." *Ethnos*, 87: 211–222.

Guerdali, Amal, and Søren K. Nielsen. 2018. "Amalie besvimede for fire år siden under en piercing: Nu må hun vente på at få kørekort." *DR Nyheder*, October 22, 2018, Regionalt section.

Gunnarson, Martin. 2016. *Please be patient: A cultural phenomenological study of haemodialysis and kidney transplantation care.* Media-Tryck.

Gupta, Akhil. 2018. "The future in ruins: Thoughts on the temporality of infrastructure." In Nikhil Anand, Akhil Gupta, and Hannah Appel (eds.), *The promise of infrastructure.* Duke University Press: 62–79.

Hacking, Ian. 1986. "Making up people." In Thomas C. Heller, Morton Sosna, and David E. Wellbery (eds.), *Reconstructing individualism. Autonomy, individuality, and the self in Western thought.* Stanford University Press: 222–236.

Hagemann-Nielsen, Frederik. 2020. "Danmarks kollektive dødsdom til mink går verden rundt: "Det giver grund til bekymring"." *DR Nyheder*, November 5, 2020, Udland section.

Haggerty, Kevin D., and Richard V. Ericson. 2000. "The surveillant assemblage." *British Journal of Sociology*, 51: 605–622.

Halpern, Orit. 2014. *Beautiful data: A history of vision and reason since 1945.* Duke University Press.

Halpern, Sydney A. 2004. *Lesser harms.* University of Chicago Press.

Halting Problem. 2017. "Facebook"s new motto: 'Move fast and please please please don"t break anything.'" *Medium*, May 22, 2017. https://medium.com/halting-problem /facebooks-new-motto-move-fast-and-please-please-please-don-t-break-anything -8aefdd405d15.

Hamblin, James. 2020. *Clean: The new science of skin and the beauty of doing less.* Riverhead Books.

Hand, David J. 2020. *Dark data: Why what you don't know matters.* Princeton University Press.

Harari, Yuval Noah. 2018. *Homo Deus. En kort historie om i morgen.* Lindhardt og Ringhof.

Harari, Yuval Nori. 2020. "Yuval Noah Harari: The world after coronavirus." *Financial Times*, March 20, 2020.

Hartmans, Avery, and Paige Leskin. 2020. "The rise and fall of Elizabeth Holmes, the Theranos founder whose federal fraud trial is delayed until 2021." *Business Insider,* August 11, 2020.

Hartong, Sigrid, and Annina Förschler. 2019. "Opening the black box of data-based school monitoring: Data infrastructures, flows and practices in state education agencies." *Big Data & Society*, January–June: 1–12.

Harwell, Drew. 2018. "Scarlett Johansson on fake AI-generated sex videos: 'Nothing can stop someone from cutting and pasting my image.'" *Washington Post*, December 31, 2018, Technology section.

Hastrup, Kirsten. 1994. "Anthropological Knowledge Incorporated. Discussion." In Kirsten Hastrup and Peter Hervik (eds.), *Social Experience and Anthropological Knowledge* Routledge: 224–240.

Hastrup, Kirsten. 1995. *A passage to anthropology. Between experience and theory* Routledge.

Hatch, Steven. 2016. *Snowball in a blizzard. The tricky problem of uncertainty in medicine.* Atlantic Books.

Healy, Kieran. 2017. "Fuck nuance." *American Sociological Association*, 35: 118–127.

Hecht, Jennifer Michael. 2003. *The end of the soul: Scientific modernity, atheism, and anthropology in France.* Columbia Unviersity Press.

Hecklen, Alexander 2017. "Afdelingschef om fejl i kræftkontrol: Vi er gået tilbage til papir." *DR.dk*, July 3.

Hedegaard, Metta, Øjvind Lidegaard, Charlotte Wessel Skovlund, Lina Steinrud Mørch, and Morten Hedegaard. 2014. "Reduction in stillbirths at term after new birth induction paradigm: results of a national intervention." *BMJ Open*, 4, doi: 10.1136/bmjopen-2014-005785.

Hedgecoe, Adam. 2004. *The politics of personalised medicine: Pharmacogenetics in the clinic*. Cambridge University Press.

Heick, Kamma Kronborg. 2016. "Læger får krisehjælp på grund af nyt it-system." *DR.dk*, June 14, 2016. København Section.

Heissel, Anders. 2020. "Bor flere sammen og har udsatte job: Indvandrere har markant højere risiko for at blive indlagt med corona." *DR Nyheder*, December 20, 2020, Indland section.

Henderson, R., and N. Keiding. 2005. "Individual survival time prediction using statistical models." *Journal of Medical Ethics*, 31: 703–706.

Henriksen, Anne, and Anja Bechmann. 2020. "Building trust in AI: Making predictive algorithms doable in healthcare." *Information, Communication & Society*, 23: 802–16.

Henriksen, Thomas Duus, Rikke Kristine Nielsen, Signe Vikkelsø, Frans Bévort, and Mette Mogensen. 2021. "A paradox rarely comes alone a quantitative approach to investigating knotted leadership paradoxes in SMEs." *Scandinavian Journal of Management*, 37: 101135.

Henwood, Flis, Sally Wyatt, Angie Hart, and Julie Smith. 2003. "'Ignorance is bliss sometimes': Constraints on the emergence of the 'informed patient' in the changing landscapes of health information." *Sociology of Health & Illness*, 25: 589–607.

Hildebrandt, Sybille. 2017a. "Firmaer fusker med kliniske data for generiske lægemidler." *Dagens Medicin*, November 17, 2017.

Hildebrandt, Sybille. 2017b. "Novo Nordisk har ansat specialister til at opspore fejl og fusk i kliniske studier." *Dagens Pharma*, November 30, 2017.

Hildebrandt, Sybille. 2017c. "Sundhedsplatformen: 500 klinikere foretrak Cerner frem for EPIC." *Dagens Medicin*, October 5, 2017: 5–5.

Hildebrandt, Sybille. 2017d. "Sundhedsøkonom: Sundhedsplatformens business case holder ikke." *Dagens Medicin*, July 4, 2017: 8–12.

Hill, Austin Bradford. 1965. "The environment and disease: Association or causation?." *Proceedings of the Royal Society of London. Section of Occupational Medicine*: 295–300.

Himmelstein, David, and Steffie Woolhandler. 2015. "Quality improvement: 'Become good at cheating and you never need to become good at anything else.'" *Health Affairs Blog*: 1–6.

Hjertholm, Peter, Kaare Rud Flarup, Louise Mahncke Guldbrandt, and Peter Vedsted. 2017. "The completeness of chest X-ray procedure codes in the Danish National Patient Registry." *Clinical Epidemiology*, 9: 151–156.

Hochschild, Arlie Russell. 1979. "Emotion work, feeling rules, and social structure." *American journal of sociology*, 85: 551–575.

Hoeyer, Klaus. 2005. "Studying ethics as policy: The naming and framing of moral problems in genetic research." *Current Anthropology*, 46: 71–90.

Hoeyer, Klaus. 2016. "Bioeconomy, moral friction and symbolic law." In Bart van Klink, Britta van Beers and Lonneke Poort (eds.), *Symbolic legislation theory and developments in biolaw*. Springer: 161–176.

Hoeyer, Klaus. 2019. *Hvem skal bruge sundhedsdata—og til hvad?* Informations Forlag.

Hoeyer, Klaus, Susanne Bauer, and Martyn Pickersgill. 2019. "Datafication and accountability in public health: Introduction to a special issue." *Social Studies of Science*, 49: 459–475.

Hoeyer, Klaus, and Malene Bødker. 2020. "Weak data: The social biography of a measurement instrument and how it failed to ensure accountability in home care." *Medical Anthropology Quarterly*, 34: 420–437.

Hoeyer, Klaus, and Linda F. Hogle. 2014. "Informed consent: The politics of intent and practice in medical research ethics." *Annual Review of Anthropology*, 43: 347–362.

Hoeyer, Klaus Lindgaard, and Henriette Langstrup. 2021. "Datafying the patient voice: The making of pervasive infrastructures as processes of promise, ruinaiton, and repair." In Susi Geiger (ed.), *Healthcare activism: Markets, morals, & the collective good*. Oxford University Press: 116–139.

Hoeyer, Klaus, and Richard Tutton. 2005. "'Ethics was here': studying the language-games of ethics in the Case of UK Biobank." *Critical Public Health*, 15: 385–397.

Hoeyer, Klaus, and Sarah Wadmann. 2020. "'Meaningless work': How the datafication of health reconfigures knowledge about work and erodes professional judgement." *Economy and Society*, 49: 433–454.

Hoeyer, Klaus, and Brit Ross Winthereik. 2022. "Knowing, unknowing, and re-knowing." In Maja Hojer Bruun, Ayo Wahlberg, Rachel Douglas-Jones, Cathrine Hasse, Klaus Hoeyer, Dorthe Brogård Kristensen, and Brit Ross Wintereik (eds.), *Palgrave handbook of the anthropology of technology*. Springer: 217–236.

Hoffman, Anna Lauren. 2018. "Making data valuable: Political, economic, and conceptual bases of big data." *Philosophy & Technology*, 31: 209–212.

Hoffman, Bjørn. 2020. "The first casualty of an epidemic is evidence." *Journal of Evaluation in Clinical Practice*, 26: 1344–1346.

Hoffmaster, Barry. 2001. *Bioethics in social context* Temple University Press.

Hogle, Linda F. 1995. "Standardization across non-standard domains: The case of organ procurement." *Science, Technology, & Human Values*, 20: 482–500.

Hogle, Linda F. 2016. "Data-intensive resourcing in healthcare." *BioSocieties*, 11: 372–393.

Hogle, Linda F. 2018. "Intersections: Global perspectives on stem cell technologies." In Aditya Bharadwaj (ed.), *Global perspectives on stem cell technologies*. Palgrave Macmillan.

Hogle, Linda F. 2019. "Accounting for accountable care: Value-based population health management." *Social Studies of Science*, 49: 556–582.

Hollands, Gareth J, David P French, Simon J Griffin, A Toby Prevost, Stephen Sutton, Sarah King, and Theresa M Marteau. 2016. "The impact of communicating genetic risks of disease on risk-reducing health behaviour: systematic review with meta-analysis," *BMJ*, 352: 1–11.

Holm, Søren, and Søren Madsen. 2009. "Informed consent in medical research—a procedure stretched beyond breaking point?" In Oonagh Corrigan, John McMillan, Kathleen Liddell, Martin Richards and Charles Weijer (eds.), *The limits of consent*. Oxford University Press: 11–24.

Holm, Søren, and Thomas Ploug. 2017. "Big data and health research—the governance challenges in a mixed data economy." *Journal of Bioethical Inquiry*, 14: 515–525.

Holmberg, Christine, Christine Bischof, and Susanne Bauer. 2013. "Making predictions: Computing populations." *Science, Technology, & Human Values*, 38: 398–420.

Holm-Petersen, Christina, Sarah Wadmann, and Natascha Belén Vejen Andersen. 2015. "Styringsreview på hospitalsområdet. Forslag til procedure og regelforenkling." Copenhagen.

Hood, Christopher. 1991. "A public management for all seasons?." *Public Administration*, 69: 3–19.

Hood, Leroy, and Mauricio Flores. 2012. "A personal view on systems medicine and the emergence of proactive P4 medicine: Predictive, preventive, personalized and participatory." *New Biotechnology*, 29: 613–624.

Hood, Leroy, Jennifer C. Lovejoy, and Nathan D. Price. 2015. "Integrating big data and actionable health coaching to optimize wellness." *BMC Medicine*, 13: 1–4.

Horowitz, Mark, William Yaworsky, and Kenneth Kickham. 2019. "Anthropology's science wars: Insights from a new survey." *Current Anthropology*, 60: 674–698.

Howe, Cymene, Jessica Lockrem, Hannah Appel, et al. 2016. "Paradoxical infrastructures: Ruins, retrofit, and risk." *Science, Technology, & Human Values*, 41: 547–565.

Hunt, Linda M., Hannah S. Bell, Allison M. Baker, and Heather A. Howard. 2017. "Electronic health records and the disappearing patient." *Medical Anthropology Quarterly*, 31: 403–421.

Hurlbut, J. Benjamin, Sheila Jasanoff, and Krishnau Saha. 2020. "Constitutionalism at the nexus of life and law." *Science, Technology & Human Values*, 45: 979–1000.

Hutchinson, Elenor, Susan Nayiga, Christine Nabirye, Lilian Taaka, and Sarah G Staedke. 2018. "Data value and care value in the practice of health systems: A case study in Uganda." *Social Science & Medicine*, 211: 123–130.

Hyysalo, Sampsa, Torben Elgaard Jensen, and Nelly Oudshoorn. 2016. "Introduction to the New Production of Users." in Sampsa Hyysalo, Torben Elgaard Jensen, and Nelly Oudshoorn (eds.), *The new production of users: Changing innovation collectives and involvement strategies*. Routledge. 1–42.

Højer, Lise. 2016. "It-system svækker stadig Riget." *DR.dk*, December 7.

Højer, Lise, and Anne Sophie Flach. 2017. "Psykiatrien: It-system stjæler tid fra psykiatriske patienter." *DR.dk*, September 7.

Højgaard, Liselotte. 2017. *Hvordan får vi verdens bedste sundhedsvæsen?* Informations Forlag.

Høybye-Mortensen, Matilde. 2015. "Decision-making tools and their influence on caseworkers' room for discretion." *British Journal of Social Work*, 45: 600–615.

Haase, Christoffer Bjerre, Margaret Bearman, John Brodersen, Klaus Hoeyer, and Torsten Risor. 2020. "'You should see a doctor', said the robot: Reflections on a digital diagnostic device in a pandemic age." *Scandinavian Journal of Public Health*, 49: 33–36.

Haase, Christoffer Bjerre, John Brandt Brodersen, and Jacob Bülow. 2022. "Sarcopenia: Early prevention or overdiagnosis?" *BMJ*, 376: e052592.

Ihde, Don. 2002. *Bodies in technology.* University of Minnesota Press.

Iliadis, Andrew, and Federica Russo. 2016. "Critical data studies: An introduction." *Big Data & Society*, July–December: 1–7.

Illmer, Andreas. 2021. "Singapore reveals Covid privacy data available to police." *BBC News*, January 5, 2021, Asia section. https://www.bbc.com/news/world-asia-55541001.

Ingold, Tim. 2018. *Anthropology: Why it matters.* Polity Press.

Islam, Saiful, Tonmoy Sarkar, Sazzad Hossain Khan, et al. 2020. "COVID-19-related infodemic and its impact on public health: A global social media analysis." *American Journal of Tropical Medicine & Hygiene*, 103: 1–9.

Jackson, Michael. 1996. "Introduction: Phenomenology, radical empiricism, and anthropological critique." In Michael Jackson (ed.), *Things as they are: New directions in phenomenological anthropology.* Indiana University Press: 1–50.

Jackson, Michael. 2002a. "Biotechnology and the Critique of Globalisation." *Ethnos*, 67: 141–154.

Jackson, Michael. 2002b. "Familiar and foreign bodies: A phenomenological exploration of the human-technology interface." *Journal of the Royal Anthropological Society*, 8: 333–346.

Jackson, Steven J. 2017. "Speed, time, infrastructure: Temporalities of breakdown, maintenance, and repair." In Judy Wajcman and Nigel Dodd (eds.), *The sociology of speed: Digital, organizational, and social temporalities.* Oxford University Press: 169–185.

Jacobsen, Steffen. 2018. *Hvis de lige vil sidde helt stille, Frue. Dr. Jacobsen er ny på afdelingen.* København: Lindhardt og Ringhof.

James, William. 1950 [1890]. *The principles of psychology.* Dover Publications.

Jasanoff, Sheila. 1987. "Cultural aspects of risk assessment in Britain and the United States." In Branden B. Johnson and Vincent T. Covello (eds.), *The social and cultural construction of risk.* D. Reidel Publishing Company: 359–392.

Jasanoff, Sheila. 2012a. "Product, process, or programme: Three cultures and the regulation of biotechnology." In *Science and public reason.* Routledge: 23–58.

Jasanoff, Sheila. 2012b. "Restoring reason." In *Science and public reason.* Routledge. 59–77.

Jasanoff, Sheila, and Sang-Hyun Kim. 2013. "Sociotechnical imaginaries and national energy policies." *Science as Culture*, 22: 189–196.

Jasanoff, Sheila, and Ingrid Metzler. 2020. "Borderlands of life: IVF embryos and the law in the United States, United Kingdom, and Germany." *Science, Technology & Human Values*, 45: 1001–37.

Jaton, Florian. 2017. "We get the algorithms of our ground truths: Designing referential databases in digital image processing." *Social Studies og Science*, 47: 811–840.

Jaton, Florian. 2020. *The Constitution of Algorithms. Ground-truthing, Programming, Formulating*. The MIT Press.

Jensen, Andreas Ebbesen. 2020a. "Internettet er både grøn livline og overset klimasynder." *Energiforum Danmark*, April 2020.

Jensen, Anja M. B. 2022a. "Making it happen: Data practices and the power of diplomacy among Danish organ transplant coordinators." *BioSocieties*, https://doi.org/10.1057/s41292-021-00267-z.

Jensen, Casper Bruun, and Brit Ross Winthereik. 2013. *Monitoring movements in development aid. recursive partnerships and infrastructures* MIT Press.

Jensen, Henrik Bjerregaard, and Lars Hulbæk. 2019. "MedCom på 25 år—hvad har vi lært?" In Christian Nøhr, Pernille Bertelsen, Søren Vingtoft and Stig Kjær Andersen (eds.), *Digitalisering af det danske sundhedsvæsen. Øjenvidneberetninger fra nøgleaktører*. Syddansk Universitetsforlag: 184–200.

Jensen, Jens Winther, Annette Settnes, Steen Lund Jensen, Dorte Damgaard, Lars Lund, and Per Pfeiffer. 2021. "De kliniske kvalitetsdatabaser er solidt grundlag for udvikling af den faglige kvalitet i sundhedsvæsenet." *Dagens Medicin*, Debbat section: 30–31.

Jensen, Karsten Klint, Louise Whiteley, and Peter Sandøe. 2018. *RCR—A Danish textbook for courses in responsible conduct of research*. Department of Food and Resource Economics, University of Copenhagen.

Jensen, Mark Birkedal. 2020b. "FMK Dosisdispensering—Hvad, hvordan og for hvem?" Københavns Universitet.

Jensen, Torben Elgaard. 2021. "Inskription. Fra ting til tegn." In Irina Papazu and Brit Ross Winthereik (eds.), *Aktørnetværksteori i Praksis*. DJØF's Forlag: 49–66.

Jerak-Zuiderent, Sonja, and Roland Bal. 2011. "Locating the worths of performance indicators: Performing transparencies and accaountabilities in health care." In Ann Rudinow Sætnan, Heidi Mork Lomell, and Svein Hammer (eds.), *The mutual construction of statistics and society*. Routledge Taylor & Francis Group: 224–245.

Jespersen, Annette, and Rasmus Dyrberg Hansen. 2018. "Sprællevende Steen blev erklæret død: Der er ingen erfaring med folk, der dør og genopstår,", *DR. dk*, May 4.

Jewson, N. D. 2009. "The disappearance of the sick-man from medical cosmology, 1770–1870." *International Journal of Epidemiology*, 38: 622–633.

JFK21. 2021. "JFK21—Partiprogam." JFK21, https://jfk21.dk/omjfk21 (accessed June 15, 2021).

Jirotka, Marina, Charlotte P. Lee, and Gary M. Olson. 2013. "Supporting scientific collaboration: Methods, tools and concepts." *Computer Supported Coorperative Work*, 22: 667–715.

Johansen, Venke Frederike, and Therese Marie Andrews. 2016. "On challenges to the private-public dichotomy." *Social Theory & Health*, 15: 66–83.

Johansson, Jennifer Viberg, Heidi Beate Bentzen, Nisha Shah, et al. 2021. "Preferences of the public for sharing health data: Discrete choice experiment." *JMIR Medical Informatics*, 9: e29614.

Jones, Kerina H., Graeme Laurie, Leslie Stevens, Christine Dobbs, David V. Ford, and Nathan Lea. 2017. "The other side of the coin: Harm due to the non-use of health-related data." *International Journal of Medical Informatics*, 97: 43–51.

Jordan, Tim. 2015. *Information politics*. Pluto Press.

Jørgensen, Isabella Friis, and Søren Brunak. 2021. "Time-ordered comorbidity correlations identify patients at risk of mis- and overdiagnosis." *npj Digital Medicine*, 4: 1–10.

Kahneman, Daniel, and Gary Klein. 2009. "Conditions for intuitive expertise." *American Psychologist*, 64: 515–526.

Kahneman, Daniel, Olivier Sibony, and Cass R. Sunstein. 2021. *Noise: A flaw in human judgment*. William Collins.

Kane, Beverley, and Daniel Z Sands. 1997. "Guidelines for the clinical use of electronic mail with patients." *Journal of American Medical Informatics Association*, 5: 104–111.

Kant, Immanuel. 2017 [1787]. *Critique of pure reason*. Green Bird Publications.

Karlsson, Christopher Due. 2021. "Ny mand i spidsen for Novo Nordisks digitale produkter: Fokus vil være på både intern og ekstern udvikling." *MedWatch*, September 10, 2021, Medicin & Biotek section.

Kaufman, Sharon R. 2015. *Ordinary medicine: Extraordinary treatments, longer lives, and where to draw the line*. Duke University Press.

Kaye, Jane, Edgar A. Whitley, David Lund, Michael Morrison, Harriet Teare, and Karen Melham. 2015. "Dynamic consent: A patient interface for twenty-first-century research networks." *European Journal of Human Genetics*, 23: 141–146.

Kaziunas, Elizabeth, Silvia Lindtner, Mark S. Ackerman, and Joyce M. Lee. 2018. "Lived data: Tinkering with bodies, code, and care work." *Human-Computer Interaction*, 33: 49–92.

Kaźmierska, Kaja. 2020. "Ethical aspects of social research: Old concerns in the face of new challenges and paradoxes. A reflection from the field of biographical method." *Qualitative Sociology Review*, XVI: 118–135.

Kemm, John. 2006. "The limitations of 'evidence-based' public health." *Journal of Evaluation in Clinical Practice*, 12: 319–324.

Kielgast, Nis, Alexander Hecklen, and Simone C. Møller. 2021. "2241 dødsattester afslører: Så mange døde egentlig af corona." *DR Nyheder*, May 17, 2021, Indland section.

Kierkegaard, Patrick. 2013. "eHealth in Denmark: A case study." *Journal of Medical Systems*, 37: 1–10.

Kieser, Alfred. 1997. "Rhetoric and myth in management fashion." *Organization*, 4: 49–74.

Kingod, Natasja, and Bryan Cleal. 2019. "Noise as dysappearance: Attuning to a life with type 1 diabetes." *Body & Society*, 25: 55–75.

Kingori, Patricia. 2013. "Experience everyday ethics in context: frontline data collectors perspectives and practices of bioethics." *Social Science and Medicine*, 98: 361–370.

Kitchin, Rob. 2014. *The data revolution: Big data, open data, data infrastructures & their consequences*. SAGE.

Kitchin, Rob. 2021. *Data lives: How data are made and shape our world*. Bristol University Press.

Kjærgaard, Johan, Janne Lehmann Knudsen, and Anne Frølich. 2008. "Virkemidler til regulering af faglig adfærd." In Janne Lehmann Knudsen, Mads Ellegaard Christensen and Bente Hansen (eds.), *Regulering af kvalitet i det danske sundhedsvæsen*. Nyt Nordisk Forlag: 63–91.

KMD Analyse, and Dagens Medicin. 2017. *Population health management: Deling af Patientdata*. KMD Analyse.

Knox, Hannah. 2022. "Technology, Environment and the Ends of Knowledge." In Maja Hojer Bruun, Ayo Wahlberg, Cathrine Hasse, Klaus Hoeyer, Dorte Brogård Kristensen, and Brit R. Winthereik (eds.), *Palgrave handbook of the anthropology of technology*. Palgrave Macmillan: 237–253.

Knudsen, Janne Lehmann, Mads Ellegaard Christensen, and Bente Hansen. 2008. "Fra decentral til central regulering af kvalitet i sundhedsvæsenet—en introduktion." In Janne Lehmann Knudsen, Mads Ellegaard Christensen and Bente Hansen (eds.), *Regulering af kvalitet i det danske sundhedsvæsen*. Nyt Nordisk Forlag: 15–28.

Knudsen, Jeppe Kyhne 2020. "Når mor går over tid: Antallet af dødfødte børn i Danmark er fordoblet siden 2015." *DR Nyheder*, December 24, 2020, Kroppen section.

Knudsen, Morten. 2011. "Forms of inattentiveness: The production of blindness in the development of a technology for the observation of quality in health services." *Organization Studies*, 32: 963–989.

Koch, Lene. 2006. "Past futures: On the conceptual history of eugenics—a social technology of the past." *Technology Analysis and Strategic Management*, 18: 329–344.

Koopman, Colin, Patrick Jones, Valérie Simon, Paul Showler, and Mary McLevey. 2021. "When data drive health: An archaeology of medical records technology." *BioSocieties*: 1–23.

Korsby, Trine Mygind, and Anthony Stavrianakis. 2021. "Object exchange." In Andrea Ballestero and Brit Ross Winthereik (eds.), *Experimenting with ethnography: A companion to analysis*. Duke University Press: 82–93.

Kragh-Furbo, Mette, Joann Wilkinson, Maggie Mort, Celia Roberts, and Adrian Mackenzie. 2018. "Biosensing networks: Sense-making in consumer genomics and ovulation tracking." In Rebecca Lynch and Conor Farrington (eds.), *Quantified lives and vital data. Exploring health and technology through personal medical devices*. Palgrave Macmillan: 47–96.

Krasnik, Mark. 2021. "Kvalitetsdatabaser skal løse basale problemer, før hospitaler kan sammenlignes." *Dagens Medicin*, April 30, 2021: 32–33.

Kraus, Rebecca S. 2011. *Statistical déjà vu: The National Data Center proposal of 1965 and its decendants.* US Census Bureau.

Kristensen, Benedikte Møller, John Brandt Brodersen, and Alexandra Brandt Ryborg Jønsson. 2022. "The tyranny of numbers: How e-health record transparency affects patients' health perceptions and conversations with physicians." *Medicine, Anthropology, Theory* 9: 1–25.

Kristensen, Dorthe Brogård, Charlotte Bredahl Jacobsen, and Signe Pihl-Thingvad. 2017. "Perception and translation of numbers: the case of a health campaign in Denmark." *Critical Public health*, 28: 460–471.

Kristensen, Dorte Brogård, and Carolin Prigge. 2018. "Human/technology associations in self-tracking practices." In Btihaj Ajana (ed.), *Self-tracking: Empirical and philosophical investigations.* Palgrave Macmillan: 43–59.

Kristensen, Dorte Brogård, and Minna Ruckenstein. 2018. "Co-evolving with self-tracking technologies." *New Media & Society*, 20: 3624–3640.

Kristensen, Victor Emil. 2019. "Læger: Problemer består efter opdatering af Sundhedsplatformen." *Dagens Medicin*, February 1, 2019: 4–5.

Krogh, Andreas, Chris Lehmann, and Katrine Falk Lønstrup. 2021. "Coronaprotester giver næring til nye partier." *Altinget.dk*, March 8, 2021, Civilsamfund section.

Krogh, Martine Amalie. 2020. "Regeringens corona-app forbudt for alle ansatte i Udenrigsministeriet." *Information*, July 16, 2020, section Nyheder.

Krogh, Simon. 2016. "Anticipating organizational change: A study of the pre-implementation phase of Sundhedsplatformen." Copenhagen Business School.

Krumholz, Harlan M. 2014. "Big data and new knowledge in medicine: The thinking, training, and tools needed for a learning health system." *Health Affairs*, 33: 1163–1170.

Kwet, Michael. 2019. "Digital colonialism: US empire and the new imperialism in the Global South." *Race & Class*, 60: 3–36.

König, Gerhard, Pandian Sokkar, Niclas Pryk, et al. 2021. "Rational prioritization strategy allows the design of macrolide derivatives that overcome antibiotic resistance." *PNAS*, 118: e2113632118.

Lakoff, George, and Mark Johnson. 1980. *Metaphors we live by.* University of Chicago Press.

Lambert, Helen. 2006. "Accounting for EBM: Notions of evidence in medicine." *Social Science and Medicine*, 62: 2633–2645.

Lane, Christopher. 2007. *Shyness: How normal behavior became a sickness.* Yale University Press.

Lange, Anita. 2017. *The population and housing census in a register based statistical system.* Census and Statistics Department of the Government of Hong Kong.

Lange, Lasse. 2017. "Vil man have en styrelse for kontrol og straf eller en styrelse for patientsikkerhed?" *Dagens Medicin*, March 11, 2017: 12–13.

Langhoff, Tue Odd, Mikkel Hvid Amstrup, Peter Mørck, and Pernille Bjørn. 2018. "Infrastructure for healthcare: From synergy to reverse synergy." *Health Informatics Journal*, 24: 43–53.

Langstrup, Henriette. 2013. "Chronic care infrastructures and the home." *Sociology of Health & Illness*, 35: 1008–1022.

Langstrup, Henriette. 2018. "Patient reported data and the politics of meaningful data work." *Health Informatics Journal*, 25: 567–575.

Langstrup, Henriette, and Tiago Moreira. 2021. "Infrastructuring experience: what matters in patient-reported outcome data measurement?." *BioSocieties*. https://link .springer.com/article/10.1057/s41292-020-00221-5.

Langstrup, Henriette, and Brit Ross Winthereik. 2010. "Producing alternative objects of comparison in healthcare: Following a web-based technology for asthma treatment through the lab and clinic." In Thomas Scheffer and Jörg Niewöhner (eds.), *Thick comparison: Reviving the ethnographic aspiration*. Brill: 103–128.

Larkin, Brian. 2013. "The politics and poetics of infrastructure." *Annual Review of Anthropology*, 42: 327–343.

Larsen, Jakob Bjerg, Niels Christian Hirsch, Louise Broe, Camilla Lund-Cramer, and Signe Poulsen. 2020. *Sundhedsdata som fundament for effektbaserede aftaler*. Videnscenter for Life Science.

Larsen, Johan Blem, and Nicolas Stig Nielsen. 2018. "Direktør for udskældt sundhedsplatform fik bonus på 100.000 kroner." *DR Nyheder*, February 19, 2018, Politik section.

Larsson, Stefan. 2017. "Sustaining legitimacy and trust in a data-driven society." *Ericsson Technology Review*, 94: 40–49.

Latour, Bruno. 1986. "The powers of association." In John Law (ed.), *Power, action and belief—a new sociology of knowledge?* Routledge and Keagan Paul: 264–280.

Latour, Bruno. 1993. *We have never been modern*. Harvard University Press.

Latour, Bruno. 2014. "Drawing things together." In Michael Lynch and Steve Woolgar (eds.), *Representation in scientific practice*. MIT Press: 19–68.

Lau, Sofie Rosenlund, Marie Kofod Svensson, Natasja Kingod, and Ayo Wahlberg. 2021. "Carescapes unsettled: COVID-19 and the reworking of 'stable illnesses' in welfare state Denmark." In Lenore Manderson, Nancy J. Burke and Ayo Wahlberg (eds.), *Viral loads: Anthropologies of urgency in the time of COVID-19*. UCL Press: 324–342.

Laudon, Kenneth C. 1986. *Dossier society*. Columbia University Press.

Lawton, Julia, Naureen Ahmad, Elizabeth Peel, and Nina Hallowell. 2007. "Contextualising accounts of illness: Notions of responsibility and blame in white and South Asian respondents' accounts of diabetes causation." *Sociology of Health & Illness*, 29: 891–906.

Lee, Crystal, Tanya Yang, Gabrielle Inchoco, Graham M. Jones, and Arvind Satyanarayan. 2021. "Viral visualizations: How coronavirus skeptics use orthodox data practices to promote unorthodox science online." *CHI: Conference on Human Factors in Computing Systems*, May 8–13: 1–17.

Lee, Francis. 2015. "Purity and interest. On relational work and epistemic value in the biomedical sciences." in Isabelle Dussauge, Claes-Fredrik Helgesson and Francis Lee (eds.), *Values in the life sciences & medicine*. Oxford University Press. 207–224.

Lee, Francis, and Lotta Björklund Larsen. 2019. "How should we theorize algorithms? Five ideal types in analyzing algorithmic normativities." *Big Data & Society*, July–December: 1–6.

Lehmann, Chris. 2021. "Chef i Sundhedsdatastyrelsen efter corona: Den digitale acceleration kan vende sundhedsvæsenet på hovedet." *Altinget*, June 6, 2021, Sundhed section.

Lengen, Samuel. 2017. "Beyond the conceptual framework of oppression and resistance: Creativity, religion and the Internet in China." In Stefania Travagnin (ed.), *Religion and media in China: Insights and case studies from the mainland, Taiwan and Hong Kong* Routledge: 19–34.

Leonelli, Sabina. 2012a. "Classificatory theory in data-intensive science: The case of open biomedical ontologies." *International Studies in the Philosophy of Science*, 26: 47–65.

Leonelli, Sabina. 2012b. "Introduction: Making sense of data-driven research in the biological and biomedical sciences." *Studies in History and Philosophy of Biological and Biomedical Sciences*, 43: 1–3.

Leonelli, Sabina. 2014. "What difference does quantity make? On the epistemology of Big Data in biology." *Big Data & Society*, April–June: 1–11.

Leonelli, Sabina. 2016. *Data-centric biology. A philosphical study*. University of Chicago Press.

Lévi-Strauss, Claude. 1966 translation [1962]. *The savage mind* (La pensée sauvage). University of Chicago Press.

Levin, Nadine. 2019. "Big data and biomedicine." In Maurizio Meloni, John Cromby, Des Fitzgerald, and Stephanie Lloyd (eds.), *Palgrave handbook of biology and society*. Palgrave Macmillan: 663–681.

Lewis, Marianne A., and Wendy K. Smith. 2014. "Paradox as a metatheoretical perspective: Sharpening the focus and widening the scope." *Journal of Applied Behavioral Science* 50: 127–149.

Lewis, Sara. 2016. "Director of NIMH leaves for Google. Does early intervention promote recovery?" *Anthropology News*, 57: 17.

Liang, Fan, Vishnupriya Das, Nadiya Kostyuk, and Muzammil M. Hussain. 2018. "Constructing a data-driven society: China's social credit system as a state surveillance infrastructure." *Policy & Internet*, 10: 415–453.

Lidegaard, Øjvind, Lone Krebs, Olav Bennike Bjørn Petersen, Nis Peter Damm, and A. Tabor. 2020. "Are the Danish stillbirth rates still record low? A nationwide ecological study." *BMJ Open*, 10.

Lie, Anne Kveim, and Jeremy A. Greene. 2020. "From Ariadne's thread to the labyrinth itself: Nosology and the infrastructure of modern medicine." *New England Journal of Medicin*, 382: 1273–1277.

Lievevrouw, Elisa, Luca Marelli, and Ine Van Hoyweghen. 2021. "The FDA's standard-making process for medical digital health technologies: Co-producing technological and organizational innovation." *BioSocieties*.

LIF. 2020. *Indspil fra Lif: Rammevilkår for styrket innovation i Dansk Life Science*. LIF.

Lindblom, Charles E. 1959. "The science of 'muddling through'" *Public Administration Review*, 19: 79–88.

Lindenius, Erik. 2009. *Guldgruvan som försvann? En mediestudie av konflikten kring UmanGenomics och Medicinska biobanken 2001–2006*. Umeå Universitet. Dissertation

Lindholm, Henrik, and Steffen Lerche. 2019. "En beretning fra de private leverandører." In Christian Nøhr, Pernille Bertelsen, Søren Vingtoft and Stig Kjær Andersen (eds.), *Digitalisering af det danske sundhedsvæsen. Øjenvidneberetninger fra nøgleaktører*. Syddansk Universitetsforlag: 146–155.

Lipsky, Michael. 1980. *Street-level bureaucracy—the dilemmas of the individual in public services*. Russel Sage Foundation.

Lipworth, Wendy, Paul H. Mason, Ian Kerridge, and John PA Ioannidis. 2017. "Ethics and epistemology in big data research." *Bioethical Inquiry*, 14: 489–500.

Liu, Huan, Fred Morstatter, Jiliang Tang, and Reza Zafarani. 2016. "The good, the bad, and the ugly: Uncovering novel research opportunities in social media mining." *International Journal of Data Science and Analytics*, 1: 137–143.

Liu, Yanjun, Shiyong Xu, and Bainan Zhang. 2020. "Thriving at work: How a paradox mindset influences innovative work behavior." *Journal of Applied Behavioral Science*, 56: 347–366.

Lomborg, Stine, Henriette Langstrup, and Tariq Osman Andersen. 2020. "Interpretation as luxury: Heart patients living with data doubt, hope, and anxiety." *Big Data & Society*, January–June: 1–13.

Loukissas, Yanni Alexander. 2019. *All data are local: Thinking critically in a data-driven society*. MIT Press.

Luhmann, Niklas. 1999. *Tillid—en mekanisme til reduktion af social kompleksitet*. Hans Reitzels Forlag.

Lund, Lars Christian, Jesper Hallas, Henrik Nielsen, et al. 2021. "Post-acute effects of SARS-CoV-2 infection in individuals not requiring hospital admission: A Danish population-based cohort study." *Lancet Infection*, 21: 1373–1382.

Lupton, Deborah. 2016a. "The diverse domains of quantified selves: Self-tracking modes and dataveillance." *Economy and Society*, 45: 101–122.

Lupton, Deborah. 2016b. "Foreword: Lively devices, lively data and lively leisure studies." *Leisure Studies*, 35: 709–711.

Lupton, Deborah. 2017. "How does health feel? Towards research on the affective atmosphere of digital health." *Digital Health*, 3: 1–11.

Lupton, Deborah. 2020. *Data selves*. Polity Press.

Lupton, Deborah, and Sarah Maslen. 2017. "Telemedicine and the senses: a review." *Sociology of Health & Illness*, 39: 1557–1571.

Lupton, Deborah, Clare Southerton, Marianne Clark, and Ash Watson. 2021. *The face mask in COVID times: A sociomaterial analysis*. De Gruyter.

Lury, Celia, and Sophie Day. 2019. "Algorithmic personalization as a mode of individuation." *Theory, Culture & Society*, 36: 17–37.

Luscher, Lotte S., and Marianne Lewis. 2008. "Organizational change and managerial sensemaking: Working through paradox." *The Academy of Management Journal*, 51: 221–240.

Lyneborg, Anna Olejasz. 2019. "Social work in the Danish digitalized welfare state—and the use of digital technologies for professional konwledge in child services." In John Storm Pedersen and Adrian Wilkinson (eds.), *Big data: Promise, application and pitfalls*. Edward Elgar Publishing: 224–244.

Lynteris, Christos. 2018. "Plague masks: The visual emergence of anti-epidemic personal protection equipment." *Medical Anthropology*, 37: 442–457.

Lyon, David. 2019. "Surveillance capitalism, surveillance culture and data politics." In Didier Bigo, Engin Isin and Evelyn Ruppert (eds.), *Data politics: Worlds, subjects, rights*. Routledge: 64–77.

Lyotard, Jean-François. 1984. *The postmodern condition: A report on knowledge*. University of Minnesota Press.

Löfgren, Karl, and William Webster. 2019. "Big data in government: The case of 'smart cities.'" In John Storm Pedersen and Adrian Wilkinson (eds.), *Big data: Promise, application and pitfalls*. Edward Elgar Publishing. 133–148.

Maach, Maja. 2016. "Regionrådsformand efter chefs protestopsigelse: Det er trygt at føde på Riget." *DR.dk*, November 30, 2016.

Mackenzie, Donald. 2021. *Trading at the speed of light: How ultrafast algorithms are transforming financial markets*. Princeton University Press.

Madsen, Anders Koed, Mikkel Flyverbom, Martin Hilbert, and Evelyn Ruppert. 2016. 'Big Data: Issues for an International Political Sociology of Data Practices', *International Political Sociology*, 10: 275–296.

Maguire, James, Henriette Langstrup, Peter Danholt, and Christopher Gad. 2020. "Engaging the data moment: An introduction." *STS Encounters*, 11: 2–21.

Maguire, James, and Brit R. Winthereik. 2021. "Digitalising the state: Data centres and the power of exchange,", *Ethnos*, 86: 530–551.

Mainz, Jan, and Paul D. Bartels. 2014. "Kvalitetsudvikling i sundhedsvæsenet anno 2025." In Kjeld Møller Pedersen and Niels Christian Petersen (eds.), *Fremtidens Hospital*. Munksgaard: 203–216.

Malacinski, Leny. 2020. "Manden, der ikke kan begraves." *Weekendavisen*, August 28, 2020, Samfund section: 4–5.

Manderson, Lenore, Mark Davis, Chip Colwell, and Tanja Ahlin. 2015. "On secrecy, disclosure, the public, and the private in anthropology." *Current Anthropology*, 56: S183–S90.

March, James G., and Johan P. Olsen. 1976. "Organizational choice under ambiguity." In James G. March and Johan P. Olsen (eds.), *Ambiguity and choice in organizations*. Universitetsforlaget: 10–23.

Marcus, George E. 2021. "The para-site in ethnographic research projects." In Andrea Ballestero and Brit Ross Winthereik (eds.), *Experimenting with ethnography: A companion to analysis*. Duke University Press: 41–52.

Marcussen, M and K Ronit (eds.) 2010. Globaliseringens udfordringer. Politiske og administrative modeller under pres. Copenhagen: Hans Reitzels Forlag.

Markel, Howard, Harvey B. Lipman, Alexander Navarro, Alexandra Sloan, Joseph R. Michalsen, Alexandra Minna Stern, and Martin S. Cetron. 2007. "Nonpharmaceutical interventions implemented by US cities during the 1918–1919 influenza pandemic." *JAMA*, 298: 644–654.

Markus, M. Lynne. 2001. "Toward a theory of knowledge reuse: Types of knowledge reuse situations and factors in reuse success." *Journal of Management Information Systems*, 18: 57–93.

Marmot, Michael, Tony Atkinson, John Bell, Carol Black, Patricia Broadfoot, Julia Cumberlege, Ian Diamond, Ian Gilmore, Chris Ham, Molly Meacher, and Geoff Mulgan. 2010. "Fair Society, Healthy Lives." London: University College London. 1–34.

Martani, Andrea, David Shaw, and Bernice Simone Elger. 2019. "Stay fit or get bit—ethical issues in sharing health data with insurers' apps." *Swiss Medical Weekly*, 149: w20089.

Martin, Aryn, and Michael Lynch. 2009. "Counting things and people: The practices and politics of counting." *Social Problems*, 56: 243–66.

Martin, Emily. 2013. "The potentiality of ethnography and the limits of affect theory." *Current Anthropology*, 54: 149–158.

Mason, Katherine A. 2018. "Quantitative care: Caring for the aggregate in US academic population health sciences." *American Ethnologist*, 45: 201–213.

Mattingly, Cherly. 2010. *The paradox of hope: Journeys through a clinical borderland.* University of California Press.

Mau, Steffen. 2019. *The metric society: On the quantification of the social.* Polity Press.

Mauss, Marcel. 2007. "Techniques of the body." In Margaret Lock and Judith Farquhar (eds.), *Beyond the body proper: Reading the anthropology of maternal life.* Duke University Press: 50–68.

Mayer-Schönberger, Viktor, and Kenneth Cukier. 2013. *Big data: A revolution that will transform how we live, work and think.* John Murray.

Mayo, Elton. 2003 [1933]. *The human problems of an industrial civilization.* Routledge.

McDonald, Aleecia M, and Lorrie Faith Cranor. 2008. "The cost of reading privacy policies." *I/S: A Journal of Law and Policy for the Information Society*, 4: 540–565.

Mcfall, Liz. 2019. "Personalizing solidarity? The role of self-tracking in health insurance pricing." *Economy and Society*, 48: 52–76.

McGoey, Linsey. 2010. "Pharmaceutical controversies and the performative value of uncertainty." *Science as Culture*, 18: 151–164.

McKinsey & Company. 2016. *Värdet av digital teknik i den svenska vården.* McKinsey & Company.

McMahon, Aisling, Alena Buyx, and Barbara Prainsack. 2019. "Big data governance needs more collective responsibility: The role of harm mitigation in the governance of data use in medicine and beyond." *Medical Law Review*, 28: 155–182.

Meng, Xiao-Li. 2018. "Statistical paradises and paradoxes in big data (I): Law of large populations, big data paradox, and the 2016 US presidential election." *Annals of Applied Statistics*, 12: 685–726.

Mercier, Hugo. 2020. *Not born yesterday: The science of who we trust and what we trust.* Princeton University Press.

Merleau-Ponty, Maurice. 2002. *Phenomenology of perception.* Routledge.

Merry, Sally Engle. 2016. *The seductions of quantification: Measuring human rights, gender violence, and sex trafficking.* University of Chicago Press.

Mertens, Mayli, Owen C. King, Michel J. A. M. van Putten, and Marianne Boenink. 2021. "Can we learn from hidden mistakes? Self-fulfilling prophecy and responsible neuroprognostic innovation." *Journal of Medical Ethics]*, http://dx.doi.org/10.1136/medethics-2020-106636.

Merton, Robert K. 1968. "The self-fulfilling prophecy." In *Social theory and social structure.* The Free Press: 475–490.

Meyer, Eric T, and Ralph Schroeder. 2015. *Knowledge machines: Digital transformations of the sciences and humanities.* MIT Press.

Meyer, Harris. 2020. "HHS eases HIPAA enforcement on data releases during COVID-19." *Modern Healthcare*, April 2, 2020, Law & Regulation section.

Michael, Mike. 2015. "Ignorance and the epistemic choreography of method." In Matthias Gross and Linsey McGoey (eds.), *Routledge international handbook of ignorance studies* Routledge and Taylor & Francis Group: 84–91.

Middleton, Alexandra. 2022. "The datafication of pain: Trials and tribulations in measuring phantom limb pain." *BioSocieties*, 17: 123–144.

Milan, Stefania, Emiliano Treré, and Silvia Masiero. 2021. "Introduction: COVID-19 seen from the land of otherwise." In Stefania Milan, Emiliano Treré and Silvia Masiero (eds.), *COVID-19 from the margins: Pandemic invisibilities, policies and resistance in the datafied society.* Institute of Network Cultures: 14–22.

Miller, Peter, and Nikolas Rose. 2008. *Governing the present: Administering economic, social and personal life.* Polity Press.

Mills, C. Wright. 2000 1959. *The sociological imagination.* Oxford University Press.

Ministry of Foreign Affairs, Ministry of Health, Ministry of Business and Growth, et al. 2018. *The heart of life sciences for research and business.* Ministry of Foreign Affairs of Denmark.

Miron-Spektor, Ella, Francesca Gino, and Linda Argote. 2011. "Paradoxical frames and creative sparks: Enhancing individual creativity through conflict and integration." *Organizational Behavior and Human Decision Processes*, 116: 229–240.

Miron-Spektor, Ella, Amy Ingram, Joshua Keller, Wendy K. Smith, and Marianne W. Lewis. 2018. "Microfoundations of organizational paradox: The problem is how we think about the problem." *Academy of Management Journal*, 61: 26–45.

Mirzaei-Fard, Marcel. 2020. "Corona-appen er udkommet: Her er, hvad den kan." *DR Nyheder*, June 18, 2020, Teknologi section.

Mirzaei-Fard, Marcel, and Line Gudnitz Rønø Baun. 2019. "46 fik forkert mængde blodtryksmedicin på grund af fejl i Sundhedsplatformen." *DR Nyheder*, February 10, 2019, København section.

Mirzaei-Fard, Marcel, and Peter Led Korsgaard. 2019. "Udskældt it-system blev opdateret—to uger senere kan lægerne ikke mærke forskel." *DR Nyheder*, February 16, 2019, København section.

Moerenhout, Tania, Gary S. Fischer, and Ignaas Decvisch. 2020. "The elephant in the room: A postphenomenological view on the electronic health record and its impact on the clinical encounter." *Medicine, Health Care and Philosophy*, 23: 227–236.

Mol, Annemarie. 2002. *The body multiple: Ontology in medical practice*. Duke University Press.

Moore, Phoebe V. 2018. *The quantified self in precarity: Work, technology and what counts*. Routledge.

Moreira, Tiago. 2004. "Coordination and embodiment in the operating room." *Body & Society*, 10: 109–129.

Moreira, Tiago. 2019. "Devicing future populations: problematizing the relationship between quantity and quality of life." *Social Studies of Science*, 49: 118–137.

Moriera, Tiago, and Paolo Palladino. 2011. "'Population laboratories' or 'laboratory populations'? Making sense of the Baltimore Longitudinal Study of Aging, 1965–1987." *Studies in History and Philosophy of Biological and Biomedical Sciences*, 42: 317–327.

Morrison, Cecily, Matthew Jones, Rachel Jones, and Alain Vuylsteke. 2013. "'You can't just hit a button': An ethnographic study of strategies to repurpose data from advanced clinical information systems for clinical process improvement." *BMC Medicine*, 11: 1–8.

Morrison, Michael. 2017. "Infrastructural expectations: Exploring the promise of the international large-scale induced pluripotent stem cell banks." *New Genetics and Society*, 36: 66–83.

Mortensen, Henny, and Lukas Seier Dencher. 2018. "Læge siger op i protest over it-system: Sundhedsplatformen har ødelagt min arbejdsglæde." *DR Nyheder*, June 1, 2018, Sjælland section.

Mortensen, Klaus Ulrik. 2018. "Nyt forslag om datasamkørsel: Nu skal arbejdsløse med sociale problemer opspores." *Altinget*, April 20, 2018

Moynihan, Ray, Iona Heath, and David Henry. 2002. "Selling sickness: The pharmaceutical industry and disease mongering." *BMJ*, 324: 886–891.

Mozur, Paul, Raymond Zhong, and Aaron Krolik. 2020. "In coronavirus fight, China gives citizens a color code, with red flags." *New York Times*. https://www.nytimes.com/2020/03/01/business/china-coronavirus-surveillance.html.

Mulkay, Michael. 1993. "Rhetorics of hope and fear in the great embryo debate." *Social Studies of Science*, 23: 721–742.

Muller, Jerry Z. 2018. *The tyranny of metrics*. Princeton University Press.

Munk, Linda Svenstrup 2020. "Antallet af dødfødte børn efter termin er fordoblet efter fald i igangsættelser efter terminen." Rigshospitalet, https://www.rigshospitalet

.dk/presse-og-nyt/nyheder/nyheder/Sider/2020/december/antallet-af-doedfoedte
-boern-efter-termin-er-fordoblét-efter-fald-i-igangsaettelser-efter-terminen.aspx
(accessed January 7, 2021).

Murphy, Michelle. 2017. *The economization of life*. Duke University Press.

Møller, Naja Holten, Claus Bossen, Kathleen H. Pine, Trine Rask., and Gina Neff. 2020. "Who does the work of data?." *ACM Interactions*, 27: 52–55.

Møllerhøj, Jakob, and Robin Engelhardt. 2013. "Systembiologi: Et eksempel på udfordringer." *Ingeniøren*, February 22, 2013: 1–3.

Möllers, Norma. 2021. "Making digital territory: Cybersecurity, techno-nationalism, and the moral boundaries of the state." *Science, Technology & Human Values*, 46: 112–138.

Nagesh, Ashitha. 2020. "Coronavirus: US funerals move to live-streaming." *BBC News*, March 17, 2020, World section. https://www.bbc.com/news/world-us-canada -51935266.

Nair, Vijayanka. 2021. "Becoming data: Biometric IDs and the individual in 'digital India.'" *Journal of the Royal Anthropological Insitute*, 27: 26–42.

Nathan, Ida. 2017. "#DetKuHaVæretMig: Sundhedsminister får 13.625 underskrifter mod lægedom." *DR.dk*, December 1.

Negroponte, Nicholas. 1995. *Being digital*. Vintage Books.

Nelson, Wendy, Valerie F. Reyna, Angela Fagerlin, Isaac Lipkus, and Ellen Peters. 2008. "Clinical implications of numeracy: Theory and practice." *Annals of Behavioral Medicine*, 35: 261–274.

Nettleton, Sarah, Roger Burrows, and Ian Watt. 2008. "Regulating medical bodies? The consequences of the 'modernisation' of the NHS and the disembodiment of clinical knowledge." *Sociology of Health & Illness*, 30: 333–48.

Newell, Sue, Maxine Robertson, and Jacky Swan. 2001. "Management fads and fashions." *Organization*, 8: 5–15.

Nhør, Christian, Søren Vingtoft, and Pernille Bertelsen. 2019. "Digitalisering af den danske sundhedssektor." In Christian Nøhr, Pernille Bertelsen, Søren Vingtoft and Stig Kjær Andersen (eds.), *Digitalisering af det danske sundhedsvæsen. Øjenvidneberet-ninger fra nøgleaktører*. Syddansk Universitetsforlage. 7–23.

Nissen, Christian S. 2009. "Vi har sejret ad helvede til—men var det godt alt sammen?" In Christian S. Nissen (ed.), *På Ministerens Vegne*. Hanelshøjskolens Forlag. 207–238.

Nissenbaum, Helen. 2011. "A contextual approach to privacy online." *Dædalus, the Journal of the American Academy of Arts & Sciences*, 140: 32–48.

Nordfalk, Francisca. 2015. *Forskerbeskyttelsen i Danmark 1995–2014*. Københavns Universitet. Kandidat: 1–79.

Nordfalk, Francisca. 2021a. *Enabling national research populations: A study of the Danish newborn dried blood spot samples*. Department of Public Health. Copenhagen, University of Copenhagen. Ph.D.

Nordfalk, Francisca. 2021b. "The mutual enablement of research data and care: How newborn babies become a national research population." *Science & Technology*

Studies, (online first): 1–14, https://sciencetechnologystudies.journal.fi/article/view/98655.

Nordfalk, Francisca, and Claus Thorn Ekstrøm. 2019. "Newborn dried blood spot samples in Denmark: The hidden figures of secondary use and research participation." *European Journal of Human Genetics* 27: 203–210.

Nordfalk, Francisca, and Klaus Hoeyer. 2020. "The rise and fall of an opt-out system." *Scandinavian Journal of Public Health*, 48: 400–404.

Nordfalk, Francisca, Maria Olejaz, and Klaus Hoeyer. 2022. "The unique and the universal: Analyzing the interplay between regulatory organization, researchers and research participants in data making." *Engaging Science, Technology, and Society*, 8: 8–28.

NordForsk. 2014. *Joint Nordic registers and biobanks: A goldmine for health and welfare research*. NordForsk.

Nordic Committee on Bioethics. 2014. *Legislation on biotechnology in the Nordic countries—an overview 2014*. Nordic Committee on Bioethics.

Norup, Mark Lindved 2019. "Dreng eller pige? For Charlie var det en befrielse endelig at få et cpr-nummer, der matchede kønnet." *DR Nyheder*, July 30, 2019, Indland section.

Novas, Carlos. 2006. "The political economy of hope: Patients' organizations, science and biovalue." *BioSocieties*, 1: 289–305.

Nørmark, Dennis, and Anders Fogh Jensen. 2019. *Pseudo-arbejde. Hvordan vi fik travlt med at lave ingenting*. Gyldendal.

Oakley, Tim. 2010. "The issue of meaninglessness." *The Monist*, 93: 106–122.

Obar, Jonathan A. 2017. "Big data and *The Phantom Public*: Walter Lippmann and the fallacy of data privacy self-management." *Big Data & Society*, July–December: 1–16.

Olesen, Jes. 2018. *Det Syge Væsen. Hvordan det kan helbredes*. Saxo Publish.

Olsen, Jan Kyrre Berg, Evan Selinger, and Søren Riis. 2008. "Introduction." In Jan Kyrre Berg Olsen, Evan Selinger and Søren Riis (eds.), *New waves in philosophy of technology* Palgrave Macmillan: 1–9.

Olsen, Leigh, Anne, Dara Aisner, and J. Michael McGinnis. 2007. *The learning healthcare system: Workshop summary*. National Academies Press.

Olsen, Theis Lange. 2021. "Stifter af 'Men In Black' står frem: 'Der foregår en heksejagt på os lige nu'." *DR Nyheder*, January 26, 2021, Indland section.

O'Neil, Cathy. 2016. *Weapons of math destruction: How big data increases inequality and threatens democracy*. Allen Lane.

O'Reilly, Jessica, Cindy Isenhour, Pamela McElwee, and Ben Orlove. 2020. "Climate change: Expanding anthropological possibilities." *Annual Review of Anthropology*, 49: 13–29.

Oreskes, Naomi. 2019. *Why trust science?* Princeton University Press.

Organisation for Economic Co-operation and Development (OECD). 2013. *Exploring the economics of personal data: A survey of methodologies for measuring monetary value*. OECD Publishing.

Organisation for Economic Co-operation and Development (OECD). 2021. "Tax revenues continue increasing as the tax mix shifts further towards corporate and consumption taxes." OECD, http://www.oecd.org/newsroom/tax-revenues-continue-increasing-as-the-tax-mix-shifts-further-towards-corporate-and-consumption-taxes.htm (accessed January 12, 2021).

Organisation of Economic Co-operation and Development (OECD), and European Union. 2018. "Health at a Glance: Europe 2018: State of Health in the EU Cycle." Paris, OECD.

O'Riordan, Kate. 2017. *Unreal objects—digital materialities, technoscientific projects and political realities*. Pluto Press.

Østrup Vallgård, Finn, Jørgen Jørgensen, and Jesper Zwisler. 2020. *Fornyelse eller kollaps? En kritik og gentænkning af offentlig styring*. Samfundslitteratur.

Oudshoorn, Nelly, and Trevor Pinch. 2003. "Introduction: How users and non-users matter." In Nelly Oudshoorn and Trevor Pinch (eds.), *How users matter—the co-construction of users and technologies*. MIT Press: 1–25.

Outsideren. 2020. "Outsiderens spørgeskemaundersøgelse: Psykisk sårbare trives under Corona-krisen." *Outsideren*, April 19, 2020.

Outzen, Mads. 2020. "Se hele pressemødet: Mette Frederiksen åbner for forsigtig exitstrategi." *Altinget*, March 30, 2020.

Oxlund, Bjarke. 2012. "Living by numbers: The dynamic interplay of asymptomatic conditions and low cost measurement technologies in the cases of two women in the Danish provinces." *Suomen Antropologi*: 1–21.

PA Consulting. 2019. "Analyse af virksomheder og forskeres behov og barrierer for adgang til offentlige sundhedsdata." København, PA Consulting: 1–52.

Palmgren, Juni. 2017. *Nordic biobanks and registers. A basis for innovative research on health and welfare* NordForsk.

Pálsson, Gísli. 2002. "The life of family trees and the "Book of Icelanders"." *Medical Anthropology*, 21: 337–367.

Pálsson, Gísli, and Paul Rabinow. 2001. "The Icelandic genome debate." *Trends in Biotechnology*, 19: 166–171.

Pariser, Eli. 2011. *The filter bubble*. Penguin.

Parsons, Talcott. 1951. *The social system*. Free Press of Glencoe.

Parton, Nigel. 2008. "Changes in the form of knowledge in social work: From the 'social' to the 'informational'?." *British Journal of Social Work*, 38: 253–269.

Pasquale, Frank. 2015. *The black box society—the secret algorithms that control money and information*. Harvard University Press.

Pedersen, John Storm. 2019a. "Data-driven management in practice in the digital welfare state." In John Storm Pedersen and Adrian Wilkinson (eds.), *Big data. Promise, application and pitfalls*. Edward Elgar Publishing: 200–223

Pedersen, Lene Ærbo. 2019b. "Fælles Medicinkort—samarbejde gjorde forskellen." In Christian Nøhr, Pernille Bertelsen, Søren Vingtoft and Stig Kjær Andersen (eds.),

Digitalisering af det danske sundhedsvæsen. Øjenvidneberetninger fra nøgleaktører. Syddansk Universitetsforlag.

Pedersen, Merete, Mette Klarlund, Søren Jacobsen, Anders J. Svendsen, and Morten Frisch. 2004. "Validity of rheumatoid arthritis diagnoses in the Danish National Patient Registry." *European Journal of Epidemiology*, 19: 1097–1103.

Peeters, Rik, and Marc Schuilenburg. 2021. "The algorithmic society: An introduction." In Marc Schuilenburg and Rik Peeters (eds.), *The algorithmic society: Technology, power, and knowledge.* Routledge: 1–15

Pellegrino, Giuseppina, and Alessandro Mongili. 2014. "The boundaries of information infrastructures: An introduction." In Giuseppina Pellegrino and Alessandro Mongili (eds.), *Information infrastructure(s): Boundaries, ecologies, multiplicity.* Cambridge Scholars Publishing: xix-xlvi

Petersen, Alan. 2019. *Digital health and technological promise: A sociological inquiry* Routledge.

Petersen, Alan, and Claire Tanner. 2015. "Between hope and evidence: How community advisors demarcate the boundary between legitimate and illegitimate stem cell treatments." *Health*, 19: 188–206.

Petersen, Michael Bang. 2021. "COVID lesson: Trust the public with hard truths." *Nature*, 598: 237.

Petersson, Jesper, and Christel Backman. 2021. "Off the record: The invisibility work of doctors in a patient-accessible electronic health record information service." *Sociology of Health & Illness*, 43: 1270–1285.

Petersson, Lena. 2019. "Paving the way for transparency. How eHealth technology can change boundaries in healthcare." Lund University.

Petryna, Adriana. 2002. *Life exposed: Biological citizens after Chernobyl.* Princeton University Press.

Petryna, Adriana. 2005. "Ethical variability: Drug development and globalizing clinical trials." *American Ethnologist*, 32: 183–197.

Phanareth, Klaus, Niels Rossing, and Søren Vingtoft. 2019. "Telemedicinske alternativer i Danmark." In Christian Nøhr, Pernille Bertelsen, Søren Vingtoft and Stig Kjær Andersen (eds.), *Digitalisering af det danske sundhedsvæsen. Øjenvidneberetninger fra nøgleaktører.* Syddansk Universitetsforlag.

Piantadosi, Steven, David P. Byar, and Sylvan B. Green. 1988. "The ecological fallacy." *American Journal of Epidemiology*, 127: 893–904.

Piasecki, Jan, Ewa Walkiewicz-Żarek, Justyna Figas-Skrzypulec, Anna Kordecka, and Vilius Dranseika. 2021. "Ethical issues in biomedical research using electronic health records: A systematic review." *Medicine, Health Care and Philosophy*, 24: 633–658.

Pickersgill, Martyn. 2019a. "Acces, accountability, and the proliferation of psychological therapy: On the introduction of the IATP initiative and the transformation of mental healthcare." *Social Studies of Science*, 49: 627–650.

Pickersgill, Martyn. 2019b. "Psychiatry and the sociology of novelty: Negotiating the US National Institute of Mental Health 'Research Domain Criteria' (RDoC)." *Science, Technology & Human Values*, 44: 612–633.

Pine, Kathleen H. 2019. "The qualculative dimension of healthcare data interoperability." *Health Informatics Journal*, 25: 536–548.

Pine, Kathleen H., and Claus Bossen. 2020. "Good organizational reasons for better medical records: The data work of clinical documentation integrity specialists." *Big Data & Society*, July–December: 1–13.

Pine, Kathleen H., Christine Wolf, and Melissa Mazmanian. 2016. "The work of reuse: Birth certificate data and healthcare accountability measurements." *iConference 2016 proceedings*, 2016: 1–10.

Pinel, Clémence. 2020. "When more data means better results: Abundance and scarcity in research collaborations in epigenetics." *Social Science Information*, 59(1): 35–58.

Pinel, Clémence. 2021. 'Renting Valuable Assets: Knowledge and Value Production in Academic Science', *Science, Technology & Human Values*, 46: 275–97.

Pinel, Clémence, Barbara Prainsack, and Christopher McKevitt. 2020. "Caring for data: Value creation in a data-intensive research laboratory." *Social Studies of Science* 50: 175–197.

Pinel, Clémence, and Mette Nordahl Svendsen. 2021. "In search of "extra data": Making tissues flow from personal to personalized medicine." *Big Data & Society*. July–December: 1–12.

Pink, Sarah, Debora Lanzeni, and Heather Horst. 2018. "Data anxieties: Finding trust in everyday digital mess." *Big Data & Society*, January–June: 1–14.

Pisinger, Charlotta. 2013. "Tobaksindustrien: "Spred tvivl om stærk videnskabelig evidens og offentligheden vil ikke vide, hvad den skal tro"." *Bibliotek for Læger*, June: 156–181.

Plant, Sadie. 1998. *Zeros+Ones*. Fourth Estate.

Plantin, Jean-Christophe. 2019. "Data cleaners for pristine datasets: Visibility of data processors in social science." *Science, Technology & Human Values*, 44: 52–73.

Plesner, U., and L. Justesen 2021. The double darkness of digitalization: Shaping digital-ready legislation to reshape the conditions for public-sector digitalization. *Science, Technology and Human Values*, 47: 146–173.

Poirier, L., K. Fortun, B. Costelloe-Kuehn, and M. Fortun. 2020. "Metadata, digital infrastructure, and the data ideologies of cultural Anthropology." In J. Crowder, M. Fortun, R. Besara and L. Poirier (eds.), *Anthropological Data in the Digital Age*. Palgrave Macmillan: 209–237

Poirier, Lindsay. 2021. "Data, Knowledge Practices, and Naturecultural Worlds: Vehicle Emissions in the Anthropocene." In Maja Hojer Bruun, Ayo Wahlberg, Rachel Douglas-Jones, Cathrine Hasse, Klaus Lindgaard Hoeyer, Dorthe Brogård Kristensen and Brit Ross Winthereik (eds.), *The Palgrave Handbook of the Anthropology of Technology*. Palgrave Macmillan: 273–306

Polanyi, Michael. 1966. *The tacit dimension.* University of Chicago Press.

Pollitt, Christopher, Stephen Harrison, George Dowswell, Sonja Jerak-Zuiderent, and Roland Bal. 2010. "Performance regimes in health care: Institutions, critical junctures and the logic of escalation in England and the Netherlands." *Evaluation,* 16: 13–29.

Pollock, Neil, and Robin Williams. 2010. "The business of expectations: How promissory organizations shape technology and innovation." *Social Studies of Science,* 40: 525–548.

Pols, Jeannette, Dick Willems, and Margunn Aanestad. 2019. "Making sense with numbers: Unravelling ethico-psychological subjects in practices of self-quantification." *Sociology of Health and Illness,* 41: 98–115.

Poole, Marshall Scott, and Andrew van de Ven. 1989. "Using paradox to build management and organization theories." *Academy of Management Review,* 14: 562–578.

Porter, Roy. 1999. *The greatest benefit to mankind: A medical history of humanity from antiquity to the present.* Fontana Press.

Poster, Mark. 1990. *The mode of information. Poststructuralism and social context.* Polity Press.

Pottegård, Anton, Kasper Bruun Kristensen, Mette Reilev, et al. 2020. "Existing data sources in clinical epidemiology: The Danish COVID-19 cohort." *Clinical Epidemiology,* 12: 875–881.

Potts, Jamaica. 2002. "At least give the natives glass beads: An examination of the bargain made between Iceland and deCODE Genetics with implications for global bioprospecting." *Virginia Journal of Law and Technology,* 7: 1–40.

Power, Michael. 1997. *The audit society. Rituals of verification* Oxford University Press.

Power, Michael. 2020. "Playing and being played by the research impact game." In Mario Biagioli and Alexandra Lippman (eds.), *Gaming the metrics: Misconduct and manipulation in academic research.* MIT Press: 57-66

Powers, Benjamin. 2020. "Privacy advocates are sounding alarms over coronavirus surveillance." CoinDesk, https://www.coindesk.com/privacy-advocates-are-sounding-alarms-over-coronavirus-surveillance.

Prainsack, Barbara. 2017. *Personalized medicine—empowered patients in the 21st century?* New York University.

Prainsack, Barbara. 2019. "Logged out: Ownership, exclusion and public value in the digital data and informative commons." *Big Data & Society,* January–June: 1–15.

Prainsack, Barbara. 2020. "The political economy of digital data: Introduction to the special issue." *Policy Studies Journal,* 41: 439–446.

Prainsack, Barbara, and Alena Buyx. 2017. *Solidarity in biomedicine and beyond.* Cambridge University Press.

Price, Nathan D., Andrew T Magis, John C Earls, et al. 2017. "A wellness study of 108 individuals using personal, dense, dynamic data clouds." *Nature Biotechnology,* 35: 747–756.

Privacy International. 2020. "Germany: Deutsche Telekom gives user location data to Robert-Koch Institute." *Privacy International*, March 17, 2020.

Proctor, Robert N. 2008. "Agnotology—a missing term to describe the cultural production of ignorance and its study." In Robert N Proctor and Londa Schiebinger (eds.), *Agnotology—the making and unmaking of ignorance*. Stanford University Press: 1–33.

Qvarsell, Roger. 1986. *I Framtidens Tjänst. Ur Folkemmets Idéhistoria*. Gidlunds: Malmö.

Rabeharisoa, Vololona, Michel Callon, Angela Marques Filipe, João Arriscado Nunes, Florence Paterson, and Frédéric Vergnaud. 2014. "From 'politics of numbers' to 'politics of singularisation': Patients' activism and engagement in research on rare diseases in France and Portugal." *BioSocieties*, 9: 194–217.

Rabeharisoa, Vololona, Tiago Moreira, and Madeleine Akrich. 2014. "Evidence-based activism: Patients', users' and activists' groups in knowledge society." *BioSocieties*, 9: 111–128.

Race, Kane. 2009. *Pleasure consuming medicine: The queer politics of drugs*. Duke University Press.

Rahman, Hatim A. 2021. "The invisible cage: Workers' reactivity to opaque algorithmic evaluations." *Administrative Science Quarterly*, 66: 945–988.

Rajan, Kaushik Sunder. 2003. "Genomic capital: Public cultures and market logics of corporate biotechnology." *Science as Culture*, 12: 87–121.

Rajan, Kaushik Sunder. 2006. *Biocapital. The constitution of postgenomic life*. Duke University Press.

Rapp, Rayna. 2011. "Chasing science: Children's brains, scientific inquiries, and family labors." *Science, Technology, & Human Values*, 36: 662–684.

Rasmussen, Lars Igum. 2016. "Danmark er et diagnosesamfund." *Politiken*, March 27, 2016: 4–6.

Ratner, Helene, and Evelyn Ruppert. 2019. "Producing and projecting data: Aesthetic practices of government data portals." *Big Data & Society*, July–December: 1–16.

Raz, Aviad. 2004. "'Important to test, important to support': Attitudes toward disability rights and prenatal diagnosis among leaders of support groups for genetic disorders in Israel." *Social Science & Medicine*, 59: 1857–1866.

Reardon, Jenny. 2017. *The postgenomic condition: Ethics, justice & knowledge after the genome*. University of Chicago Press.

Redaktionen. 2016. "Har taget imod alle kronprinsessens børn—nu siger han op i protest." *TV2 Nyheder*, November 29, 2016.

Redaktionen. 2018. "Lægeoprør vokser: 6000 protestunderskrifter på få dage". http://sundhedspolitisktidsskrift.dk/nyheder/581-laegeopror-vokser-5-650-protest-underskrifter-pa-fa-dage.html.

Redaktionen. 2020. "Her er Mette Frederiksens historiske tale." *Sundhedspolitisk Tidsskrift*, March 12, 2020, Nyheder section.

Regeringen. 2014. "Jo før—jo bedre: Tidlig diagnose, bedre behandling og flere gode leveår for alle." Sundhedsministeriet.

Regeringen. 2021. "Strategi for life science." Regeringen.

Regeringen, Finansministeriet, Erhvervsministeriet. 2019. "National Strategi for kunstig intelligens." Erhvervsministeriet.

Riles, Annelise. 2006. "Introduction." In Annelise Riles (ed.), *Documents.* University of Michigan Press: 1–38

Riles, Annelise. 2013. "Market collaboration: Finance, culture, and ethnography after neoliberalism." *American Anthropologist,* 115: 555–569.

Rittel, Horst W. J., and Melvin M. Webber. 1973. 'Dilemmas in a General Theory of Planning', *Policy Sciences,* 4: 155–69.

Ritzau. 2017. "Sundhedsplatformen: Nu skal lægesekretærerne tilbage." *DenOffentlige .dk,* November 28, 2017, Infrastruktur section.

Roberton, Timothy, Emily D. Carter, Victoria B. Chou, et al. 2020. "Early estimates of the indirect effects of the COVID-19 pandemic on maternal and child mortality in low-income and middle-income countries: A modelling study." *Lancet Global Health,* 8: E901–E908.

Roberts, Celia, Adrian Mackenzie, and Maggie Mort. 2019. *Living data. Making sense of health biosensing.* Bristol University Press.

Roeser, Sabine. 2012. "Risk communication, public engagement, and climate change: A role for emotions." *Risk Analysis,* 32: 1033–1040.

Røhl, Ulrik Bisgaard Ulsrod, and Jeppe Agger Nielsen. 2019. "Sundhedsplatformen i modvind: En analyse af aktørernes teknologiforståelser i danske medier." *Samfundslederskab i Skandinavien,* 34: 178–206.

Rose, Dale, and Stuart Blume. 2003. "Citizens as users of technology: An exploratory study of vaccines and vaccination." In Nelly Oudshoorn and Trevor Pinch (eds.), *How users matter: The co-construction of users and technology.* MIT Press: 103-132

Rose, Nikolas. 1999. *Powers of freedom. Reframing political thought.* Cambridge University Press.

Rose, Nikolas. 2007. *The politics of life itself: Biomedicine, power, and subjectivity in the twenty-first century* Princeton University Press.

Rosenberg, Daniel. 2013. "Data before the fact." In Lisa Gitelman (ed.), *"Raw data" is an oxymoron.* MIT Press: 15-40

Rosenhan, David L. 1973. "On being sane in insane places." *Science,* 179: 250–258.

Rothenberg, Albert. 1996. "Janusian process in scientific creativity." *Creativity Research Journal,* 9: 207–231.

Rothman, David J. 1991. *Strangers at the bedside: A history of how law and bioethics transformed medical decision making.* BasicBooks.

Rothman, Kenneth J., and Sarah Greenland. 2005. "Hill"s criteria for causality." *Encyclopedia of biostatistics:* 1–4.

Røvik, Kjell-Arne. 1996. "Deinstitutionalization and the logic of fashion." In Barbara Czarniawska and Guje Sevón (eds.), *Translating organizational change.* Walter de Gruyter: 139-172

Rowley, Olivia. 2017. *Analysis: Pricing of goods and services on the deep & dark web* Flashpoint.

Ruckenstein, Minna, and Julia Granroth. 2020. "Algorithms, advertising and the intimacy of surveillance." *Journal of Cultural Economy*, 13: 12–24.

Ruckenstein, Minna, and Natasha Dow Schüll. 2017. "The datafication of health." *Annual Review of Anthropology*, 46: 261–278.

Rufo, Rebecca Zapatochny. 2012. "Use of change management theories in gaining acceptance of telemedicine technology." *Critical Care Nursing*, 35: 322–327.

Ruppert, Evelyn. 2012. "The governmental topologies of database devices." *Theory, Culture & Society*, 29: 116–136.

Ruppert, Evelyn, Engin Isin, and Didier Bigo. 2017. "Data politics." *Big Data & Society*, July–December: 1–7.

Sadowski, Jathan. 2019. "When data is capital: Datafication, accumulation, and extraction." *Big Data & Society*, January–June: 1–12.

Salokannel, Marjut. 2017. "Ethical review, data protection and biomedical research in the Nordic countries: A legal perspective." NordForsk.

SAS Institute. 2017. *Datadrevet ledelse i det danske sundhedsvæsen—inspiration til en forandringsproces. Rapport om visioner for og indsigt i datadrevet ledelse i sundhedssektoren.* SAS Institute.

Sauder, Michael, and Wendy Nelson Espeland. 2009. "The discipline of rankings: Tight coupling and organizational change." *American Sociological Review*, 74: 63–82.

Schad, Jonathan. 2016. "Paradox research in management science: Looking back to move forward." *Academy of Management Annals*, 10: 5–64.

Schicktanz, Silke, and Aviad Raz. 2012. "Responsibility revisited." *Medicine Studies*, 3: 129–130.

Schicktanz, Silke, and Mark Schweda. 2012. "The diversity of responsibilty: The value of explication and pluralization." *Medicine Studies*, 3: 131–145.

Schiermer, Bjørn. 2020. "Corona og kroppens kollektivitet." In Ole B. Jensen and Nikolaj Schultz (eds.), *Det epidemiske samfund*. Hans Reitzels Forlag: 133–146

Schmidt, Morten, Sigrun Alba Johannesdottir Schmidt, Kasper Adelborg, Jens Sundbøll, Vera Ehrenstein, and Henrik Toft Sørensen. 2019. "The Danish health care system and epidemiological research: from health care contacts to database records." *Clinical Epidemiology*, 11: 563–591.

Schmidt, Morten, Sigrun Alba Johannesdottir Schmidt, Jakob Lynge Sandegaard, Vera Ehrenstein, Lars Pedersen, and Henrik Toft Sørensen. 2015. "The Danish National Patient Registry: A review of content, data quality, and research potential." *Clinical Epidemiology*, 7: 449–489.

Schneble, Christophe Olivier, Bernice Simone Elger, and David Martin Shaw. 2020. "All our data will be health data one day: The need for universal data protection and comprehensive consent." *Journal of Medical Internet Research*, 22: e16879.

Schuilenburg, Marc, and Rik Peeters. 2021. "Understanding the algorithmic society. Concluding thoughts." In Marc Schuilenburg and Rik Peeters (eds.), *The algorithmic society: Technology, power, and knowledge*. Routledge: 193–200

Schulte, Fred, and Erika Fry Fortune. 2019. "Death by 1.000 clicks: Where electronic health records went wrong." *Kaiser Health News*, March 18, 2019: 1–35.

Schultz, Kåre, Allan Flyvbjerg, Anders Thelborg, et al. 2017. "Life science i verdensklasse. Anbefalinger fra regeringens vækstteam for life science." Erhvervsministeriet.

Schwennesen, Nete. 2017. "When self-tracking enters physical rehabilitation: From 'pushed' self-tracking to ongoing affective encounters in arrangements of care." *Digital Health*, 3: 1–8.

Schwennesen, Nete. 2019. "Algorithmic assemblages of care: Imaginaries, epistemologies and repair work." *Sociology of Health & Illness*, 41: 176–192.

Scullen, Steven E., and Michael K. Mount. 2000. "Understanding the latent structure of job performance ratings." *Journal of Applied Psychology*, 85: 956–70.

Sebhatu, Abiel, Karl Wennberg, Stefan Arora-Jonsson, and Staffan I. Lindberg. 2020. "Explaining the homogeneous diffusion of COVID-19 nonpharmaceutical interventions across heterogeneous countries." *PNAS*, 117: 21201–21208.

Sedgwick, Eve Kosofsky. 2003. "Paranoid reading and reparative reading; or, you're so paranoid, you probably think this introduction is about you." In Eve Kosofsky Sedgwick, Michéle Aina Barale, Jonathan Goldberg, and Michael Moon (eds.), *Touching feeling: Affect, pedagogy, performativity*. Duke University Press: 123–151.

Seeman, Melvin. 1975. "Alienation studies." *Annual Review of Sociology*, 1: 91–123.

Selinger, Evan. 2006. "Introduction." In Evan Selinger (ed.), *Postphenomenology: A critical companion to Ihde*. State University of New York Press: 1–10

Senn, Stephen. 2015. "Mastering variation: Variance components and personalised medicine." *Statistics in Medicine*, 35: 966–977.

Severinsen, Marianne Tang, Søren Risom Kristensen, Kim Overvad, Claus Dethlefsen, Anne Tjønneland, and Søren Paaske Johnsen. 2010. "Venous thromboembolism discharge diagnoses in the Danish National Patient Registry should be used with caution." *Journal of Clinical Epidemiology*, 63: 223–228.

Shah, Sooraj. 2020. "Amazon plots a course into the healthcare industry." *BBC News*, Business section.

Shanahan, Murray. 2015. *The technological singularity*. MIT Press.

Sharon, Tamar. 2016. "The Googlization of health research: From disruptive innovation to disruptive ethics." *Personalized Medicine*, 13: 563–574.

Sharon, Tamar, and Dorion Zandbergen. 2016. "From data fetishism to quantifying selves: Self-tracking practices and the other values of data." *New Media & Society*, 19: 1695–1709.

Sharp, Lesley A. 2019. *Animal ethos: The morality of human-animal encounters in experimental lab science*. University of California Press.

Shaw, Ian, Margaret Bell, Ian Sinclair, et al. 2009. "An exemplary scheme? An evaluation of the Integrated Children's System." *British Journal of Social Work*, 39: 613–626.

Sheikh, Aziz, Harpreet S. Sood, and David W. Bates. 2015. "Leveraging health information technology to achieve the 'triple aim' of healthcare reform." *Journal of the American Medical Informatics Association*, 22: 849–856.

Shklovski, Irina, Emily Troshynski, and Paul Dourish. 2015. "Mobile technologies and the spatiotemporal configurations of institutional practice." *Journal of the Association for Information Science and Technology*, 66: 2098–2115.

Shore, Cris, and Susan Wright. 1999. "Audit culture and anthropology: Neo-liberalism in British higher education." *Journal of the Royal Anthropological Institute*, 5: 557–575.

Shore, Cris, and Susan Wright. 2001. "Changing institutional contexts: New managerialism in the rise of UK higher education PLC." *Anthropology in Action*, 8: 14–21.

Sigurdsson, Skúli. 2001. "Yin-yang genetics, or the HSD deCODE controversy." *New Genetics and Society*, 20: 103–118.

Simmel, Georg. 1950. "The secret society." In Kurt H Wolf (ed.), *The sociology of Georg Simmel*. Free Press: 345-376.

Sismondo, Sergio. 2008. "Pharmaceutical company funding and its consequences: A qualitative systematic review." *Contemporary Clinical Trials*, 29: 109–113.

Sjönell, Göran, and John Brodersen. 2009. "Mammografiscreening i Sverige—en kontroversiel historie." In Lotte Hvas, John Brodersen and Birgitta Hovelius (eds.), *Kan sundhedsvæsenet skabe usundhed? Refleksioner fra almen praksis*. Månedsskrift for Praktisk Lægegerning: 143–152

Skovgaard, Lea Larsen, and Klaus Hoeyer. 2022. "Data authority: Public debate about personalized medicine in Denmark," *Public Understanding of Science*, 31: 590–607.

Skovgaard, Lea Larsen, Sarah Wadmann, and Klaus Hoeyer. 2019. "A review of attitudes towards the reuse of health data among people in the European Union: The primacy of purpose and the common good." *Health Policy*, 123: 564–571.

Skøtt, Ole, Lars Melholt Rasmussen, Torben Kruse, et al. 2015. *Personlig Medicin og Individualiseret Behandling*. Danske Regioner.

Slayton, Rebecca. 2021. "Governing uncertainty or uncertain governance? Information security and the challenge of cutting ties." *Science, Technology & Human Values*, 46: 81–111.

Smith, Gavin. 2018. "Data doxa: The affective consequences of data practices." *Big Data & Society*, 5: 1–15.

Snowden, Edward. 2019a. *Permanent record*. Macmillan.

Snowden, Frank M. 2019b. *Epidemics and society. From the Black Death to the present.* Yale University Press.

Sokolowski, Robert. 2000. *Introduction to phenomenology*. Cambridge University Press.

Son, Hugh. 2021. "Haven, the Amazon-Berkshire-JP Morgan venture to disrupt health care, is disbanding after 3 years." *CNBC*, January 4, 2021, Finance section.

Spear, Brian B., Margo Heath-Chiozzi, and Jeffrey Huff. 2001. "Clinical application of pharmacogenetics." *TRENDS in Molecular Medicine*, 7: 201–204.

Star, Susan Leigh. 1991. "The sociology of the invisible: The primacy of work in the writings of Anselm Strauss." In David R. Maines (ed.), *Social organization and social process: Essays in honor of Anselm Strauss*. Aldine De Gruyter: 265–283

Star, Susan Leigh, and Karen Ruhleder. 1996. 'Steps Toward an Ecology of Infrastructure: Design and Access for Large Information Spaces', *Information Systems Research*, 7: 111–34.

Stark, Luke. 2018. "Algorithmic psychometrics and the scalable subject." *Social Studies of Science*, 48: 204–231.

Statsrevisorerne. 2022. *5 statslige myndigheders efterlevelse af 20 tekniske minimumskrav til it-sikkerheden*. Statsrevisorerne.

Statsrevisorerne and Rigsrevisionen. 2018. *Beretning om Sundhedsplatformen*. Folketinget.

Statsrevisorerne, and Rigsrevisionen. 2020. "Beslutningsfasen i statslige it-projekter." Statsrevisorerne, Rigsrevisionen.

Statt, Nick. 2019. "This AI startup claims to automate app making but actually just uses humans." *The Verge*, August 14, 2019.

Steen-Andersen, Anne Mette. 2017. "Else Smith: 'Gentænk sundhedsvæsenet!'" *Dagens Medicin*, January 20, 2017: 4–5.

Stegenga, Jacob. 2018. *Medical nihilism*. Oxford University Press.

Sterckx, Sigrid, Vojin Rakic, Julian Cockbain, and Pascal Borry. 2015. "'You hoped we would sleep walk into accepting the collection of our data': Controversies surrounding the UK care.data scheme and their wider relevance for biomedical research." *Medicine, Health Care and Philosophy*, 19: 177–190.

Stewart, Rosemary. 1967. *Managers and their jobs*. Macmillan.

Storeng, Katerini T, and Dominique P Behage. 2017. "'Guilty until proven inncent': The contested use of maternal mortality indicators in global health." *Critical Public health*, 27: 163–176.

Strasser, B. J. 2019. *Collecting Experiments. Making Big Data Biology*. University of Chicago Press.

Strathern, Marilyn. 2004. "Global and local context." In Lawrence Kalinoe and James Leach (eds.), *Rationales of ownership. transactions and claims to ownership in contemporary Papua New Guinea*. Sean Kingston Publishing: 107–127

Strathern, Marilyn. 2007. "Measures of usefulness: A diatribe." In Bridget Somekh and Thomas A. Schwandt (eds.), *Knowledge production: Research work in interesting times*. Routledge: 9–23

Strauss, Anselm L., Shizuko Fagerhaugh, Barbara Suczek, and Carolyn Wiener. 1997. "Articulation work." In Anselm Strauss, Shizuko Fagerhaugh, Barbara Suckzek and Carolyn Wiener (eds.), *Social organization of medical work*. Transaction Publishers.

Strochlic, Nina, and Riley D. Champine. 2020. "How some cities 'flattened the curve' during the 1918 flu pandemic." *National Geographic*, March 27, 2020, History & Culture section.

Sullivan, Noelle. 2017. "Multiple accountabilities: Development cooperation, transparency, and the politics of unknowing in Tanzania's health sector." *Critical Public health*, 27: 193–204.

Sundheds-og Ældreministeriet. 1994. "Bekendtgørelse om optikervirksomhed." In *BEK nr 817 af 14/09/1994*. Copenhagen: Sundheds-og Ældreministeriet.

Sundheds-og Ældreministeriet, and Danske Regioner. 2016. *Personlig medicin til gavn for patienterne*. Copenhagen: Sundheds-og Ældreministeriet.

Sundheds-og Ældreministeriet, KL, and Danske Regioner. 2018. *Nationale mål for sundhedsvæsenet*. Copenhagen: Sundheds-og Ældreministeriet.

Sustainable Development Solutions Network. 2020. *World happiness report*. Sustainable Development Solutions Network.

Svendsen, Mette N. 2011. "Articulating potentially: Notes on the delineation of the blank figure in human embryonic stem cell research." *Cultural Anthropology*, 26: 414–437.

Svendsen, Mette N. 2022. *Near human: Border zones of species, life, and belonging*. Rutgers University Press.

Svenningsen, Signe. 2004. *Den Elektroniske Patientjournal*. Handelshøjskolens Forlag.

Swierstra, Tsjalling, and Sophia Efstathiou. 2020. "Knowledge repositories. In digital knowledge we trust." *Medicine, Health Care and Philosophy*, 23: 543–47.

Sætnan, Ann Rudinow. 2018. "The haystack fallacy, or why Big Data provides little security." In Ann Rudinow Sætnan, Ingrid Schneider and Nicola Green (eds.), *The politics of Big Data: Big Data, Big Brother?* Routledge: 21–36

Sætnan, Ann Rudinow, Heidi Mork Lommel, and Svein Hammer. 2011. "Introduction. By the very act of counting—the mutual construction of statistics and society." In Ann Rudinow Sætnan, Heidi Mork Lomell and Svein Hammer (eds.), *The mutual construction of statistics and society*, Routledge and Taylor & Francis Group: 1–21

Sætnan, Ann Rudinow, Ingrid Schneider, and Nicola Green. 2018. "The politics of Big Data: Principles, policies, practices." In Ann Rudinow Sætnan, Ingrid Schneider and Nico Green (eds.), *The politics of Big Data: Big Data, Big Brother?* Routledge: 1-18

Søgaard, Jes 2021. "Når ønsketænkning afgør sagen." In Niels Bentzon and Jacob Rosenberg (eds.), *Destruktiv Digitalisering. En debatbog om Sundhedsplatformen 2016– 2021*. FADL's Forlag: 207–218

Sørensen, Henrik Toft. 2013. "Sudbøsagen. Artikler i førende tidsskrifter på fabrikerede data." *Bibliotek for Læger*, June 2013: 110–118.

Sørensen, Ninna Nyberg. 2020. "Coronavirus og migration" In Ole B. Jensen and Nikolaj Schultz (eds.), *Det epidemiske samfund*. Hans Reitzels Forlag: 101–116

Sørensen, Tea Krogh. 2016. "Læger advarer: Alvorlige it-problemer er fortsat til fare for patienter." *Jyllands-Posten*. July 31.

Tanner, Adam. 2017. *Our bodies, our data: How companies make millions selling our medical records*. Beacon Press.

Tarkkala, Heta, Ilpo Helén, and Karoliina Snell. 2018. "From health to wealth: The future of personalized medicine in the making." *Future*, 109: 142–152.

Taussig, Karen-Sue. 2009. *Ordinary genomes: Science, citizenship, and genetic identities.* Duke University Press.

Taussig, Karen-Sue, Klaus Hoeyer, and Stefan Helmreich. 2013. "The anthropology of potentiality in biomedicine: An introduction to Supplement 7." *Current Anthropology*, 54: 3–14.

Taylor, Charles. 1994. "The politics of recognition." In David Theo Goldberg (ed.), *Multiculturalism: A critical reader.* Blackwell: 75–106.

Taylor, Frederick Winslow. 1998. *The principles of scientific management.* Dover Publications.

Taylor, Linnet. 2017. "Safety in numbers? Group privacy and big data analytics in the developing world." In Linnet Taylor, Luciano Floridi and Bart van der Sloot (eds.), *Group privacy.* Springer: 13–36.

Taylor, Linnet. 2020. "The price of certainty: How the politics of pandemic data demand an ethics of care." *Big Data & Society*, July–December: 1–7.

Taylor, Linnet, Luciano Floridi, and Bart van der Sloot. 2017. "Introduction: A new perspective on privacy." In Linnet Taylor, Luciano Floridi and Bart van der Sloot (eds.), *Group privacy.* Springer: 1–13

Taylor-Alexander, Samuel. 2016. "Ethics in numbers: Auditing cleft treatment in Mexico and beyond." *Medical Anthropology Quarterly*, 31: 385–402.

Tegmark, Max. 2017. *Life 3.0.* Penguin Books.

Thompson, W. (Lord Kelvin). 1891. "Electrical units of measurement." In *Popular lectures and addresses.* Cambridge University Press. 73–136

Thorgeirsdóttir, Sigrídur. 2004. "The controversy on consent in the Icelandic database case and narrow bioethics." In Gardar Árnason, Salvör Nordal and Viljálmur Árnason (eds.), *Blood and data: Ethical, legal and social aspects of human genetic databases.* Reykjavik: University of Iceland Press: 67–77

Thylstrup, Nanna Bonde. 2021. "Error." in Nanna Bonde Thylstrup, Daniela Agostinho, Annie Ring, Cathrine D'Ignazio and Kristin Veel (eds.), *Uncertain Archives - Critical Keywords for Big Data.* The MIT Press: 191–200.

Timmermans, Stefan, and Marc Berg. 1998. "Introduction: The politics of standardization." In *The gold standard.* Temple University Press: 294–316

Timmermans, Stefan, and Mara Buchbinder. 2013. "Potentializing newborn screening." *Current Anthropology*, 54: 26–35.

Tomašev, Nenad, Xavier Glorot, Jack W. Rae, et al. 2019. "A clinically applicable approach to continous prediction of future acute kidney injury." *Nature*, 572: 116–119.

Topol, Eric. 2010. *Deep Medicine: How Artificial Intelligence Can Make Healthcare Human Again.* Basic Books.

Topol, Eric. 2015. *The Patient Will See You Now.* Basic Books.

Torenholt, Rikke, and Henriette Langstrup. 2021. "Between a logic of disruption and a logic of continuation: Negotiating the legitimacy of algorithms used in automated clinical decision making." *Health*, 2021: 1–19.

Torenholt, Rikke, Lena Saltbæk, and Henriette Langstrup. 2020. "Patient data work: Filtering and sensing patient-reported outcomes." *Sociology of Health & Illness*, 42: 1379–1393.

Transparency International. 2020. *Corruption Perceptions Index 2019*. Transparency International.

Trauttmansdorff, Paul, and Ulrike Felt. 2021. "Between infrastructural experimentation and collective imagination: The digital transformation of the EU border regime." *Science, Technology, & Human Values* (online first): 1–28.

Trier, Troels. 2016. "Dronning Margrethe: Nationalstaten betyder stadig meget for danskerne." *DR.dk.*

Tsing, Anna Lowenhaupt. 2015. *The mushroom at the end of the world*. Princeton University Press.

Tufte, Edward. 2020. *Seeing with fresh eyes meaning space data truth*. Graphics Press LLC.

Tupasela, Aaro. 2017a. "Data-sharing politics and the logics of competition in biobanking." In Vincenzo Pavone and Joanna Goven (eds.), *Bioeconomics: Life, technology, and capital in the 21st century*. Palgrave Macmillan: 187-206

Tupasela, Aaro. 2017b. "Populations as brands in medical research: Placing genes on the global genetic atlas." *BioSocieties*, 12: 47–65.

Tupasela, Aaro. 2021a. "Data hugging in European biobank networks." *Science as Culture*: 1–22.

Tupasela, Aaro. 2021b. *Populations as brands: Marketing national resources for global markets*. Palgrave Macmillan.

Tupasela, Aaro, Karoliina Snell, and Jose A. Cañada. 2015. "Constructing populations in biobanking." *Life Sciences, Society and Policy*, 11: 1–18.

Tupasela, Aaro, Karoliina Snell, and Heta Tarkkala. 2020. "The Nordic data imaginary." *Big Data & Society*, January–June: 1–13.

Tutton, Richard. 2017. "Multiplanetary imaginaries and utopia: The case of Mars One." *Science, Technology & Human Values*, 43: 518–539.

Tutton, Richard. 2020. "Sociotechnical imaginaries and techno-optimism: Examining outer space utopias of Silicon Valley." *Science as Culture*, 30: 416–439.

Tønder, Lars. 2020. "Biopolitikkens dobbelthed: Om magt og magtesløshed i det epidemiske samfund." In Ole B. Jensen and Nikolaj Schultz (eds.), *Det epidemiske samfund*. Hans Reitzels Forlag: 55–70

US Congress. 2009. "American Recovery and Reinvestment Act of 2009." Washington, DC.

US Food and Drug Administration. 2019. "Digital Health Innovation Action Plan." US Food and Drug Administration.

US Food and Drug Administration. 2013. *Paving the way for personalized medicine: FDA's role in a new era of medical product development*. US Food and Drug Administration.

US Food and Drug Administration, US Department of Health and Human Services, Center for Devices and Radiological Health, and Center for Biologics and Research.

2017. *Use of real-world evidence to support regulatory decision-making for medical devices.* US Food & Drug Administration.

United Nations. 2020. *E-government survey 2020: Digital government in the Decade of Action for Sustainable Development.* Department of Economic and Social Affairs, United Nations.

United Nations Secretary-General's Independent Expert Advisory Group on a Data Revolution for Sustainable Development. 2014. *A world that counts.* UN Secretary General's Independent Expert Advisory Group.

Vallee, Mickey. 2020. "Doing nothing does something: Embodiment and data in the COVID-19 pandemic." *Big Data & Society,* January–June: 1–12.

Vallgårda, Signild. 1992. *Sygehuse og sygehuspolitik i Danmark—Et bidrag til det specialiserede sygehusvæsens historie 1930–1987.* Jurist- og Økonomforbundets Forlag.

Vallgårda, Signild. 2003. *Folkesundhed som Politik. Danmark og Sverige fra 1930 til i Dag* Aarhus Universitetsforlag.

van der Geest, Sjaak, Susan Reynolds Whyte, and Anita Hardon. 1996. "The anthropology of pharmaceuticals: A biographical approach." *Annual Review of Anthropology,* 25: 153–178.

van der Niet, Anneke G., and Alan Bleakley. 2020. "Where medical education meets artificial intelligence: 'Does technology care?'" *Medical Education,* 55: 30–36.

van Dijck, José. 2013. *The culture of connectivity: A critical history of social media.* Oxford University Press.

van Dijck, José, Thomas Poell, and Martijn De Wall. 2018. *The platform society: Public values in a connective world.* Oxford University Press.

van Dijk, Jan. 2020. *The digital divide.* Polity Press.

van Eijk, Gwen. 2021. "Algorithmic reasoning. The production of subjectivity through data." In Marc Schuilenburg and Rik Peeters (eds.), *The algorithmic society: Technology, power, and knowledge.* Routledge. 119-134

Varga, Tibor V., Feifei Bu, Agnete S. Dissing, et al. 2021. "Loneliness, worries, anxiety, and precautionary behaviours in response to the COVID-19 pandemic: A longitudinal analysis of 200,000 Western and Northern Europeans." *Lancet Regional Health—Europe.* 2: 1–9.

Varga, Tibor V., Kristoffer Niss, Angela C. Estampador, Catherine B. Collin, and Pope L. Moseley. 2020. "Association is not prediction: A landscape of confused reporting in diabetes—A systematic review.." *Diabetes Research and Clinical Practice,* 170: 1–10.

Venkatraman, Vinay, Priya Mani, and August Ussing. 2015. "Mapping the healthcare data landscape in Denmark." Leapcraft.

Verbeek, Peter-Paul. 2011. *Moralizing technology: Understanding and designing the morality of things.* Chicago University Press.

Verghese, Abraham. 2008. "Culture shock—Patient as icon, icon as patient." *New England Journal of Medicine,* 359: 2748–2751.

Verran, Helen. 2021. "Writing an ethnographic story in working toward responsibly unearthing ontological troubles." In Andrea Ballestero and Brit Ross Winthereik (eds.), *Experimenting with ethnography: A companion to analysis*. Duke University Press: 235–245

Vestager, Margrethe. 2020. *Proposal for a regulation of the European Parliament and of the Council on European data governance (Data Governance Act)*. European Commission: COM(2020) 767 final.

Vezyridis, Paraskevas, and Stephen Timmons. 2017. "Understanding the care.data conondrum: New information flows for economic growth." *Big Data & Society*, January–June: 1–12.

Vezyridis, Paraskevas, and Stephen Timmons. 2021. "E-Infrastructures and the divergent assetization of public health data: Expectations, uncertainties, and asymmetries." *Social Studies of Science*, 51: 606–627.

Videbæk, Klaus. 2020. "Mand og døtre sagde farvel til Linda: "Hvis vi kun havde været ti, havde det ikke været til at bære"." *DR Nyheder*, March 23, 2020, Nordjylland section.

Videbæk, Klaus, Martin Geertsen, and Trine Dam. 2019. "Kø ved lægen uden grund: Data fra sundhedsapps og ure skaber bekymrede patienter." *DR.dk*, September 8.

Vikkelsø, Signe. 2005. "Subtle redistribution of work, attention and risks: Electronic patient records and organisational consequences." *Scandinavian Journal of Information Systems*, 17: 3–30.

Vincent, Bernadette Bensaude. 2014. "The politics of buzzwords at the interface of technoscience, market and society: The case of 'public engagement in science.'" *Public Understanding of Science*, 23: 238–253.

Vindegaard, Nina, and Michael Eriksen Benros. 2020. "COVID-19 pandemic and mental health consequences: Systematic review of the current evidence." *Brain, Behavior, and Immunity*, 89: 531–542.

Vitebsky, Piers. 1993. "Is death the same everywhere? Contexts of knowing and doubting." In Mark Hobart (ed.), *An anthropological critique of development: The growth of ignorance*. Routledge: 100–115

Vogt, Henrik, Sara Green, and John Brodersen. 2018. "Precision medicine in the clouds." *Nature Biotechnology*, 36: 678–680.

Vogt, Henrik, Sara Green, Claus Thorn Ekstrøm, and John Brodersen. 2019. "How precision medicine and screening with big data could increase overdiagnosis." *BMJ*, 363: 1–3.

Wachter, Robert. 2017. *The digital doctor: Hope, hype, and harm at the dawn of medicine's computer age*. McGraw-Hill Education.

Wadmann, Sarah. 2014a. "Physician–industry collaboration: Conflicts of interest and the imputation of motive." *Social Studies of Science*, 44: 531–554.

Wadmann, Sarah. 2014b. *Preventive tensions: Governing clinical research and treatment practices in contemporary cardiovascular medicine in Denmark*. University of Copenhagen.

Wadmann, Sarah, Mette Hartlev, and Klaus Hoeyer. 2022. "The life and death of confidentiality: A historical analysis of the flows of patient information." *BioSocieties* (online first).

Wadmann, Sarah, and K. Hoeyer. 2018. "Dangers of the digital fit: Rethinking seamlessness and social sustainability in data-intensive healthcare." *Big Data & Society*, January–June: 1–13.

Wadmann, Sarah, Christina Holm-Petersen, and Charlotta Levay. 2018. "'We don't like the rules and still we keep seeking new ones': The vicious circle of quality control in professional organizations." *Journal of Professions and Organization*, 6: 17–32.

Wadmann, Sarah, and Betina Højgaard. 2020. "Real-world evidence ved lægemiddelgodkendelse." *Ugeskrift for Læger*, 182: 1–9.

Wadmann, Sarah, Sarah Johansen, Ane Lind, Hans Okkels Birk, and Klaus Hoeyer. 2013. "Analytical perspectives on performancebased management: An outline of theoretical assumptions in the existing literature." *Health Economics, Policy and Law*, 8: 511–527.

Wadmann, Sarah, and Kirstine Zinck Pedersen. 2020. "Den økonomisk ansvarlige læge i krisetider: Konstituering af lægerollen i 1930erne og 1970erne." *Tidsskrift for Arbejdsliv*, 22. årgang: 72–88.

Wahlberg, Ayo. 2009. "Serious disease as kinds of living." In Susanne Bauer and Ayo Wahlberg (eds.), *Contested categories. Life sciences in society*. Routledge: 89–111

Wahlberg, Ayo. 2018a. *Good quality: The routinization of sperm banking in China*. University of California Press.

Wahlberg, Ayo. 2018b. "The vitality of disease." In Maurizio Meloni, John Cromby, Des Fitzgerald and Stephanie Lloyd (eds.), *Palgrave handbook of biology and society*. Palgrave Macmillan: 727–748

Wahlberg, Ayo, Nancy J. Burke, and Lenore Manderson. 2021. "Viral loads." In Lenore Manderson, Nancy J. Burke and Ayo Wahlberg (eds.), *Viral loads: Anthropologies of urgency in the time of COVID-19*. UCL Press: 1–23

Wahlberg, Ayo, and Nikolas Rose. 2015. "The governmentalization of living: Calculating global health." *Economy and Society*, 44: 60–90.

Wajcman, Judy. 2015. *Pressed for time*. University of Chicago Press.

Wajcman, Judy. 2019. "The digital architecture of time management." *Science, Technology & Human Values*, 44: 315–337.

Wakefield, Jane. 2017. "Google DeepMind's NHS deal under scrutiny." *BBC News*, March 17.

Walford, Antonia. 2021. "Data—ova—gene—data." *Journal of the Royal Anthropological Insitute*, 27: 127–141.

Wang, Laura Friis. 2017. "En læge glemte at skrive notat—det kan føre til et mere bureaukratisk sundhedssystem." *Information*, October 10, 2017: 6–7.

Warzel, Charlie. 2019. "The fake Nancy Pelosi video hijacked our attention. just as intended.." *New York Times*, May 26, 2019, Opinion section.

Weber, Max. 1947a. *From Max Weber: Essays in sociology*. Oxford University Press.

Weber, Max. 1947b. "Science as a vocation." In H. H. Gerth and C. Wright Mills (eds.), *From Max Weber: Essays in sociology*. Oxford University Press: 129–156

Weber, Max. 2003a. "Det Legitime Herredømmes Tre Rene Typer." In Heine Andersen, Hans Henrik Bruun and Lars Bo Kaspersen (eds.), *Udvalgte Tekster—Bind 2*. Hans Reitzels Forlag: 173–188

Weber, Max. 2003b. "Herredømmets Sociologi; 2. afsnit: Det Bureaukratiske Herredømmes Væsen, Forudsætninger og Udvikling." In Heine Andersen, Hans Henrik Bruun and Lars Bo Kaspersen (eds.), *Udvalgte Tekster—Bind 2*. Hans Reitzels Forlag: 63–112

Webster, Frank. 2002. *Theories of the information society*. Routledge.

Weible, Christopher M., Daniel Nohrstedt, Paul Cairney, et al. 2020. "COVID-19 and the policy sciences: Initial reactions and perspectives." *Policy Sciences*, 53: 225–241.

Weiner, Kate, Catherine Will, Flis Henwood, and Rosalind Williams. 2020. "Everyday curation? Attending to data, records and record keeping in the practices of self-monitoring." *Big Data & Society*, January–June 1–15.

Weiskopf, Nicole Gray, and Chunhua Weng. 2012. "Methods and dimensions of electronic health record data quality assessment: enabling reuse for clinical research." *Journal of the American Medical Informatics Association*, 20: 151.

Weiss, Carol Hirschon. 1986. "Research and policy-making: A limited partnership." In Frank Heller (ed.), *The use and abuse of social science*. SAGE: 214–235

Wells, H. G. 1938. *World brain*. Methuen & Co. Limited.

White, Mary Terrell. 1999. "Making responsible decisions: An interpretive ethic for genetic decisionmaking." *Hastings Center Report*, 29: 14–21.

Whyte, Susan Reynolds, Sjaak Van der Geest, and Anita Hardon. 2003. *Social lives of medicines*. Cambridge University Press.

Widdows, Heather, and Sean Cordell. 2011. "Why communities and their goods matter: Illustrated with the example of Biobanks.." *Public Health Ethics*, 4: 14–25.

Wiener, Anne. 2020. *Uncanny valley: A memoir*. MCD.

Wiener, Carolyn L. 2000. *The elusive quest: Accountability in hospitals*. Aldine De Gruyter.

Wiener, Carolyn L., and Jeanie Kayser-Jones. 1989. "Defensive work in nursing homes: Accountability gone amok." *Social Science & Medicine*, 28: 37–44.

Wienroth, Matthias, Louise Lund Holm Thomsen, and Anna Marie Høstgaard. 2020. "Health technology identities and self. Patients' appropriation of an assistive device for self-management of chronic illness." *Sociology of Health & Illness*, 42: 1077–1094.

Wikan, Unni. 1992. "Beyond the words: The power of resonance." *American Ethnologist*, 19: 460–482.

Wilson, Mark. 2020. "The story behind "flatten the curve," the defining chart of the coronavirus." *Fast Company*, March 13, 2020.

Winthereik, Brit R. 2010. "The project multiple: Enactments of systems development." *Scandinavian Journal of Information Systems*, 22: 1–16.

Winthereik, Brit Ross. 2003. "'We fill in our working understanding": On codes, classifications and the production of accurate data." *Methods of Information in Medicine*, 42: 489–496.

Winthereik, Brit Ross. 2004. "Klassifikationer og Kodningsarbejde: Praktiserende Lægers Oversættelse af Kliniske Oplysninger til Data i EPJ." In Signe Vikkelsø and Sidsel Vinge (eds.), *Hverdagens Arbejde og Organisering i Sundhedsvæsnet*. Handelshøjskolens Forlag: 213–232

Winthereik, Brit Ross, Irma van der Ploeg, and Marc Berg. 2007. "The electronic patient record as a meaningful audit tool: Accountability and autonomy in general practitioner work." *Science, Technology & Human Values*, 32: 6–25.

Winthereik, Brit Ross, and Signe Vikkelsø. 2005. "ICT and integrated care: Some dilemmas of standardising inter-organisational communication." *Computer Supported Coorperative Work*, 14: 43–67.

Wise, Jacqui. 2016. "Activity trackers, even with cash incentives, do not improve health." *BMJ*, 355: i5392.

Wittgenstein, Ludwig. 2001. *Philosophical investigations: The German text with a revised English translation*. Blackwell.

Wolf, Adam. 2017. *Sundhedens digitale transformation*. Danske Regioner.

World Economic Forum, and Government of Denmark. 2018. *Memorandum of understanding between World Economic Forum and Government of Denmark*. World Economic Forum.

World Health Organization (WHO). 2020. *ApartTogether survey*. WHO.

Wounters, Paul. 2020. "The mismeasurement of quality and impact." In Mario Biagioli and Alexandra Lippman (eds.), *Gaming the metrics: Misconduct and manipulation in academic research*. MIT Press: 67–75.

Wyatt, Sally. 2017. "Making policies for open data: Experiencing the technological imperative in the policy world." *Science, Technology & Human Values*, 42: 320–324.

Wyatt, Sally. 2018. "Addiction: Apt metaphor for over)use of digital technology?" Humboldt Institute for Internet and Society (HIIG).

Wyatt, Sally. 2022. "Critical (big) data studies." In Daryl Cressman (ed.), *The neccessity of critique: Andrew Feenberg and the philosophy of technology*. Springer (in press)

Wynne, Brian. 1992. "Public understanding of science research: New horizons or hall of mirrors?" *Public Understanding of Science*, 1: 37–43.

Žižek, Slavoj. 2020. *Pandemic! COVID-19 shakes the world*. Polity Press.

Zuboff, Shoshana. 1989. *In the age of the smart machine: The future of work and power*. Basic Books.

Zuboff, Shoshana. 2019. *The age of surveillance capitalism: The fight for a human future at the new frontier of power*. Public Affairs.

Zurita, Laura, and Christian Nøhr. 2004. "Patient opinion—EHR assessment from the users' perspective." *MEDINFO*, 11: 1333–1336.

INDEX

Page numbers followed by f and t indicate figures and tables, respectively.